101 Foods
That Could
Save Your Life!

1-18-08

101 Foods That Could Save Your Life!

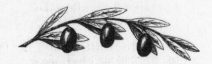

DAVID W. GROTTO, RD, LDN

Foreword by Marianne Smith Edge, MS, RD, LD, FADA

BANTAM BOOKS

The information found in this book is intended to help guide you toward healthier eating choices, but is not intended to replace the services of a qualified medical professional. Seek medical attention if you suspect that you have a health challenge.

Any mention of an organization, product, service, company, or professional does not imply endorsement by either the author or the publisher. Any adverse effect arising from the use or misuse of the information from this book is the sole responsibility of the reader and not that of the author or the publisher.

101 FOODS THAT COULD SAVE YOUR LIFE!
A Bantam Book / January 2008

Published by Bantam Dell
A Division of Random House, Inc.
New York, New York

Cover design by Tom McKeveny
Cover images copyright © 2007 by Stockbyte/Getty Images

Book design by Helene Berinsky

Library of Congress Cataloging-in-Publication Data
Grotto, David W.
101 foods that could save your life! / by David W. Grotto;
foreword by Marianne Smith Edge.
p. cm.
Includes bibliographical references and index.
ISBN 978-0-553-38432-1 (trade pbk. : alk. paper)
1. Nutrition.   2. Natural foods.   3. Diet therapy.   I. Title.
II. Title: One hundred one foods that could save your life!
III. Title: One hundred and one foods that could save your life!
RA784.G765 2008
613.2—dc22   2007028783

978-0-553-38432-1

Printed in the United States of America
Published simultaneously in Canada

www.bantamdell.com

BVG 10 9 8 7 6 5 4 3

To my wife, Sharon, for her unwavering support and love

To my mother, Eileen, who watches over me from above

CONTENTS

ACKNOWLEDGMENTS

This book would not have been possible without the help of my wonderful research assistants Traci Beierwaltes, RD; Jessica Colletta, MS, RD; Katherine Finn, MPH, RD; Jill Stiens, MS, RD; and Anne Marie Van Vossen, RD. Thanks to Julie Moreshi and Julie Davis from Benedictine University who helped me find many of these talented professionals. Thanks to Doris Acosta and her amazing public relations team, my fellow spokespersons, and countless others from the American Dietetic Association for their support, encouragement, and dedication to the message of positive nutrition.

Immense gratitude to Vicki Dieter, my daughter's fifth-grade English teacher, who instilled a passion in her—and me along with her—to write! Thanks also to my wonderful literary agent, Rick Broadhead, whose spare-no-prisoners approach fortunately whipped my proposal into shape and guided it into the very talented hands of my editor, Philip Rappaport, who masterfully made *101 Foods* come to life! Thank you also to all of the wonderful folks at Bantam Dell who made this book a reality.

Thank you to the many colleagues, friends, and family members, especially my father and mother-in-law, who worked behind the scenes and offered me great advice and encouragement during my maiden voyage as an author.

To my incredibly wonderful and loving wife, Sharon, who kindly indulged me in this project, rolled up her own food-splattered sleeves, and became a partner in it, while all along keeping our family happy, healthy, and well-fed! I am also grateful to my beautiful children, Chloe, Katie, and Madison, who were so loving and supportive during the process. I am proud of the great patience and enthusiasm they showed while taste-testing and re–taste-testing an amazing number of recipes and thank them for giving me their most honest opinions!

FOREWORD

Food facts, health guide, recipe book, diet plans—all under one cover! *101 Foods That Could Save Your Life!* is truly a lifesaver. Finally, a book that not only lists "super" foods but discusses the history of the food, health benefits, and most important, how to incorporate the foods into your daily diet for maximum health benefits. Dave Grotto's emphasis on "what to eat" rather than "what not to eat" is a refreshing approach that makes it easier to commit to a lifetime of healthy eating. When one turns the pages and finds the list of lifesaving foods contains glorious fruits, herbs and spices, coffee, and yes, even chocolate—the commitment suddenly becomes one of indulgence, not drudgery. This book reinforces the importance of having a variety of foods in our diets and validates the science behind the 2005 Dietary Guidelines and MyPyramid for the increased need for fruits, vegetables, and whole grains. Along with new ways to incorporate traditional foods that we have been eating since childhood, Dave Grotto introduces us to foods that have a long history of existence but that are relatively new to many of our diets.

As a registered dietitian, I commend my colleague and friend for bringing us a fresh approach to healthy eating. I have always maintained the philosophy that if one views changing eating habits as "going on a diet" then the "going off the diet" phase will soon reappear, negating any potential health benefits. In today's world of escalating health costs and the rise of chronic disease, each of us must accept the responsibility of personal preventive health. Dave Grotto, a registered dietitian and spokesperson for the American Dietetic Association, has provided us with the guidance and knowledge to accept the challenge. With an eye to taste and enjoyment, he will teach you to add the lifesavers of powerhouse foods to your diet while slowly removing, but not necessarily eliminating, those foods with fewer benefits.

As you turn the pages of this innovative book, have a note pad ready! You will be making a list of new foods to buy, recipes to try, and health tips to follow. And I can ensure you will have numerous health tips and food facts to contribute at your next dinner party or family gathering. Join me on the journey of eating well to live well!

Here's to your health!

> Marianne Smith Edge, MS, RD, LD
> President, MSE & Associates, LLC
> President, American Dietetic Association (2003–2004)

Introduction

WHY 101 FOODS?

Life *n*.
1. The property or quality that distinguishes living organisms from dead organisms . . .
2. A manner of living.

My eighty-seven-year-old father's favorite expression is "When you wake up in the morning and both feet hit the ground, you're having a good day!" Indeed! But certainly the definition of "life" encompasses more than waking up and just existing, right? Isn't it also enjoying a life as pain-free and disease-free as possible? *That* is a truly desirable manner of living.

Sometimes it seems that our joyous holiday or regular dinner conversations revolve around nagging health ailments that constantly interfere with living. George now has gout, Grandma has diabetes, Suzy has irritable bowel syndrome, and your sister complains that she can't lose those last ten pounds (well, maybe twenty), even on the latest deprivation diet. In response and without fail, someone at that dinner table always comes up with a home remedy or a wonder food, heard about from a friend, that is sure to cure the ailment. Yes, everyone feels that they have some expertise in the field of nutrition, but whether their advice is sound or even safe to follow can be a roll of the dice. Still, there are foods that hold vast curing and ameliorative powers. You just need to know how to find them.

Seeking out simple interventions and using food as medicine has long been the approach of many cultures throughout the world. Before the advent of modern medicine, the family was dependent on a mother's intuition accompanied by her time-honored remedies as the first line of defense in preserving the family's health and well-being. Going to see the doctor at the first sniffle, cough, or other sign of distress used to be "Plan B," not "Plan A." But as utilization of modern medicine increased, the focus on using food as medicine declined. We have embraced the convenience of statin drugs for reducing cholesterol, when the inclusion of foods with innate heart-protecting properties—such as fatty fish, oats, almonds, and beans—might be just as effective. And many of the shortcuts of modern medicine are not without their costs. In fact, Americans who visit physicians following adverse reactions to medications account for well over two million physician visits each year!

This book aims to bring life-saving foods back into our health plans and to resurrect traditional medicinal uses for foods, many of which are now backed by modern science.

My Story

I've been a practicing registered dietitian for over twenty years. But my interest in nutrition first began when I was fifteen. I was battling acne, weight problems, panic attacks—and I'm sure a few other things at the time—and realized I had to make some changes if I was ever to see sixteen. I was working at a health food store at the time but ironically had very little interest in trying any of the products to help myself (except for the "natural" candy, which had all of the sugar, fat, and calories as other candy bars). I bought breakfast, lunch, and sometimes dinner at the fast food establishment across the street and started smoking. A customer who befriended me suggested that I try adding some veggies, fruit, and whole grains to my diet—not all at once but a little at a time. I figured I had nothing to lose, so I made some of the suggested changes and quickly discovered what good health really felt like.

Over the years, as I became healthier and more intrigued about nutrition, I did a lot of reading on the subject. More and more customers started asking me for my advice on overcoming health hurdles that they were treating medically without success. I was dispensing advice to my customers, but didn't have the credentials to back up what I was saying. I decided to pursue a degree in nutrition and became a registered dietitian.

Over the past two decades, I have worked as a nutritionist in conventional and integrative medical centers and in private practice. I've helped patients recover from multiple drug addictions; reverse heart disease; prevent and fight cancer; improve mental, physical, and sexual performance, even when challenged with diseases including multiple sclerosis, Parkinson's, and Alzheimer's; and become pregnant—all through good nutrition practices.

Though I enjoyed meeting with patients and their families, I had always desired to get out my positive health message to the greatest number of people possible. In 1990, I was asked to host a live, nutrition-focused radio show called *Let's Talk Health, Chicago,* which aired in four states and ran for over ten years. Then in 2000, I was asked to be a national spokesperson for the American Dietetic Association, an organization representing over 67,000 food and nutrition experts. Because I was experienced in both conventional nutrition and integrative medicine, and had also had the experience of interviewing hundreds of experts and answering the questions of thousands of listeners, they felt I could help consumers sort out confusing and often contradictory health messages regarding food and nutrition.

I have found that it is especially difficult for men to change their eating habits, so I was thrilled when I was asked to be on the scientific advisory board for *Men's Health* magazine. I'm often asked to *spell things out* for guys in simple terms—"eat this, not that." Bachelors do well with "black and white" and once married, that decision-making process often defaults to their wives. Women not only understand the importance of taking care of themselves and seeking regular medical attention, they also tend to be the caretakers of men too. My male clients have found that a simpler approach—a 101 Foods approach that keeps an eye on good taste and ample portions—has worked out best for them and their families, too. Through my work with thousands of individuals I found that focusing on restricting less healthy food choices didn't always work when trying to get my patients to make lasting changes. Even my most motivated patients could give up their favorite foods and follow a "perfect" diet . . . for a while. They would try restrictive dietary plans if there was an obvious payoff, but eventually they would all come to me with the same questions: "Can't I cheat just once in a while? Will I really be hurting myself?" I had always thought that an all-or-nothing approach was best and that half measures wouldn't benefit my patients. I assumed if I gave them an inch, they would take a mile. "Cheating" could only spell disaster, and they would eventually revert back to harmful habits. But fond remembrances of foods-gone-by left my patients yearning for the old days. They felt deprived and often resented that they couldn't enjoy their favorite foods anymore. Frequently, they pressed me to produce proof that adding just a few unhealthy favorites back into their diet was really going to derail their efforts, hoping I would come up empty-handed. In fact, I often did.

I came to the revelation that limiting quantities of less-than-optimal foods was a possibility, but writing them out of the book of life, permanently, was definitely not an option. Not only did I have to deal with my patients' taste preferences that had evolved over a lifetime but many of my patients faced external pressure from family members who didn't have the same motivation to abandon their favorite foods. So, more times than not, these "dietary insurgents," like candy bars and french fries, hung around—lurking behind kitchen cabinets or closed refrigerator doors, or worse yet, taking up temporary residence in the gleeful mouths of family members. Not surprisingly, I found that my patients didn't want to admit that despite my warnings they had worked many of these foods back into their diets.

Change came more easily when I eased up on the restrictions. Soon I was known as "Let's-make-a-deal Dave." My patients proved that they were able to maintain their efforts longer, stabilize their weights, sustain blood pressures within acceptable ranges, and meet a host of other markers of good health even while allowing the occasional indulgence in their diets. I started to see a pattern. Many were focusing on including "lifesavers" or "powerhouse" foods in their diets *while* decreasing, but not abandoning, foods that had little health benefit. It finally dawned on me: Healthy eating didn't have to be black and white—gray works just fine too!

Ironically, in the summer of 2006, while writing this book, I became my own patient. For over a year, I became so focused on extolling the virtues of eating properly and exercising that I slowly but surely typed myself out of a healthy lifestyle. It seemed with each keystroke, my gut and butt got bigger, while I was giving advice to make everyone else's smaller. My wake-up call came when I was asked to coach Chicago firefighters in a cholesterol-reduction program. I found out that firefighters were at much greater risk of dying from a heart attack than they would ever be from putting out fires, so I was only too happy to help. As an act of solidarity, I had my own cholesterol drawn, only to discover that I had my own four-alarm fire coursing through my veins—a cholesterol level of 238! That did it for me. But instead of my previous "nutrition smack-down" approach, I decided to slowly modify my diet by adding in the very foods you will read about throughout this book. After thirty days of simple changes, without any help from cholesterol-lowering medication or any radical diet, my cholesterol came crashing down to 168—a whopping seventy points in just thirty days. And I lost ten pounds to boot!

I begin every morning with a good-size bowl of oatmeal topped with chopped almonds, figs, cranberries, and cherries swimming in soy milk. I eat salmon and sardines and drink coffee and green tea. I started exercising thirty minutes every day and have continued this program ever since.

I've come across many foods that have had profound effects on my health and the health of my patients—foods that offer hope of eventually reducing or even replacing drug therapies to control conditions like high blood pressure, elevated blood lipids, and even diabetes. I saw digestive disorders, poor sexual performance, diminished cognitive function, low energy levels, and others among an endless list of health challenges improve because of simple but healing foods. There are foods that not only literally save lives, but that are delicious and enjoyable too.

Many of the life-saving foods that are featured in this book are common everyday foods that you may have eaten all of your life but whose contribution to your health you have taken for granted. Your introduction to them may have started when your mother encouraged you to eat all of your vegetables because they would help you to grow up to be big and strong. Or perhaps you discovered that she was using a little extra garlic in the hopes that its healing properties might ward off colds and flu. But Mom was also given the ultimate task of making good-for-you foods taste great. She knew that unless it tasted good there was very little chance you would continue to eat your "medicine." My goal, like hers, is to show you how to integrate healthy foods into your diet in a way that makes nutritious eating easy and delicious.

The Science of "Half Measures"

Small changes that don't involve a complete lifestyle or dietary overhaul can have a significant impact on the quality of your daily life. Simple life-affirming actions, such as walking a few extra steps, thinking positive thoughts, and incorporating a handful of optimal foods into the daily diet are just a few of the well-researched choices that we can all make to battle many of today's common health challenges. Yes, it sounds too good to be true, but the proof has been documented by leading researchers, such as Barbara Rolls, a leading obesity researcher from Penn State University and author of *Volumetrics*. In a study of 200 overweight and obese women and men, Dr. Rolls found that those who added two servings of a low-calorie, dense vegetable soup to their diet lost fifty percent more weight than those subjects who ate a less nutritious snack that provided the same calories as the soup. Also, including foods like whole grain breakfast cereals and other whole grain food items are associated with keeping healthy and trim. And the examples go on and on.

The 101 Foods

You may be wondering how I came up with these 101 foods. For starters, I turned in part to the concept of "nutrient density." Adam Drewnowski, director of the Center for Public Health Nutrition at the University of Washington, is one of many researchers who have been tackling the challenge of developing a system for consumers that clearly shows which foods are the healthiest. He developed a method based on a nutrients-per-calorie basis, meaning those foods that contain the most nutrition for the fewest calories. Dr. Drewnowski reviewed over 360 different foods and assigned a naturally nutrient-rich (NNR) score to each one based on the content of fourteen key nutrients. However, his system doesn't take phytochemical density into account. Phytochemicals are plant compounds that offer important health benefits but are not considered "nutrients" like vitamins and minerals. I have also incorporated phytochemical density into my analysis. A comprehensive chart in Appendix B features the phytochemicals that you will often see mentioned when I review the benefits of the 101 foods. Finally, I reviewed the scientific literature for exciting new research on the healing properties of foods. If a food was shown to improve health, regardless of its nutrient or phytochemical content, I included it in the list of the 101 foods. Also keep in mind that I don't claim that these are the quintessential or the only 101 foods that could save your life. Nutritional science is ever evolving and we find out new benefits to foods all of the time—but be assured, the foods I have chosen in this book are worthy of residence in your grocery cart and your stomach!

Because the science of nutrition is always progressing, I made the decision not to limit my criteria of evaluating the 101 foods to only the gold standard of human clinical trials but instead expanded it to all levels of evidence. I am a firm supporter of evidence-based nutrition but unfortunately, randomized, crossover, placebo-controlled, human trials and meta-analyses (reviews of several studies) are few and far between in the study of nutrition. For example, in 2007, a meta-analysis containing 149,000 participants appeared in the journal *Nutrition, Metabolism & Cardiovascular Diseases* and showed that consuming 2.5 servings of whole grains daily was associated with a twenty-one percent reduction in risk of cardiovascular disease. Exciting stuff! The lead researcher suggested, based on this new evidence, that a doubling of effort should be made by policy-makers, scientists, and clinicians to spread the good news. Considering heart disease is the number one killer of Americans, that sounds like a good idea. My patients want to know what they can do to save their lives now. If I waited until a meta-analysis came by as incentive to "double my efforts" in espousing the benefits of a healthy diet, I suspect many of my patients wouldn't be here today. I didn't want them to hesitate one moment in deciding to add more fruits, vegetables, nuts, or whole grains into their diet. Why wait? Today's possibility may be tomorrow's probability and there is certainly no downside to eating healthy foods!

You Can Write Your Own Prescription with the 101 Foods

FIRST, EAT OPTIMALLY . . .

It was important to me before ever typing a word that this be a valued resource of great foods rather than another deprivation "diet book." According to the latest surveys, one thing is abundantly clear: You're tired of being told what to do, and I can't blame you! You won't see "don't do this or don't do that" anywhere in this book. This book celebrates food. I'll leave the demonizing of this protein or that dairy product to others. But make no mistake, I do have an ultimate goal in mind: to encourage you to eat and live "optimally." I define the food portion of optimal living as a diet that is calorie-controlled, is abundant in varied and intense-colored fruits and vegetables, is whole grain–focused, contains appropriate levels and type of fats, and emphasizes low-fat dairy and reduced animal protein intake while increasing healthier, plant-based proteins, such as beans.

Think of this book as a starting point for improving your health, no matter what your health challenge. According to Dr. James Hill from the University of Colorado, a leading researcher in obesity, even if your ultimate goal is to lose weight, just keeping your present weight stable is a great start. Try introducing a few new foods your first week. The sample menu plan at the back of this book shows how easy and delicious adding in can be, and you can trim down portion sizes to tailor things to a calorie level that's right for you. Try a few more new foods the next week and the week after that. Eventually, you will find that many of your new foods have become replacements for foods less beneficial to your health. And then you will achieve a lasting program built on my simple equation: *doability + taste = sustainability.*

If you really want to "put the pedal to the metal" and maximize the health benefits of the 101 foods, you need to embrace the power of synergy. As you have discovered from my story, eating a bowl of oats every day can be an effective method for lowering cholesterol. But adding nuts like almonds, walnuts, and pistachios, along with some cranberries and cherries, all submerged in some soy milk, takes that bowl to a whole new level. When it's coupled with a diet that includes lean proteins, low-fat dairy products, and vegetables, with an eye on limiting saturated-fat foods like bacon, sausage, and butter, along with moderate physical activity, the cholesterol-reducing power is awesome!

101 FOODS IS SOUND NUTRITION

Your body needs it all—carbohydrates, protein, fats, vitamins, minerals, enzymes, and plant chemicals. You could buy bottles of dietary supplements and try to do your best to replicate what a healthy diet contains, but isn't eating food that contains all of the building blocks of health naturally a lot simpler and better-tasting? Bottom line—no dietary supplement on the market today comes close to providing the life-saving properties of the 101 foods. Proper supplementation can play an important role in maintaining or improving health but it doesn't compare to the healing-power capacity of food! Each food group serves an important function in the body, keeping you healthy and strong.

Carbo the magnificent: Carbohydrates give us energy. They're the fuel on which the human body runs. The fruits, vegetables, and whole grains that I feature do a great job of providing the right amount and right type of carbohydrates your body demands.

Keeping lean with protein: Protein helps repair the tissues of our body. In general, the American diet provides more than enough protein to meet our needs. Beans, soy, fish, and whey are the featured protein champions in this book. You may ask, "Can't lean cuts of beef, chicken, pork, and so forth fit well into this program?" Sure! In fact, some of the recipes contain some of these animal protein sources as ingredients. But I wanted to feature these special protein foods for two reasons: We don't eat enough of them and these protein foods have special value-added attributes which I will explain later.

Chewing the fat: All fats are not created equal. Some contribute to heart disease and others work to fight it and other diseases too. Fat provides taste and satisfaction, and keeps you feeling full longer. It also is a vehicle for transporting fat-soluble vitamins, such as vitamins A, D, E, and K, that boost and protect your immune system, build strong bones, and regulate blood flow into your cells.

All the rest: Vitamins, minerals, enzymes, and phytochemicals (plant chemicals) are as important to your body as carbs, protein, and fat. Food provides these nutrients in the right proportion.

Add it all together: The USDA Dietary Guidelines for Americans is the best and most credible resource for eating a healthy diet. The dietary icon that came from those guidelines is the latest food pyramid, otherwise known as "MyPyramid." The new pyramid shows that all food groups are important in a healthy diet.

What You Will See in This Book

101 Foods That Could Save Your Life! will reveal that many of the delicious foods that we often reserve for those special occasions, like cranberries and sweet potatoes, need to be invited back on a more regular basis. You will also be introduced to more unfamiliar foods like the super-nutritious grains teff, quinoa, and amaranth, along with antioxidant-rich fruits like açaí from Brazil and goji berries from China. There is a wide world of healthy and delicious foods from which to select. Every food entry includes the following sections so that you can decide which foods will make the best additions to your diet.

WHAT'S THE STORY?

Each featured food has a story unto itself. Here you will find interesting background information that may include what plant kingdom the food belongs to, where its natural habitat is located, and how it is commonly consumed. Also accompanying every food entry are entertaining factoids such as: Did you know . . . Amazon Indians used guava fruit to remedy sore throats, digestive challenges, and vertigo, and to regulate menstrual periods?

"A SERVING OF FOOD LORE . . ." AND "WHERE IS IT GROWN?"

Did you ever wonder where coffee beans originated? You might be surprised to learn that South America, where most coffee beans come from now, was not the original place of origin. This section answers such questions as "How did the kiwi make its way from the Yangtze River Valley of northern China to New Zealand and the United States?" "What stops did it make along the way?" "Who are the major suppliers today?"

WHY SHOULD I EAT IT?

This section starts off with the nutritional value, just one of many important reasons for adding the powerhouse foods into your diet. Then I'll cover the prominent vitamins and minerals unique to the featured food and explain how this food can improve your health.

HOME REMEDIES

Did mom really know best? She was giving cranberry juice to her kids to help fight urinary tract infections long before there was science to support its effectiveness. All she knew was that it worked! This section features many claims for the healing properties of the 101 foods that may not have been exhaustively studied . . . yet!

THROW ME A LIFESAVER!

This section references many research reports, from cell studies to animal studies to the granddaddy of them all, human clinical trials. Some of the studies show that there are unique properties to the 101 foods. Other research supports the value of including a food with a shared nutrient or group of nutrients held in common with other foods. You can also match up foods in the index that meet a common health challenge and then you will be on your way to a tailored approach!

TIPS ON USING THE 101 FOODS

Researchers at Gerber Foods found that a substantial number of toddlers didn't eat ANY fruits or vegetables but did eat their fair share of candy, french fries, and hot dogs. Not a big surprise, but it does raise the question, "Hey . . . who's the boss here?" I know what you are saying: "I tried several times to get my child to eat fruits and vegetables but they simply won't eat them." My advice to you is to try and try again! These same researchers found that a new food may need to be reintroduced as many as seventeen times before a child will include it in their core group of favorites. Don't give up! But to make your life easier, I have included helpful, tasty tips along with important selection, storage, and food safety recommendations to maximize your family's eating experience with the 101 foods.

THE RECIPE . . .

To help you jump right in with the 101, I've included one top-notch recipe for each food. The recipes are from award-winning chefs who know how to combine great taste and good health. I've also gathered recipes from noted dietitians, celebrities, family, and friends. Most of the recipes were written especially with children in mind and were tested on my family and neighbors. The focus here is on the great natural taste of the powerhouse foods, and easy preparation.

BREAK IT DOWN . . .

Each recipe has been analyzed for calories, fat, saturated fat, carbohydrates, sugars, fiber, sodium, and protein using the top-rated recipe software program, Food Processor by ESHA. All recipes contain virtually zero grams of synthetic trans fats.

How and Where to Shop for the 101 Foods

I've put together a list of name-brand suggestions for you to try at my website: www.101FoodsThatCouldSaveYourLife.com. The list is called

"Dave's Raves" and I will be updating it often to keep you on top of many tasty, convenient ways to enjoy *101 Foods*. These are items that either my family or my patients have tried and enjoyed. This list is by no means exhaustive, but it's certainly a good start! You may also check out the many websites that I found helpful while researching the origin, history, and benefits of the powerhouse foods. These sites are included in the References section beginning on page 369. And, I've included my one-week sample menu plan (Appendix A) to help you get started.

Perhaps the two main dilemmas you will face along your path of the 101 foods are which food you will try first and where you will keep this book! Will it be kept among the cookbooks? Health and diet books? Resource guides? On your green tea/coffee table for all to enjoy? No matter where you decide to keep it, I hope you will consult this book often as you prepare your next meal and create the menu for your next holiday feast.

The 101 Foods

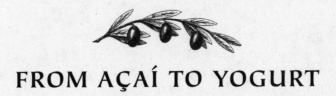

FROM AÇAÍ TO YOGURT

Açaí *(Euterpe oleracea)*

ORAC ATTACK!

Did you know . . . the antioxidant capacity or "ORAC" value for a four-ounce portion of Açaí is 6576? That is more than blueberries, strawberries, and red wine combined!

What's the Story?

Açaí (pronounced *ah-sigh-ee*) berries are produced by a palm tree grown in the floodplain areas of the Amazon River in Brazil. Theye have a unique taste—like wildberries with a hint of slightly bitter chocolate—yum! The berry, about the same size as a blueberry, is ninety-five percent seed. The seeds are discarded, leaving the skin alone for açaí products.

A Serving of Food Lore . . .

In the Amazon, açaí palms cover an area equivalent to half the size of Switzerland. Açaí is a primary food staple of Amazon River communities. It is served as a beverage and is a main part of the meal, much in the same way as bread or rice in other cultures. In the city of Belém in Brazil, more of the fruit is drunk than milk—an estimated 200,000 liters of açaí juice is consumed daily among a population of 1.3 million.

Where Is Açaí Grown?

Açaí is unique to the Amazon rainforests of Brazil and commercial production of the berry is found mainly near the city of Belém.

Why Should I Eat Açaí?

Surprisingly for a fruit, the vast majority of the calories come from fat: A four-ounce serving of pure açaí contains about 100 calories and six grams of fat. However, it is rich in anti-inflammatory omega-9 fats and also contains little sugar. Açaí contains essential fatty acids, iron, calcium, fiber, vitamin A, and other antioxidants.

Scientists have discovered that açaí is rich in anthocyanins, a special group of plant chemicals believed to have many health benefits. In fact, açaí contains ten times more anthocyanins than is found in an equal serving of red wine. Anthocyanins in açaí make up only about ten percent of the total antioxidants contained within this amazing little berry.

Açaí also contains phytosterols, a plant component known to reduce cholesterol, treat symptoms associated with benign prostatic hyperplasia (swollen prostate), and help protect the immune system from physical stress.

Home Remedies

SEXUAL PERFORMANCE: Açaí combined with guarana syrup is a popular drink in Brazil. One of the reported benefits from drinking the concoction is improved sexual performance.

BEAUTY: Dr. Nicholas Perricone mentions in his anti-aging books that açaí has beautifying properties.

Throw Me a Lifesaver!

CANCER: Utilizing a test tube study, University of Florida researchers found powerful antioxidant compounds in açaí that greatly reduced cell proliferation and enhanced apoptosis (programmed cell death) in human leukemia cells.

Tips on Using Açaí

SELECTION AND STORAGE:
- Açaí comes in juice, frozen pulp, bottled smoothies, and powder forms that are all readily available at most health food stores and

grocery markets. Due to their highly perishable nature, fresh açaí berries are only available in Brazil.
- Look for flash-pasteurized açaí products which preserve açaí's antioxidants and beautiful purple color.

PREPARATION AND SERVING SUGGESTIONS:
- Heating açaí may diminish some of its antioxidants.
- Açaí can be used to make sauces and jams.
- The pulp can be added into smoothies or beverages, spooned over cereal, added to yogurt, or eaten alone.

Brazilian-Style Açaí Bowl
by Royce Gracie
Servings: 2 • Prep time: 5 minutes

Royce Gracie is an international star in the sport of jujitsu and has a long family history of using açaí for improved performance. Royce's grandfather, Carlos, opened Brazil's first jujitsu academy and began to incorporate açaí into his own diet and those of his students many years ago. Our family loves this recipe over yogurt, ice cream, pancakes . . . you name it! All four ingredients are powerhouse foods.

INGREDIENTS:
2 100-gram packs Sambazon   *1 organic banana*
    original açaí pulp   *1 teaspoon organic honey*
4 ounces organic apple juice

DIRECTIONS:
Blend all the ingredients in a blender until thickened. Top with organic granola and additional organic honey to taste.

BREAK IT DOWN . . .
Calories: 190; Total fat: 5g; Saturated fat: 1g; Cholesterol: 0mg; Sodium: 10mg; Total carbs: 44g; Fiber: 2g; Sugar: 34g; Protein: 3g.

Agave *(Agavaceae)*

¿DÓNDE ESTÁ, AGAVE?

Did you know . . . at the turn of this century, tequila production had risen so dramatically that the blue agave plant (also used to make agave nectar) was on the verge of extinction?

What's the Story?

There are over three hundred species of agave plants. *Tequilana,* or blue agave, is the most widely known and available. The name *agave* is of Greek origin and means "noble" or "illustrious." Agave goes by many other names including maguey, mescal, lechuguilla, amole, and century plant. Though over 200 million blue agave plants are grown in several regions of Mexico, only a small percentage of them are used for agave nectar production.

The heart of the plant is often referred to as the "piña," or pineapple, which holds the naturally sweet juice used for both tequila and nectar production. The juice can either become "dark," "amber," or "light," depending on the processing. Unfiltered dark agave has a stronger flavor, while the light variety, which has had the solids removed, has a more refined flavor. The liquid is then heated to make concentrated syrup, much like maple sap is heated to create maple syrup, with a consistency a little thinner than honey.

A Serving of Food Lore . . .

Agaves were cultivated for centuries by Native Americans. In the seventeenth century, the Portuguese and Spaniards brought agaves back to Europe from the Americas. The Spaniards are actually credited with fermenting the juices from the agave and creating what we now know as tequila. Another fermented beverage made from agave was called *pulque,* made by Native Americans for use in religious ceremonies. Agave nectar has become increasingly popular as an alternative sweetener to sugar in the United States.

Where Is Agave Grown?

The agave plant is native to arid and tropical regions from the southern United States to northern South America, and throughout the Caribbean. The agave has long been cultivated in hilly regions of Mexico.

Why Should I Eat Agave?

Agave syrup (or nectar) is about ninety percent fructose, a form of natural sugar found in fruit. Fructose does not impact blood glucose (glycemic) levels as dramatically as other sweeteners such as cane sugar. Even better, because fructose is sweeter than table sugar, less is needed in your recipes. Agave also contains a complex form of fructose called *inulin*. A type of friendly bacteria called *bifidobacteria* digests inulin to produce short-chain fatty acids that have been shown to fight colon cancer. Agave also contains *sapogenins*, which have anti-inflammatory and anticancer properties.

Home Remedies

Mexican folklore has revered agave and considered it sacred for its ability to purify the body and soul. Ethopians have used agave branches as natural toothbrushes, while the Aztecs treated wound infections with concentrated sap.

Throw Me a Lifesaver!

ANTI-INFLAMMATORY: An animal study found those who were treated with an extract from agave leaves orally and topically had less inflammation than the control group.

ANTIMICROBIAL: Agave has been found to contain special substances that greatly reduce the growth of yeasts, mold, and life-threatening bacteria.

CANCER-KILLING ACTIVITY: Human cell studies have found that saponin and other compounds in agave can interrupt the life cycle of cancer cells.

Tips on Using Agave

SELECTION AND STORAGE:
- This sweetener is sometimes called "nectar" and sometimes called "syrup." It is one and the same.
- Agave comes in light, amber, and dark syrup sold in bottles.
- Unopened, agave syrup has approximately a three-year shelf life.

PREPARATION AND SERVING SUGGESTIONS:
- In recipes, use about twenty-five percent less of this nectar than of table sugar. Three-quarter cup of agave nectar should equal 1 cup of table sugar. For most recipes this rule works well.
- Reduce your oven temperature by 25 degrees.
- When substituting this sweetener in recipes, reduce your liquid slightly, sometimes as much as one-third less.
- Agave nectar can be combined with artificial sweeteners to lessen their aftertaste.
- It can be used as a substitute for honey or sugar in baking.

Sharon's Simple Berry Sauce
by Sharon Grotto
Servings: 4 • Prep and cooking time: 35 minutes

Our kids love to pour this berry sauce on their toaster waffles and pancakes or use it as an easy way to add fruit and sweetness to a smoothie. Simple to make but oh so good! This recipe contains two powerhouse ingredients.

INGREDIENTS:

1 10-ounce package frozen mixed
   organic berries
¼ cup agave syrup

1 teaspoon vanilla extract
½ cup water

DIRECTIONS:
Combine frozen berry blend, agave syrup, vanilla extract, and water in a saucepan. Cook over low heat until the frozen berries are defrosted. Bring to boil. Let simmer uncovered until sauce thickens, about 20 to 30 minutes. Serve over pancakes, waffles, French toast, or anything that you want to taste "berry good."

BREAK IT DOWN . . .

Calories: 95; Total fat: 0g; Saturated fat: 0g; Cholesterol: 0mg; Sodium: 75mg; Total carbs: 24g; Fiber: 1g; Sugar: 21g; Protein: 0g.

Almonds *(Prunus dulcis)*

WEDDED ALMOND BLISS

Did you know . . . the traditional wedding favor of five candied almonds (Jordan almonds) originated in Italy in the 1350s? They represent the five attributes of a happy marriage: health, wealth, happiness, fertility, and longevity.

What's the Story?

Almonds are the seeds of a fruit tree that is a relative of the rose family. Most commercially grown almond trees are grafted to the stumps of peach trees (rootstock), making them more resistant to pests. *Prunus dulcis,* meaning "sweet almond," is the commonly consumed version of almonds. "Bitter" almond contains a toxic chemical called hydrocyanic acid that can be deadly to humans if eaten raw. When heated, this chemical is destroyed, making the bitter almond safe to consume. Sweet almonds, the most consumed tree nuts in the United States, comprise sixty-two percent of the nut market.

A Serving of Food Lore . . .

Almonds originated in central Asia and have been cultivated in the Mediterranean since Biblical times. The Bible spoke of Aaron's rod that blossomed and bore almonds, using them as a symbol to represent divine approval by God. The almond also symbolized virginity and was often used as a marriage blessing. The Egyptians left almonds in King Tut's tomb to provide nourishment to him in the afterlife. In 1700, Franciscan padres brought the almond tree to California from Spain. By the turn of the twentieth century, the almond industry was firmly established in the Sacramento and San Joaquin areas of California.

Where Are They Grown?

The United States provides eighty-eight percent of worldwide almond production with California growing the bulk of the U.S. supply. They are also grown in Spain, Turkey, Greece, and Italy.

Why Should I Include Them?

A small handful of almonds (one ounce or 23 almonds) contains 160 calories and is a good source of protein and fiber. This same amount supplies thirty-five percent of the daily value (DV) for vitamin E and twenty percent DV of magnesium, and is a good source of calcium and iron. Almonds contain a variety of antioxidants including the flavonoids quercetin and kaempferol, which may prevent cancer cell growth and oxidation of LDL ("bad") cholesterol, attributed to increased risk for heart disease.

Home Remedies

Almonds have been used in hopes of curing cancer, ulcers, and corns, and reducing symptoms associated with consuming too much alcohol.

Throw Me a Lifesaver!

OBESITY: A 2006 study in the *American Journal of Clinical Nutrition* found that women who had eaten a serving of almonds had higher levels of cholecystokinin (a hormone associated with satiety from eating fat-containing foods) in their systems than men did. In practical terms this means that while almonds may leave both women and men with a feeling of "satisfaction," women may stay full longer. There is ongoing research into the effects of the act of "chewing" on satiety hormone release. For example, researchers at King's College in London found that almonds appear to help block absorption of carbohydrates, block their own fat from being absorbed, and improve satiety in both men and women. According to a 2003 study in the *International Journal of Obesity*, subjects who added eighty-four grams (about three handfuls) of almonds to a low-calorie diet enhanced weight loss when compared to a low-fat, low-calorie diet alone. The diet that included almonds produced greater and longer sustained weight loss.

HEART HEALTH: A study published in the *American Journal of Clinical Nutrition* (*AJCN*) showed that eating a combination of heart-healthy foods that includes almonds can help reduce LDL or "bad" cholesterol levels as much as a first-line statin drug. Loma Linda University was the first to demonstrate that eating almonds raises vitamin E levels in the bloodstream. Participants who ate almonds reduced their total cholesterol by five percent and lowered their LDL or "bad" cholesterol by nearly seven percent. In 2003, the Food and Drug Administration approved a limited health claim for almonds saying that consuming them may reduce the risk of heart disease. Dr. David Jenkins of the University of Toronto found that eating a healthy diet that included almonds reduced inflammation by about the same level as taking Lovastatin, a popular statin drug for fighting heart disease. The almond-rich diet not only lowered cholesterol but it also lowered C-reactive protein, a leading marker of inflammation and an independent risk factor for heart disease.

ALZHEIMER'S: Mice with an Alzheimer's-like disease were fed an almond-rich diet. After four months, those animals who ate the almond-rich diet did much better on memory tests than those fed the usual chow. The diet also reduced the number of Alzheimer deposits in the rodent brains.

COLON CANCER: A study from the University of California, Davis, found that almonds had a significant effect on the prevention of colon cancer in rats.

Tips on Using Almonds

SELECTION AND STORAGE:

A KERNEL OF TRUTH?

Consumer, beware! Make sure you are buying "the real McCoy." Many imported almonds are not almonds at all—they're apricot kernels! They may look similar but the taste and health benefits of real almonds are second to none.

- Look for almonds in the shell that don't rattle when you shake them. Rattling may be a sign that the almonds are old.

- Fresh almonds are white throughout. One that is yellow or has a honeycomb look to it may mean the nut has turned rancid.
- Green almonds are available for three weeks in the spring. They have a fuzzy green hull and a jellylike center. They are great on a salad or plain with a dash of sea salt.
- Look in the baking aisle, the snack aisle, and the produce section of the supermarket for many types of almonds. Look for one-ounce snack packs of whole almonds, or other on-the-go containers. Choose slivered, sliced, chopped, or ground almonds to use in recipes.
- Store in a cool, dry, dark place.
- Unopened, containers of almonds can be kept in the refrigerator or a cool pantry for up to two years. Once opened, they should be kept in an airtight container and consumed within three months.

PREPARATION AND SERVING SUGGESTIONS:
- Roasting almonds before serving them brings out their rich flavor.
- Sprinkle sliced almonds on granola, cold cereal, or yogurt for breakfast or for a healthy anytime snack.
- Spread almond butter on an English muffin or toast. Almond butter, sold by the jar, is available next to peanut butter, jams, and jellies at many supermarkets and health food stores.
- Use almond milk in breakfast smoothies or on cereal. You'll find it in an unrefrigerated box next to the soy milk section at the supermarket.
- Munch on some almond trail mix or snack mix.
- Roast whole almonds with kosher salt and a variety of herbs, such as rosemary, thyme, curry powder, cumin, cinnamon, or cardamom for some kick.
- Add slivered almonds to rice, couscous, other grain dishes, and pasta.
- Use ground almond meal for a healthy "breading" for fish or poultry.

Berry & Almond Pizza

Courtesy of the Almond Board of California

Servings: 2 • Prep and cooking time: 15 minutes

All five ingredients in this recipe are powerhouse foods.

INGREDIENTS:

1 (6-inch) whole wheat pita
3 tablespoons almond butter
⅓ cup fresh berries

1 tablespoon slivered or sliced almonds, roasted
1 teaspoon agave syrup or honey

DIRECTIONS:

Toast pita. Spread with almond butter, and sprinkle with fresh berries and almonds. Drizzle agave syrup or honey over top. Cut in half and serve.

BREAK IT DOWN . . .

Calories: 280; Total fat: 17g; Saturated fat: 1.5g; Cholesterol: 0mg; Sodium: 170mg; Total carbs: 29g; Fiber: 5g; Sugar: 7g; Protein: 8g.

Amaranth (*Amaranthus*)

"IDOL" GRAIN

Did you know . . . Aztec people used to make idols out of amaranth, honey, and human blood, and then eat them? Cortés thought this practice was an abomination and burned their amaranth fields to the ground. Amaranth had all but disappeared and was not rediscovered until several centuries later.

What's the Story?

Amaranth, also known as *Chinese spinach* or *pigweed*, is a plant that is valued for its culinary as well as its cosmetic properties. There are about sixty varieties of amaranth plants in existence today. Amaranth seeds are quite small, about the size of sesame seeds, and are typically yellow to cream in color. The flavor of amaranth seeds is a combination of sweet and nutty with a somewhat crunchy texture when cooked. The leaves of the edible varieties of amaranth taste very similar to spinach.

A Serving of Food Lore . . .

Amaranth, often referred to as the "ancient grain of the Aztecs," dates back some 8,000 years. It is thought to be the main grain consumed by the Aztecs before they were conquered by Spain. Amaranth was revered for its nutritional superiority and was hailed as the fuel of warriors. It was also prized as an offering pleasing to Montezuma due to its great nutrition and healing powers.

Where Is Amaranth Grown?

China is the largest producer of the grain today. Amaranth is also culti-vated in Mexico, Central America, and in recent years, regions of the United States such as Colorado, Illinois, and Nebraska.

Why Should I Eat Amaranth?

Amaranth ranks highest in protein per serving out of all of the grains. It contains the essential amino acid lysine, which is deficient in all other grains. Added to other grains, amaranth actually completes their incom-plete proteins. Amaranth also has one of the highest fiber contents among the grains. Of all the grains, only quinoa ranks higher in iron than ama-ranth. It is also a good source of calcium, magnesium, and folate. It con-tains the cholesterol-lowering, cancer-fighting phytochemical squalene.

Home Remedies

Flowers from the amaranth plant are used to treat toothaches and fevers in Peru. A popular rum drink in Ecuador called "aguardiente" is made out of amaranth flowers and is thought to help "cleanse the blood" and regu-late a woman's monthly cycle.

Throw Me a Lifesaver!

CANCER: Squalene is an antioxidant found naturally in amaranth that may halt blood supply to tumors. Shark oil, a more commonly used source of squalene, has only one percent squalene content, while the content of amaranth oil is eight percent.

BREAST CANCER PREVENTION: Research has found that a component in the amaranth seed can inhibit tumor growth in breast cancer cells.

HEART DISEASE: Though oats seem to be the undisputed cholesterol "soaker-upper" grain, amaranth appears to be almost as effective in lowering LDL cholesterol and may be a viable alternative for those who have an allergy to or simply don't like oats.

DIABETES: Amaranth has been found to aid in the prevention of hyperglycemia and may ease diabetic complications. In a study of diabetic rats, amaranth significantly decreased serum glucose, increased serum insulin levels, and normalized elevated liver function markers.

Tips on Using Amaranth

SELECTION AND STORAGE:
- Amaranth comes in flour form for use in baking. Combine with wheat flour in equal proportions to make bread dough.
- Amaranth seeds can be stored for up to six months in the refrigerator in an airtight jar or container.

PREPARATION AND SERVING SUGGESTIONS:
- Because amaranth seeds are so small, they should be rinsed with cold water in a fine meshed strainer or one lined with cheesecloth. Seeds can also be baked or steamed.
- Amaranth seeds taste better if cooked in strong-flavored liquids such as tomato juice.
- The leaves are used as a boiled or fried vegetable.
- Amaranth is an excellent thickener for soups.
- Simmer or bake amaranth along with another grain in apple juice, then serve it with fresh fruit.
- Prepare low-fat "refried" amaranth as an alternative to rice.
- You can toast amaranth seeds in a skillet and they pop like popcorn. Popped amaranth makes an excellent breading for fish or meat, or a crunchy topping for soups, salads, and casseroles.

- Boiled amaranth, when chilled, develops a gelatinous consistency that can be used to prepare fruit jams with no pectin and very little sweetener.

Amaranth Berry Pancakes
by Chef Kyle Shadix
Servings: 8 • Prep and cooking: 25 minutes

This recipe contains four powerhouse foods.

INGREDIENTS:

½ cup amaranth flour

½ cup whole wheat flour

½ cup all-purpose flour

2 teaspoons baking powder

¾ teaspoon baking soda

2 cups buttermilk or rice milk

2 large eggs

¼ cup canola oil

2½ cups fresh berries such as blueberries or strawberries

DIRECTIONS:
Mix all dry ingredients in a bowl. In separate bowl, mix buttermilk, eggs, and oil, and whisk until smooth. Let stand 5 minutes. Mix the dry and wet ingredients together. Add ½ cup of berries. If batter is too thick to pour easily, add water, 1 tablespoon at a time, to thin. Cook pancakes in skillet or on griddle, and serve with fresh berries.

BREAK IT DOWN . . .
Calories: 220; Total fat: 10g; Saturated fat: 2g; Cholesterol: 55mg; Sodium: 323mg; Total carbs: 26g; Fiber: 4g; Sugar: 6g; Protein: 8g.

Apples *(Malus domestica)*

AN APPLE A DAY . . .

Did you know . . . that the popular saying "An apple a day keeps the doctor away" came from the old English saying "To eat an apple before going to bed will make the doctor beg his bread"?

What's the Story?

Apples are members of the rose family. There are over 7,500 varieties grown throughout the world. About a hundred different varieties are grown commercially in the United States. Some of the most common types are Red and Golden Delicious, Granny Smith, Gala, Fiji, McIntosh, and Rome.

A Serving of Food Lore . . .

Apples originally came from an area between the Caspian and Black Seas around 6500 B.C. Apples were a favorite food of ancient Greeks and Romans. The Romans brought the apple to England and the English introduced it to North America. Today Americans consume, on average, about twenty pounds of apples per year.

Where Are Apples Grown?

China is the world's largest producer. The United States, Turkey, Poland, and Italy follow respectively. Apples are commercially grown in thirty-five of the fifty United States, with Washington and New York leading in production.

Why Should I Eat Apples?

If you are going to eat an apple, you should eat every part of it but the core. Almost half of the vitamin C content is just underneath the skin. Apples are rich in fiber, a source of both soluble and insoluble fiber. Over two-thirds of the fiber and almost all of the antioxidants are found in the peel. Apples are a rich source of phytochemicals such as phenoylics (chlorogenic acid and catechin), carotenoids such as beta-carotene, and flavonoids including phloridzin and quercetin (which may play a role in fighting cancer and heart disease).

Home Remedies

Apples are believed to help with stomachaches and are eaten to relieve constipation. Apple cider vinegar is used to help treat heartburn. As the story goes, if you rub a piece of an apple on a wart and bury the piece in the ground, the wart will disappear as the apple rots. Apples have been given to unmarried couples, teachers, and friends as good luck charms to drive away bad spirits and bad luck.

Throw Me a Lifesaver!

HEART HEALTH: Two apples a day may help keep heart disease at bay! Researchers found that for every ten grams of fiber added to the diet, there is a fourteen percent reduction in heart disease. A medium apple contains five grams of fiber. Another group of researchers followed men at risk for heart disease for five years. They found that the flavonoids and antioxidants in the apple skin peel may contribute to a decreased risk of developing heart disease.

CANCER: A rat study showed that the more apples they ate, the less mammary tumor growth there was. In one human cell study, apples appeared to protect cells by halting signals that cause the cancerous cells to form. In another study, of human colon cancer cells, flavonoids, associated with apples, inhibited the growth and spread of the cancerous cells.

WEIGHT LOSS: A study conducted by researchers from the State University of Rio de Janeiro found that overweight women who added three apples a day to their low-fat diet lost more weight than those women who did not add in apples.

BRAIN HEALTH: A 2005 animal study found that eating apple products may help protect against cellular damage attributed to memory loss. In another animal study, this time with mice, researchers added apple juice concentrate to their diet. The results showed that the juice concentrate prevented an increase in oxidative damage to brain tissue and decline in cognitive performance.

DIABETES: Diabetics who consumed apples had smaller spikes in glucose after eating, perhaps due to their soluble fiber content.

Tips on Using Apples

SELECTION AND STORAGE:
- Choose apples with firm, undented, shiny skin.
- Keep apples in the refrigerator after purchasing because apples ripen six to eight times faster at room temperature.
- Bruised or rotten apples give off a gas that promotes ripening of fruits, which may cause spoilage of other foods.

PREPARATION AND SERVING SUGGESTIONS:
- If you are not going to use cut apples right away, squeeze some lime, lemon, or orange juice on them to prevent browning.
- Raw apples are great for a snack and in salads.
- Apples can be baked in pies and tarts or pureed into applesauce.
- Golden Delicious, Granny Smith, and Rome are best for baking. The best salad apples are Red Delicious, Golden Delicious, and Fiji.
- Golden Delicious apples are an all-purpose apple and may be used for many cooking methods.

Apple Cranberry Fruit Salad
Courtesy of the Cranberry Marketing Committee
Servings: 8 • Prep time and cooking time: 15 minutes

This recipe contains six powerhouse foods.

INGREDIENTS:

3 apples, red and green, cored and
   chopped into 1-inch pieces
1 cup celery, sliced on bias
¾ cup cranberries, sweetened, dried
½ cup hazelnuts, toasted and
   coarsely chopped

½ cup yogurt, plain, low-fat
3 tablespoons orange juice
   concentrate, thawed
¼ teaspoon table salt

DIRECTIONS:

Mix apples, celery, cranberries, and hazelnuts in large bowl; set aside. Blend yogurt, orange juice concentrate, and salt until smooth. Pour over apple mixture and mix all ingredients together.

BREAK IT DOWN . . .

Calories: 150; Total fat: 5g; Saturated fat: 0.5g; Cholesterol: 0mg; Sodium: 110mg; Total carbs: 26g; Fiber: 4g; Sugar: 18g; Protein: 2g.

Apricots *(Prunus armeniaca L.)*

APRICOT OR NOT?

Did you know . . . seeds of the apricot grown in central Asia and around the Mediterranean are so sweet that they are often substituted for almonds?

What's the Story?

The apricot belongs to the *Rosaceae* family, which includes other tree fruits such as the apple, pear, and peach. There are approximately forty different varieties of apricots, differing in size from three-eighths of an inch to many varieties that surpass two inches, and in colors ranging from yellow to orangey red. The most prevalent varieties are the Pattersons, Blenheims, Tiltons, and Castlebrites. About half the apricot crop is canned and the remainder consists of dried, preserved, and fresh forms. If left to the effects of nature, orange apricots will turn brown within days of harvesting. Apricots stay orange-colored because they are treated with sulphur dioxide, a preserving agent. Unless you are allergic to sulphur dioxide, this ubiquitous preservative usually doesn't pose a health risk. Unsulphured (brown) versions can be found at your local health food store.

A Serving of Food Lore . . .

Cultivation of apricots dates back more than three thousand years. The botanical name for apricots suggests that the fruit originated in Armenia, yet it appears that its true origins actually lie somewhere between north-eastern China and Russia, close to the Great Wall. Apricots eventually made their way to Armenia and then onward into a greater westward expansion through Europe. Apricots were brought to the eastern United States by English settlers and to California by Spanish missionaries.

Where Are Apricots Grown?

Apricots are produced commercially in sixty-three countries. Turkey contributes over twenty percent of the world production, followed by Iran, Italy, France, Pakistan, Spain, Syria, Monaco, China, and the United States.

Why Should I Eat Apricots?

Particularly in their dried form, apricots are one of the best natural sources of vitamin A and beta-carotene. Just a handful of apricots easily meets one hundred percent of the recommended daily allowance (RDA) of beta-carotene and, depending on the variety, the carotenoid content can reach over 16,000 micrograms in just three fresh apricots. Beta-carotene, cryptoxanthin, and gamma-carotene are the predominant carotenoids. Apricots are also a good source of potassium, vitamin C, and fiber, and contain an abundance of phytochemicals such as D-glucaric acid, chlorogenic acid, geraniol, quercetin, and lycopene.

Home Remedies

As early as 502 A.D., there were reports that apricot seed, often referred to as kernels, were effective in treating cancer. Today, many people still believe that the naturally occurring toxin cyanide, found in apricot kernels, might be helpful. Apricot kernels are used to make the alternative cancer drug laetrile. Over twenty-five years ago, the National Cancer Institute claimed laetrile was an ineffective cancer treatment, yet many who seek alternative cancer treatments travel to Mexico, where laetrile remains available. In the seventeenth century, apricot oil was said to be used in England to cure ulcers. In *A Midsummer Night's Dream*, Titania lauded apricot's aphrodisiac properties.

Throw Me a Lifesaver!

VISION: Rich in vitamin A, a powerful antioxidant that prevents free radical damage to eye tissue, apricots may help to promote good vision. Researchers who studied over 50,000 registered female nurses found that those with the highest vitamin A intake reduced their risk of developing cataracts by nearly forty percent.

CANCER: The American Cancer Society states that apricots and other foods rich in carotenes may lower the risk of cancers of the larynx, esophagus, and lungs.

HEART HEALTH: Patients who had the lowest level of beta-carotene intake had almost twice the risk of having a heart attack compared to those with the highest intake. Those with the highest intake of beta-carotene had about one-third the risk of suffering a heart attack and about one-half the risk of dying from it if they did have one.

Tips on Using Apricots

SELECTION AND STORAGE:
- Look for fresh apricots that have a rich orange color and are slightly soft.
- To avoid extra calories, choose canned apricots that are packed in juice rather than in sugar syrup.
- Dried apricots come in orange (sulphured) and brown (unsulphured).
- Keep fresh apricots refrigerated as they have a short shelf life. Consume within a few days when ripe.

PREPARATION AND SERVING SUGGESTIONS:
- For use in cooking or preparing for canning, place whole apricots into boiling water for about thirty seconds, peel, pit, and halve or slice.
- Apricots can be made into wine and brandy.
- Add sliced apricots to hot or cold cereal or even to pancake batter.
- Dried apricots give a Middle Eastern flavor to chicken or vegetable stews.

Apricot-Cranberry-Mango Ice
Courtesy of the Cranberry Institute
Servings: 8 • Prep, cooking, and freezing time: 4½ hours

All five ingredients contained in this recipe are powerhouse foods.

INGREDIENTS:

1½ cups apricot nectar

1½ cups dried cranberries

2 cups (2 large) mangoes, peeled,
  pitted, pureed

⅓ cup lemon juice

2 tablespoons agave nectar

INSTRUCTIONS:

Bring cranberries and apricot nectar to boil in small saucepan. Reduce heat and simmer 3 minutes until softened. Place cranberry mixture, lemon juice, and agave in food processor and puree until blended. Place cranberry puree in small bowl. Place mango puree in separate bowl. Remove ⅔ cup cranberry puree and ⅔ cup mango puree and stir together in a separate bowl until blended. Layer in small 3-ounce paper cup, 1 tablespoon at a time: cranberry–mango mixture, mango puree, cranberry puree, mango puree, cranberry puree, and cranberry-mango mixture. Place a popsicle stick in center of mixture. Repeat to make 7 more popsicles. Freeze at least 4 hours until firm. Cut down side of cup to remove popsicle.

BREAK IT DOWN . . .

Calories: 150; Total fat: 0g; Saturated fat: 0g; Cholesterol: 0mg; Sodium: 0mg; Total carbs: 38g; Fiber: 2g; Sugar: 34g; Protein: 0g.

Artichoke *(Cynara scolymus L.)*

What's the Story?

Artichokes are actually the immature flowers of a thistle plant. The leaves
and flower buds are edible but the center isn't. Artichokes range in color
from dark purple to pale green and come in several varieties such as Green
Globe, Desert Globe, Big Heart, and Imperial Star. The "Jerusalem artichoke" is a nutritious tuber cherished for its similar taste to the artichoke
but is really a member of the magnolia family and not at all related to
Cynara scolymus L.

A Serving of Food Lore . . .

The artichoke most likely originated in the Mediterranean, possibly Sicily,
Italy. Artichokes were seen in Ancient Egyptian writings as symbols of
sacrifice and fertility and have been mentioned in Greek and Roman literature as far back as 77 A.D. In sixteenth-century Europe, the artichoke was
a favored food of royalty. It is thought to be one of the world's oldest medicinal plants. The Spanish brought it to California in 1600 but it didn't
catch on with Americans until the 1920s.

Where Are Artichokes Grown?

The largest commercial growers of artichokes are in France, Spain, Italy,
and the United States. California provides almost one hundred percent of
the U.S. artichoke crop, and Castroville, in the heart of California's
Central Coast farm country, calls itself the "artichoke center of the world."
Castroville is home to the only artichoke processing center in the United
States.

Why Should I Eat Artichokes?

Artichokes are a rich source of vitamin C, folate, dietary fiber, magnesium, and potassium. Artichokes contain the phytochemical cynarin, which aids in digestion by stimulating bile production and may also help to increase appetite. Artichokes contain the flavonoid silymarin, also found in a relative of the artichoke, milk thistle. Silymarin is thought to lend protective support to the liver and protect from heart disease by preventing LDL cholesterol from turning into the more harmful oxidative form. Artichokes ranked seventh out of the top 100 highest antioxidant-containing foods, according to a 2004 USDA study.

Home Remedies

Throughout history, Egyptians and Europeans believed that the artichoke enhanced sexual power and aided in conception. Greeks and Romans have used artichokes to promote regularity and to alleviate stomach upset. It has been said that consumption of artichokes helps "clean" the blood by detoxifying the liver and gallbladder. They have also been used to treat snakebites, anemia, edema (swelling), arthritis, and itching.

Throw Me a Lifesaver!

HIGH CHOLESTEROL: Researchers have found that artichoke leaf extract can reduce cholesterol levels in people.

CIRCULATION: In rat models, researchers have found that wild artichoke restored veins and arteries that did not have sufficient flow in them.

DIGESTIVE HEALTH: Studies conducted on guinea pigs have found that chemicals in artichokes can stop disturbances in the GI tract. The chemicals halt the intestines from spastic movement. Human studies have also found that artichoke leaf extract can significantly reduce the symptoms of irritable bowel syndrome (IBS) and dyspepsia (pain in the mid-abdominal area).

Tips on Using Artichokes

SELECTION AND STORAGE:

- When selecting artichokes you want to pick ones that feel heavy, have tightly packed leaves, and are dark green in color.
- Keep artichokes refrigerated in a plastic bag and use them within four days of purchase.

PREPARATION AND SERVING SUGGESTIONS:

- Wash artichokes well.
- Trim the stem about 1–1½" if desired. The stem is edible and does not have to be cut off. Remove damaged leaves.
- Though steaming is an option, the most common method of cooking artichokes is to place them in a pot and cover with water and a tablespoon of olive oil. Bring the water to a boil, cover the pot, and reduce to a simmer. Cook for 25 to 30 minutes.
- To eat, dip the end of the cooked leaf in either mayonnaise or a combination of olive oil, salt, and pepper. Scrape the artichoke pulp from the leaf between your teeth. Scrape off the fine fibers that lie on top of the artichoke heart and peel away any remaining outer skin to reveal the "heart." Slice and dip hearts into same mixture . . . enjoy!
- Use canned or jarred artichokes in pasta or salad for a quick, easy meal.
- Stuff the leaves with a combination of breadcrumbs, garlic, and butter. Bake for 20 to 25 minutes at 350 degrees.
- Make a great hot artichoke dip by combining artichoke, mayonnaise, salt, pepper, and water chestnuts.
- Artichoke hearts are delicious on salads, as part of a dip, or by themselves. Drizzle olive oil, cracked black pepper, and a little salt over steamed hearts.

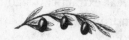

Steamed Artichoke with Cilantro Aioli
by Chef J. Hugh McEvoy

Servings: 12 • Prep and cooking time: 35 minutes

This recipe contains five powerhouse foods.

INGREDIENTS:

1 cup canola mayonnaise
¼ cup fresh cilantro, chopped
1 tablespoons fresh lime juice
1 fresh garlic clove, minced

Pinch chili pepper
Pinch black pepper
Pinch sea salt
6 fresh artichokes

DIRECTIONS:

Blend the first five ingredients in nonreactive bowl. Chill until needed. Steam artichokes in a large pot using a steamer insert or wire rack. Cook until tender when pierced with fork, about 25 minutes. Turn steamed artichokes upside down on wire rack to drain water from the leaves before serving. Serve artichokes hot. Serve cilantro aioli well chilled.

BREAK IT DOWN . . .
Calories: 147; Total fat: 15g; Saturated fat: 2g; Cholesterol: 7mg; Sodium: 205mg; Total carbs: 3g; Fiber: 3g; Sugar: 18g; Protein: 2g.

Asparagus *(Asparagaceae)*

GREEN OR WHITE—DELIGHT!

Did you know . . . white and green asparagus come from the same plant? When the spears emerge from the ground, the sunlight turns the stalks green by producing chlorophyll.

What's the Story?

Asparagus is a member of the lily family. There are approximately three hundred varieties of asparagus of which about twenty are edible. The name asparagus comes from the Greek language meaning "sprout" or "shoot." The most widely known species is the vegetable asparagus, which comes in green, white, and purple colors.

A Serving of Food Lore . . .

The Egyptians wrote about asparagus, which is believed to have originated in the Mediterranean region more than 2,000 years ago. Greeks and Romans prized asparagus for its unique flavor, texture, and alleged medicinal qualities. The Roman Empire even had an "asparagus fleet" of special ships charged with the task of gathering the finest asparagus plants in the world. In the sixteenth century, asparagus gained popularity throughout France and England and, from there, the early colonists brought it to America.

Where Is Asparagus Grown?

Wild asparagus grows in such diverse places as England, central Wisconsin, Russia, and Poland. In 2004, the top four cultivated asparagus producers were China, Peru, the United States, and Mexico.

Why Should I Eat Asparagus?

Asparagus is an excellent source of folic acid, which may help control homocysteine, a risk factor for heart disease, cancer, and cognitive dysfunction, and also may reduce birth defects. Asparagus is also a good source of vitamin C, thiamine, and vitamin B6. It is also high in rutin, a flavonoid that is thought to have anti-inflammatory properties, strengthen blood vessels, and protect against oxidative damage.

Asparagus is also high in glutathione, an antioxidant that protects cells from damage. Protodioscin is a plant chemical found in asparagus that has been found to reduce bone loss, improve sexual desire, enhance erection, and possess cancer cell–killing ability against a number of different forms of cancer. Fresh purple asparagus has a fruity flavor and is high in the phytochemical anthocyanin.

Home Remedies

The Greeks and Romans valued asparagus for medicinal uses like treating bee stings, heart ailments, dropsy, and toothaches. The fresh juice, taken in small doses, is said to act medicinally as a diuretic and laxative. Asparagus roots are used by Chinese herbalists to treat many ailments, such as arthritis and infertility. Madame de Pompadour used asparagus mixed with egg yolks, vanilla, and truffles as an aphrodisiac. Historically, asparagus has been used to treat problems involving swelling, such as arthritis and rheumatism, and may also be useful for PMS-related water retention.

Throw Me a Lifesaver!

DIGESTIVE HEALTH: Asparagus contains *inulin,* a carbohydrate that is not digested but promotes friendly bacteria in our large intestine. It also contains fructo-oligosaccharides (FOS) that promote the growth of beneficial bacteria in the colon. *Asparagine,* a phytochemical in asparagus, gives it a diuretic effect.

DIABETES: A 2006 study reported in the *British Journal of Medicine* pointed to promising news for diabetes care. Research showed that an extract of asparagus significantly increased the action of insulin by producing an eighty-one percent increase in glucose uptake in fat cells.

HEART HEALTH: When folate levels are low, blood levels of homocysteine can rise. A rise in homocysteine can significantly increase the risk for heart disease by promoting atherosclerosis. Just one serving of asparagus supplies almost sixty percent of the daily recommended intake of folate.

Tips on Using Asparagus

SELECTION AND STORAGE:
- Select bright green asparagus with closed, compact, firm tips.
- If the tips are slightly wilted, freshen them up by soaking them in cold water.
- Keep fresh asparagus moist until you intend to use it.
- Asparagus can be frozen but it is better not to defrost it before cooking.
- When you bring the asparagus home and aren't going to use it the same day, trim a little of the bottom off and store upright in a container with a little water. For longer storage, wrap spears in a paper

towel or a clean, damp tea towel, then store in a plastic bag in the crisper section of your refrigerator for up to five days.

PREPARATION AND SERVING SUGGESTIONS:
• For purees, soups, or salads, break or cut asparagus spears at the tender part and use the trimmed ends that you might otherwise discard.
• If your recipe calls for cold asparagus, plunge the stalks into cold water immediately after cooking, then remove them quickly; letting them soak too long can cause them to become soggy.
• Try fresh asparagus with lemon juice.
• Chives, parsley, chervil, savory, tarragon, or other spices melted into butter are delicious when poured over asparagus.
• Use pureed in soups, stews, creamed dishes, or sauces.

Asparagus with Fresh Citrus Dressing and Toasted Almonds
by Chef Cheryl Bell
Servings: 6 • Prep and cooking time: 10 minutes

This recipe contains five powerhouse foods.

INGREDIENTS:

2 tablespoons almonds, sliced
1½–2 pounds asparagus stalks, washed and trimmed
¼ teaspoon freshly grated orange zest

1 tablespoon orange juice
1 teaspoon fresh lemon juice
2 tablespoons extra-virgin olive oil
Kosher salt and fresh ground pepper to taste

DIRECTIONS:
Preheat oven to 375 degrees. Toast almonds in a small shallow baking dish until golden brown; 4 to 5 minutes. Steam asparagus until crisp and tender, about 4 to 5 minutes. Transfer hot asparagus to serving bowl or platter. In a small bowl, whisk together orange zest, orange juice, lemon juice, olive oil, and salt and pepper to taste. Spoon orange dressing over top of asparagus and sprinkle with almonds.

BREAK IT DOWN . . .
Calories: 90; Total fat: 6g; Saturated fat: 1g; Cholesterol: 0mg; Sodium: 10mg; Total carbs: 5g; Fiber: 2g; Sugar: 2g; Protein: 3g.

Avocado *(Persea Americana)*

PEAR-SHAPED AND GREEN-SKINNED IS IN!
Did you know . . . avocado is also called "alligator pear" because of its pear-like shape and green skin?

What's the Story?

"Avocado" is derived from the Aztec word "Ahuacuatl," which means "testicle tree." The meaning stems from the shape of the fruit (that's right . . . it's not a vegetable) and its supposed aphrodisiac qualities. Over 500 varieties of avocados are grown throughout the world but only seven are grown commercially in California. Bacon, Fuerte, Gwen, Pinkerton, Reed, Zutano, and Hass are the main types seen in most grocery stores in the United States. A small percentage of avocados consumed in the United States are imported from Mexico, Chile, and the Caribbean or come from the states of Florida, Hawaii, Louisiana, and Texas, but California accounts for over ninety percent of all avocado consumption (and the Hass in particular) in America.

A Serving of Food Lore . . .

The avocado originated in south-central Mexico, sometime between 7000 and 5000 B.C. Archaeologists in Peru discovered avocado seeds buried in Incan tombs dating back to 750 B.C. It was thought that the seed of the avocado would offer aphrodisiac qualities in the afterlife. There is evidence that avocados were cultivated in Mexico as early as 500 B.C. Florida was the first U.S. state in which avocados appeared, around 1833. In 1871, avocados became a major crop in California. Rudolf Hass planted his namesake fruit, a hybrid avocado, in La Habra, California, where it continues to flourish.

Where Are Avocados Grown?

Mexico, Chile, and the United States are the top producers of avocados. Mexico accounts for one-third of all avocado production. San Diego County, which produces forty percent of all California avocados, is often called the avocado capital of the nation.

Why Should I Eat Avocados?

Avocados contain mainly heart-healthy monounsaturated fat. In comparison with any other fruit, avocados contain more protein, potassium, magnesium, folic acid, B vitamins, vitamin E, and vitamin K. They are also rich in other nutrients and plant chemicals such as beta-sitosterol, a phytochemical that has cholesterol-lowering properties and may aid in reducing the size of the prostate gland and fighting prostate cancer too; lutein, a phytochemical that helps fight macular degeneration and inhibits prostate cancer growth; and carotenoids, which help the body to absorb fat-soluble nutrients and protect against cancer, eye problems, and heart disease.

Home Remedies

Every part of the avocado has been used at one time or another to tackle a few of life's inconveniences. Throughout the Caribbean, Mexico, and South America, the avocado has been put to use in unique ways. A powder made from avocado seeds has been used to control dandruff. Some people have chewed the seeds to reduce toothache pain, and even the skin has been used as an antibiotic for intestinal parasites and dysentery. The flesh has long been used to condition dry hair and as a soothing shaving cream.

Throw Me a Lifesaver!

GINGIVITIS AND OTHER GUM DISEASE: Test tube studies conducted on human gum tissue found that avocado helped to decrease the occurrence of gingivitis and other periodontal disease.

SKIN DISORDERS: A 2001 study in the *Journal of Dermatology* found that a cream containing vitamin B12 and avocado oil kept psoriasis outbreaks at bay longer when compared to a conventional vitamin D cream. Avocado and B12 creams are available without prescription.

HIGH CHOLESTEROL: Patients with high cholesterol were placed on a diet high in avocado for seven days. These patients showed a significant decrease in total cholesterol, LDL ("bad") cholesterol, and triglycerides. These patients also showed a significant increase in HDL ("good") cholesterol.

DIABETES: A randomized human study found that those diabetic subjects who consumed a high monounsaturated-fat diet, consisting mostly of avocados, had far better control of their blood glucose and triglycerides (elevated triglycerides contribute to heart disease) when compared with those subjects who consumed a low-fat, high-carbohydrate diet.

ARTHRITIS: A dietary supplement made from a combination of soybean and avocado oil may relieve symptoms of osteoarthritis. Four well-controlled studies have verified the effectiveness of this oil combination.

PROSTATE CANCER: Dr. David Heber, director of the UCLA Center for Human Nutrition, showed that when avocado extract was added to prostate cancer cells, cell growth was inhibited by up to sixty percent.

Tips on Using Avocados

SELECTION AND STORAGE:
- Choose avocados that are soft to the touch but not too soft.
- Hass avocados turn black when they are ripe.
- Other varieties require a slight squeeze to determine if they are ripe.
- Ripe avocados should be kept in the refrigerator.
- If the avocado is bought unripe, you can place the fruit in a paper bag until it is ripe or store it at room temperature for a few days.

PREPARATION AND SERVING SUGGESTIONS:
- Slice avocado lengthwise and twist to separate the two halves. To remove the pit, put a knife into the pit and twist. To remove the flesh, scoop it out with a spoon.
- If the avocado is not used immediately, add some lemon or lime juice to it to prevent browning.
- Place diced avocado in salads.
- Slice and add to a sandwich or place on crackers with cheese.
- Spread on bread for a butter or mayonnaise substitute.

- Brazilians add avocados to ice cream.
- Filipinos make a beverage out of pureed avocados, sugar, and milk.

Luxurious Guacamole

Adapted from *Mexican Everyday* by Rick Bayless

Servings: 6 • Prep time: 15 minutes

I tried this for the first time in Rick Bayless's restaurant, Frontera Grill, in Chicago. Simply heaven! This recipe contains six powerhouse foods.

INGREDIENTS:

2 ripe Hass avocados

1 garlic clove, finely chopped or crushed through a garlic press

½ teaspoon salt (more or less to taste)

¼ small white onion, finely chopped

½ medium tomato, chopped into ¼-inch dice

1 serrano or ½ to 1 jalapeño pepper, finely chopped (optional)

Garnish with fresh cilantro

DIRECTIONS:

Cut the avocados in half. Remove pit and scoop the avocado flesh into a medium bowl. Mash the avocado with a large fork or potato masher. Meanwhile, rinse chopped onion to prevent it from over-powering the guacamole. Pat onion well with a paper towel to re-move moisture. Stir it into the avocado along with the garlic, salt, pepper, and tomato. If not using immediately, cover with plastic wrap pressed directly on the surface of the guacamole and refriger-ate—preferably for no more than a few hours.

BREAK IT DOWN . . .

Calories: 120; Total fat: 10g; Saturated fat: 2g; Cholesterol: 0mg; Sodium: 230 mg; Total carbs: 8 g; Fiber: 6g; Sugar: 1g; Protein: 2g.

Bananas *(Musa sp.)*

HERBALLY YOURS

Did you know . . . the banana is not actually a tree but, in fact, the world's largest herb?

What's the Story?

Arabian slave traders are credited with giving the banana its popular name. In Arabic *Banan* means "finger." There are over 100 varieties of bananas but the most popular worldwide are the Apple, Silk, or Manzana; Cavendish (the most common imported variety to the United States); Cuban Red; Gros Michel; Ice Cream or Blue Java; Lady Finger; Orinoco, sometimes called "hog," "burro," or "horse" banana; Popoulu; Valery; and Williams varieties.

A Serving of Food Lore . . .

The earliest cultivation of the banana is said to have originated in Malaysia over seven thousand years ago. Bananas then traveled to India, where they were discovered by Alexander the Great in 327 B.C. and continued to travel throughout the Middle East, eventually finding their way to Africa. In 1516, a Portuguese Franciscan monk brought banana roots with him to the Canary Islands and, soon afterward, they found their way throughout the Western Hemisphere. In the early 1900s, bananas began to be imported into the United States from Cuba. The term *Banana Republics* referred to those countries' economies that were largely dependent on banana trade.

Where Are Bananas Grown?

Over 130 countries contribute to the fourth largest fruit crop in the world. The vast majority of the world production of bananas comes from countries in Latin America, followed by Southeast Asia, and a smaller contribution from Africa.

Why Should I Eat Bananas?

Bananas are a good source of vitamin C, B6, and fiber. Green bananas are an excellent source of resistant starch, which tends to be digested slower, thus not causing blood glucose to surge. Resistant starch may reduce the risk of many different types of cancer, especially colon cancer. Red bananas contain more vitamin C, beta-, and alpha-carotene than yellow bananas do. They are an excellent source of potassium, supplying about 300 to 400 milligrams per medium banana. The U.S. Food and Drug Administration (FDA) recommends eating foods rich in potassium and low in sodium, which may help reduce the risk of high blood pressure and stroke.

Home Remedies

Many cultures use banana peel for eliminating warts and also for soothing mosquito bites. Try rubbing your skin with a banana peel after an insect bite to reduce the swelling, itching, and irritation that often results after a bite. The secret may be that the enzymes within the peel are helpful in reducing inflammation. At the very least, the cool peel against hot skin feels great.

Throw Me a Lifesaver!

ULCERS: Animal research found that bananas caused the cells that line the stomach to produce a thicker protective barrier against acid. Bananas were also found to contain compounds called *protease inhibitors* that help destroy harmful bacteria such as *H. Pylori,* believed responsible for most stomach ulcers today.

DIARRHEA: Researchers tested three different groups of children with diarrhea. One group was treated with a diet that included bananas; a second group received pectin; and in the third group the children were given plain rice. The "banana group" fared best—eighty-two percent of them recovered within four days.

REDUCED KIDNEY CANCER RISK: A large population study found that women who ate bananas four to six times a week reduced their risk of developing kidney cancer by fifty percent compared to women who did not eat bananas.

Tips on Using Bananas

SELECTION AND STORAGE:

- Select full-yellow bananas if you are going to eat them within a few days.
- Use fully ripe bananas, with speckles on the peel, for baking, mixing smoothies, or in recipes that specify mashed bananas.
- Keep bananas on a fruit dish at room temperature.
- If you want the bananas to ripen faster, place the bowl in the sun or ripen in a brown paper bag with a piece of apple or a tomato overnight.
- Storing bananas in the refrigerator will delay ripening but will turn the peels black.

PREPARATION AND SERVING SUGGESTIONS:

- When peeling and slicing bananas that you won't be serving immediately, dip them into lemon, lime, or orange juice to slow browning.
- Heating enhances the taste and smell of bananas. Slightly under-ripe fruits are best for cooking, as they hold their shape better.
- Eat them raw, cooked, or frozen. Bananas can be added to baked goods, hot and cold cereals, and desserts.

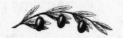

Banana-Blueberry Bread
by Nicki Anderson
Servings: 12 • Prep and baking time: 1 hour

Nothing smells or tastes as good as fresh-baked banana bread. My girls love Nicki's banana bread toasted, too. This recipe contains five powerhouse foods.

INGREDIENTS:

1½ cups bananas, mashed
¾ cup blueberries (if frozen, thaw and drain well)
⅔ cup light brown sugar
¼ cup canola oil
1 large egg white
1 large egg
1 cup all-purpose flour

¾ cup whole wheat flour
1¼ teaspoons cream of tartar
¾ teaspoon baking soda
½ teaspoon cinnamon
¼ teaspoon nutmeg
½ teaspoon salt
Cooking spray

DIRECTIONS:

Preheat oven to 350 degrees. Combine banana, brown sugar, oil, and eggs in a large bowl and mix until smooth. Combine flour, cream of tartar, baking soda, cinnamon, nutmeg, and salt in another bowl and mix thoroughly. Add flour mixture to banana mixture, stirring until moist. Add blueberries. Spoon batter into an 8 × 4 loaf pan generously coated with nonstick spray. Bake at 350 degrees for 40 minutes or until toothpick inserted comes out clean. Cool for 15 minutes before removing from pan, then cool completely on rack.

BREAK IT DOWN . . .

Calories: 132; Total fat: 5g; Saturated fat: 0.5g; Cholesterol: 18mg; Sodium: 19mg; Total carbs: 20g; Fiber: 1g; Sugar: 13g; Protein: 2g.

Barley *(Hordeum vulgare)*

BARLEY WORTH MENTIONING!
Did you know . . . the FDA now allows barley products to attach labels saying that barley "may reduce the risk of heart disease"?

What's the Story?

Barley is a member of the grass family called Poaceae. There are more than fifty different varieties of barley grown throughout the world. It is one of the main grains fed to livestock, and only a small amount is used for human consumption, mainly for beer and other foods. Barley kernels must be first polished or "pearled" to remove the inedible hull. Barley malt is a fundamental ingredient in making beer.

A Serving of Food Lore . . .

The actual origin of barley remains unknown but many researchers believe it came from China or Ethiopia. Archaeologists have discovered that barley was one of the first grains domesticated in the Fertile Crescent by Egyptians some 10,000 years ago. Christopher Columbus brought barley to North America from Spain in 1493.

Where Is Barley Grown?

The top producers are Russia, Germany, Ukraine, France, Canada, Turkey, Australia, and the United States. North Dakota contributes most of the United States' grain.

Why Should I Eat Barley?

Barley is a good source of insoluble and soluble fiber. Beta-glucans, which lower cholesterol and aid in immune function, are found in the soluble fiber portion. In fact, barley is the richest source of beta-glucans compared to any other grain. It also contains B vitamins, iron, magnesium, zinc, phosphorus, and copper, and is one of the richest sources of chromium, which is important in maintaining proper blood glucose levels. Barley is rich in antioxidants, such as selenium, quercetin, and phenolic acids, which protect against damage to human body cells, and also contains a high concentration of tocols and tocotrienols, oils that help reduce the risk of cancer and heart disease.

Home Remedies

Barley has been used in a variety of home remedies throughout the centuries. Many cures are based on preparing a beverage of the grain boiled in water for an hour. For an upset stomach, or to soothe ulcers, drink the liquid straight. Mix in lemon juice for diarrhea. Making a paste from barley, turmeric, and yogurt in equal proportions is another common preparation. The paste can be rubbed on sunburned areas of the body. The same paste, mixed with one half glass of buttermilk and the juice from half a lime, may relieve the symptoms of bladder or kidney infection.

Throw Me a Lifesaver!

CONSTIPATION AND COLON CANCER: Two rat studies showed promising results in treating vastly different illnesses. In one, constipated rats were fed barley, which increased bowel movements. In another, rats with colon cancer were fed varying high-fiber diets. The group on barley had significantly fewer tumors than the other groups.

HEART DISEASE: The beta-glucan fraction in barley, which is also found in oats and mushrooms, is associated with reducing the risk of heart disease.

DIABETES: A small human study showed promise in regulating blood glucose and improving insulin production when the subjects' diet included barley.

Don't Throw Me an Anvil!

Though barley is low in gluten, it is not gluten-free, so people with celiac disease should not use it in place of wheat.

Tips on Using Barley

SELECTION AND STORAGE:
- Whole barley comes hulled (also known as "pot barley"), pearled, cracked, flaked, and in flour forms. Barley malt, a natural sweetener made from the sprouted form of the grain, comes in either liquid or powdered varieties.
- Make sure you buy your grain from stores with high turnover. If you're unsure of its freshness, check for evidence of moisture or condensation on the packaging.
- Barley should be kept in a Ziplocked plastic bag or container with a tight lid and stored in a cool, dry place.

PREPARATION AND SERVING SUGGESTIONS:
- Rinse the grain under running water to remove dirt before cooking.
- Substitute twenty-five to fifty percent of the white wheat flour in a recipe with barley flour.
- Add hot water to cracked barley for a hot cereal.
- Add cooked barley to soups, stews, and salads.
- Adding barley flour increases soluble fiber in your diet.
- Barley flakes are easy additions to granola, muesli, cookies, and muffins.

Barley Orzo Salad
by Chef J. Hugh McEvoy
Servings: 22 • Prep and cooking time: 20 minutes

This recipe contains seven powerhouse foods.

INGREDIENTS:

2 cups pearled barley	⅛ cup Vidalia onions, chopped
2 cups orzo pasta, cooked	3 tablespoons red wine vinegar
4 cups water	¼ cup extra-virgin olive oil
½ cup fresh basil, chopped	1 teaspoon sea salt
2 cloves garlic, chopped	1 teaspoon fennel seed
Juice of ½ fresh lemon	1 teaspoon white pepper

DIRECTIONS:

Cook barley in boiling, salted water until tender—eight to ten minutes. Drain and reserve for next step. Fold herbs, onions, garlic, olive oil, lemon juice, vinegar, seeds, and spices into cooked barley. Fold cooked pasta [orzo] into mixture. Add salt and pepper to taste. Serve hot or cover and refrigerate until chilled, then serve cold as a side dish.

BREAK IT DOWN . . .

Calories: 70; Total fat: 1g; Saturated fat: 0g; Cholesterol: 0mg; Sodium: 320mg; Total carbs: 15g; Fiber: 3g; Sugar: 0g; Protein: 2g.

Basil (*Ocimum*)

LOOKING FOR LOVE?

Did you know . . . in some parts of Italy, men still wear a sprig of basil in their lapel if they are looking for a mate?

What's the Story?

Basil is an herb belonging to the mint family, *Lamiaceae.* The name is of Greek origin and means "royalty." Basil comes in many different varieties, differing in shape, size, and color. Large-leaf Italian sweet, tiny-leaf bush, thai, lemon, and African blue are the most common cooking varieties.

A Serving of Food Lore . . .

Basil origins can be traced back to India nearly 4,000 years ago. Basil was called "the Herb of Kings" by the ancient Greeks. It also has been found in Asia, Egypt, and around the Mediterranean. Some people believe that basil found growing around Christ's tomb was taken to Rome and dispersed throughout Europe. The leaf became popular in sixteenth-century England and was carried to North America by English explorers.

Where Is Basil Grown?

Basil is grown commercially in Yugoslavia, India, Mexico, Italy, Israel, Morocco, and the United States. Within the United States, California is the main producer.

Why Eat Basil?

Basil is rich in rosmarinic and caffeic acid, which are phenolic compounds with strong antioxidant properties. Other phytochemicals in basil include orientin and vicerin, flavonoids that protect cells from damage; volatile oils, such as camphor and 1,8-cineole, that have antibacterial properties; and carotenoids such as beta-carotene.

Home Remedies

Basil appears in many simple preparations. A leaf tucked over a mouth ulcer may ease the sore's pain. Try treating sore gums with a tea made from eight basil leaves in one cup of boiling water. Swish frequently with the tea. Treat an earache with the juice from ten basil leaves: With a dropper apply a drop or two into the ear canal. For hair loss or dandruff, massage the scalp with oil of basil. An hour later, wash your hair with cold water. Two to three crushed basil leaves mixed with water and rock salt may soothe indigestion. You may drink it hot or cold. A spoonful of a mixture of the juice of basil leaves and honey may help soothe a hoarse voice. At the very least you'll enjoy a delicious beverage. Basil juice may also relieve itching. Massage the juice onto the trouble area. Basil also makes an excellent bug repellent!

Throw Me a Lifesaver!

HEART HEALTH: A study conducted on rabbits found that when they ingested holy basil mixed with alcohol and water, the fatty component of cells did not become damaged as easily when exposed to stress, thus improving circulation and reducing heart disease. Another animal study found that rats who were having a heart attack and who were treated with holy basil had less damage to their heart tissue than rats who were having a heart attack and who were not treated with holy basil.

ANTIADHESION: Basil has been shown to make platelets, a component of red blood cells, less "sticky"—a process that may reduce the chance of blood clots forming.

IMMUNE RESPONSE: Rats who were administered holy basil had decreases in immune response to allergens.

ANTIBACTERIAL PROPERTIES: Oil of basil has demonstrated strong antibacterial traits, even with antibiotic-resistant types. It has been found particularly effective in killing harmful bacteria found in produce. Next time you order a salad out, ask for lots of basil.

Tips on Using Basil

SELECTION AND STORAGE:
- Choose leaves that are bright green and free from any brown or yellow spots.
- Basil only keeps a few days in the refrigerator.
- Place cut stems in water and keep them on the windowsill. Sprigs will remain fresh a week or more.
- Layer basil between sheets of waxed paper and freeze. The leaves will darken but they will retain their aroma and flavor.
- Fresh basil leaves can be covered with olive oil in an airtight container and stored in the refrigerator up to two months.
- When stored in a cool, dark, dry space, dried basil may last up to six months.

PREPARATION AND SERVING SUGGESTIONS:
- Add leaves only during the last few minutes of cooking.
- Wash fresh basil under cold running water to remove dirt.
- Chop leaves by rolling them tightly into a cigar shape and chop to desired consistency.
- Place mozzarella cheese and a fresh basil leaf on top of a tomato slice for a simple and tasty tomato salad.
- Add basil to tomato sauce, stir-fry, and pasta shortly before serving.
- Stalks of basil can be added to bottles of vinegar and olive oil for added flavor.

Basil Pistachio Pesto
by Chef J. Hugh McEvoy

Servings: 20 (a serving is ⅛ cup) • Prep time: 10 minutes

This recipe contains four powerhouse foods.

INGREDIENTS:

1 cup extra-virgin olive oil
1 cup Parmesan cheese, shredded
¾ cup dry roasted pistachios
5 fresh garlic cloves

½ teaspoon sea salt
1 teaspoon black pepper
8 cups fresh basil, chopped

DIRECTIONS:

Chill all ingredients. Combine all ingredients except cheese, salt, and pepper into a blender or food processor; blend until a smooth sauce forms. Add shredded cheese, blend until just smooth. Add salt and pepper—season to taste. Garnish with fresh, whole basil leaves. Serve immediately. Can be kept chilled; however, color and flavor fade with time.

BREAK IT DOWN . . .

Calories: 150*; Total fat: 15g; Saturated fat: 3g; Cholesterol: 3mg; Sodium: 75mg; Total carbs: 3g; Fiber: 1g; Sugar: 0g; Protein: 3g.
*⅔ cup cooked pasta + ⅛ cup pesto = 320 calories

Beans *(Phaselous vulgaris)*

BOGUS BEAN

Did you know . . . Mexican "Jumping Beans" are not actually beans at all? They are part of a seed shell that contains the larva of a small gray moth who is really behind all of the "jumping."

What's the Story?

There are over one thousand bean species, which are also known as pulses and legumes, in various cultures. Beans can be broken down into three basic categories: snap beans, which includes string and pole beans; shell beans, including lima beans and peas; and "dry" beans, which includes such varieties as black, kidney, garbanzo, Great Northern, navy, pinto, and red beans, to name a few. "Dry beans" come in both wet (i.e., canned) and dry (unhydrated) states. The term "dry" does not refer to the hydration state of the bean, but rather means that the bean variety is allowed to dry in the pod before harvesting.

A Serving of Food Lore . . .

The first evidence of beans can be traced back some 20,000 years. The lima and pinto were cultivated by Mexican and Peruvian civilizations more than 7,000 years ago. Historians are unsure whether these two beans originated in Mexico, Peru, or Guatemala. Migrating tribes brought beans throughout the Americas. Spanish explorers introduced the beans from the New World to Europe in the 1500s. From there, Spanish and Portuguese traders carried them to Africa and Asia.

Where Are Beans Grown?

The United States is the sixth-leading producer of dry edible beans, behind Brazil, India, China, Burma, and Mexico. North Dakota and Michigan lead the nation in dry bean cultivation.

Why Should I Eat Beans?

Beans count as both a vegetable and a protein source in the United States Department of Agriculture's MyPyramid food guide. They are one of the few vegetables that are rich in both protein and fiber, including both soluble and insoluble fiber to promote regularity, control cholesterol, and reduce the risk of certain cancers. Beans are an excellent source of potassium, folate, and magnesium, and are also a good source of manganese, molybdenum, and the B vitamin thiamine. Darker beans like black beans are as rich in antioxidant compounds called anthocyanins as grapes and cranberries. In fact, four out of the twenty top antioxidant-containing foods are beans. The 2005 Dietary Guidelines for Americans recommend that people consume three cups of beans per week. Unfortunately, the average American only meets one-third of that recommendation!

Home Remedies

Beans have long been a remedy for constipation as they are rich in fiber that promotes laxation.

Throw Me a Lifesaver!

LONGEVITY: A study showed that those who ate beans regularly, more so than any other food, seemed to live longer across various ethnicities.

OBESITY: According to data from the National Health and Nutrition Examination Survey of 1999–2002, bean-eaters are less obese than people who don't include beans in their daily diet.

HEART HEALTH: Years of large studies offer conclusive data linking bean consumption and heart health. Let's take a look at four of the best.
- Researchers from Arizona State University found significant reductions in total and LDL cholesterol in those subjects who simply added pinto beans to their diet.
- Following the dietary intake patterns of 16,000 middle-aged men from around the world for 25 years, a study found that higher consumption of legumes was associated with a whopping eighty-two percent reduction in risk of heart disease!
- A study of nearly 10,000 American adults found that those who ate the greatest amount of soluble fiber foods (at least 21 grams of fiber per day) had a fifteen percent reduction in risk of heart disease compared to those eating five or less grams daily.
- Beans are a main staple of the Dietary Approaches to Stop Hypertension (DASH) diet and the Portfolio diet, both effective in lowering blood pressure.

BREAST CANCER: The consumption of beans is associated with reduced risk for breast cancer in postmenopausal women.

DIABETES: Researchers compared two groups of people with type 2 diabetes who were fed different amounts of high-fiber foods. The group who ate a diet containing 50 grams of fiber a day had lower levels of both plasma glucose and insulin.

Tips on Using Beans

CLEARING THE AIR

If you are not used to eating beans and are worried about being "gassy," start off by eating smaller amounts of beans such as ¼ cup per day and increase up to ½ cup. Gas produced by eating beans is often due to a sudden introduction of fiber. Your body will adjust if you are consistent with your fiber intake and you will be less "windy" in no time!

SELECTION AND STORAGE:
- "Dry" beans come packaged or already cooked, either canned or frozen.
- If stored in a cool, dry place, dry beans can be stored for at least twelve months or longer.
- Canned beans can be stored up to twelve months.
- Cooked beans may be refrigerated for up to five days and frozen for up to six months.

PREPARATION AND SERVING SUGGESTIONS:
- You can reduce up to forty percent of sodium by rinsing canned beans or by purchasing no-salt-added versions. Rinsing beans may also reduce gas production as well!
- Use a pressure cooker to speed up the cooking time.
- Bean soup and chili are two of the most popular ways to eat beans.
- Add beans to burritos or dips to increase nutritional value and add extra flavor!
- Do not add salt or anything acidic, like tomatoes, until after the beans have been cooked, to avoid longer cooking time.

Easy Pasta Fagioli
by Christine M. Palumbo

Servings: Twelve 1-cup servings • Prep and cooking time: 45 minutes

This recipe contains eight powerhouse foods.

INGREDIENTS:

½ cup white or yellow onion, finely chopped

1 garlic clove, minced

¼ cup extra-virgin olive oil

3 cans stewed tomatoes, 14.5-ounce can

2 cans reduced-sodium chicken broth, 14-ounce can

½ cup Italian leaf parsley, chopped

1 teaspoon dried basil

1 teaspoon dried oregano

4 cans cannellini or Great Northern beans, drained and rinsed

½ pound ditalini pasta

Salt and black pepper to taste

DIRECTIONS:

Sauté onion in the olive oil. Add garlic and cook until soft. Add tomatoes, chicken broth, parsley, pepper, basil, and oregano. (If desired, lightly mash the tomatoes before adding them.) After bringing it to a boil, add the beans. Bring to a boil again, lower the heat, and simmer for ½ hour. In the meantime, boil water for the pasta. Cook the pasta and drain, reserving 2 cups of the pasta water. Add the pasta to the soup along with the pasta water. Serve with freshly grated Romano cheese along with crusty Italian bread.

BREAK IT DOWN . . .

Calories: 273; Total fat: 5g; Saturated fat: 0g; Cholesterol: 0mg; Sodium: 647mg; Total carbs: 45g; Fiber: 9g; Sugar: 7g; Protein: 12g.

Blackberries *(Rubus sp.)*

Did you know . . . American Indian women ate blackberries to prevent miscarriages?

What's the Story?

Blackberries are shrubs that belong to the rose family. As a bramble, blackberry fields produce fruit every other year. There are many types of blackberries, including: Himalaya, Marion, Silvan, Evergreen, and Black Diamond. Evergreen blackberries are the main type sold. Blackberries are often used in hybrids such as boysenberry and loganberry.

A Serving of Food Lore . . .

The Evergreen blackberry was known to have grown throughout northern Europe and was especially prominent in England centuries before settlers brought them to the eastern United States in 1850. Migratory birds helped spread the seeds westward, where they took prominence along the Pacific Coast. The Himalaya blackberry came from Germany to the United States, but its true origins can be found in Asia. This type of blackberry is quite common in the Pacific Northwest. Blackberries can be found growing in abundance on the Cascade and Sierra Mountain ranges.

Where Are Blackberries Grown?

Chile, the United States, Guatemala, Mexico, Ecuador, and Romania are the world's top growers. Oregon, California, Texas, Georgia, and Arkansas top the list in the U.S.

Why Should I Eat Blackberries?

Blackberries are high in antioxidants: An in vitro study found that blackberries had the highest antioxidant capacity when compared with blueberries, cranberries, strawberries, and raspberries. They are also rich in vitamin C, fiber, and in the phytochemicals tannin, flavonoid, and cyanidin, which have anticarcinogenic properties. Blackberries also contain catechins, such as quercetin, which is an antioxidant that can reduce the risk of heart disease and stop the action of histamine for people with allergies.

Home Remedies

A combination of distilled water and blackberries made into a drink and taken regularly in the morning is known to promote laxation. Either chewing on blackberry leaves or drinking the aforementioned beverage may help provide relief from bleeding gums and sore throats. To relieve and soothe burns, gently rub blackberry leaves on the burned area.

Throw Me a Lifesaver!

COLON AND LIVER CANCER: Human cell studies have shown that components in blackberries capture free radicals and prevent damage to liver and colon cells.

LUNG CANCER: Studies done on human lung cancer cells have shown that blackberry extracts inhibited further growth of the cancer. A rat study demonstrated for the first time that an anthocyanin extract from blackberries (cyanidin-3-glucoside) inhibited tumor promotion and metastasis (the spreading of cancer cells).

ESOPHAGEAL CANCER: Blackberries have been shown to inhibit and reduce the growth rate of esophageal cancer in laboratory rats.

Tips on Using Blackberries

SELECTION AND STORAGE:
- Look for deep, even color with a glossy look to the berries.
- Look for dents or bruising as this will cause berries to deteriorate quickly.
- Keep them refrigerated. They can only be kept for one to three days and taste best when consumed immediately.

PREPARATION AND SERVING SUGGESTIONS:
- Wash blackberries in cold water just before using. If you decide to freeze them, wash them in cold water and immediately place them in a freezer-safe container.

- Eat blackberries plain, in yogurt or cereal, or put them in a fruit salad.
- Make jellies or jams with frozen berries.
- Blackberries are great for use in pies, cookies, and bars.
- Ferment blackberry juice for homemade red wine.

Simple Blackberry Crisp
by Sharon Grotto
Servings: 8 • Prep and baking time: 40 minutes

This recipe contains five powerhouse foods.

INGREDIENTS:

4 cups blackberries, fresh or frozen
½ cup honey
3 tablespoons lemon juice
¼ cup + 1 tablespoon whole wheat
    flour
¼ cup + 1 tablespoon all-purpose
    flour
¼ cup (packed) brown sugar
½ cup old-fashioned rolled oats
4 tablespoons margarine

DIRECTIONS:

Preheat oven to 375 degrees. Combine blackberries, honey, lemon juice, and one tablespoon each of the all-purpose and whole wheat flours in a large bowl. Spray 9" pie plate with nonstick cooking spray and pour in mixture. In separate bowl, combine remaining flours, brown sugar, oats, and margarine. Mix with fork until crumbly. Sprinkle over berry mixture. Bake for 30 minutes or until golden brown.

BREAK IT DOWN . . .

Calories: 220; Total fat: 5g; Saturated fat: 1.5g; Cholesterol: 0mg; Sodium: 50mg; Total carbs: 43g; Fiber: 5g; Sugar: 27g; Protein: 3g.

Blueberries
(*Vaccinium angustifolium* [wild] &
Vaccinium corymbosum [cultivated])

HAVING THE "BLUES"

Did you know . . . Native Americans believed that blueberries had magical powers and told stories of how the Great Spirit sent "star berries" to feed children during times of famine?

What's the Story?

Blueberries belong to a group of flowering plants. The species are native to North America and eastern Asia. The two major types available in the United States are wild blueberries (lowbush) and cultivated blueberries (highbush). Wild blueberries are one of just three berries native to North America; the others are cranberries and Concord grapes.

A Serving of Food Lore . . .

Native Americans have gathered blueberries from the woods and bogs for generations and were the first to make preserves from blueberries, and to use blueberry juice to dye clothing. Colonists learned to dry blueberries from the Wampanoag Indians. Blueberry juice became an important staple for Civil War soldiers to protect themselves against scurvy.

Why Should I Eat Blueberries?

Because wild blueberries contain less water and are smaller than highbush varieties, they tend to be more nutrient-dense when comparing equal volumes. There are 1,600 wild blueberries to the pound, compared to 500 of the cultivated blueberries. Fresh blueberries have an Oxygen Radical Absorption Capacity (ORAC) value of 2400 per 100 grams. Blueberries are rich in phytochemicals such as phenolic acid, anthocyanins (the pigments that make blueberries blue), and ellagic acid, a natural compound that may inhibit tumor growth. Fresh and frozen blueberries contain high amounts of anthocyanins but very little is found in dried forms.

Home Remedies

Native Americans found that blueberries helped reduce morning sickness, coughs, and headaches. The leaves were used to make tea and were thought to help purify the blood.

Throw Me a Lifesaver!

MEMORY AND COGNITIVE FUNCTION: Animal research has shown promise for using blueberry extract in the areas of improving balance, coordination, and memory, even in those challenged with Alzheimer's disease.

CANCER: Several studies have reported promising results for compounds in blueberries as effective inhibitors of cancer. Both wild and cultivated blueberries were found to be effective in inhibiting androgen-sensitive prostate cancer.

ANTIBACTERIAL: Blueberries, like cranberries, contain compounds that prevent the bacteria responsible for urinary tract infections from attaching to the bladder wall.

HEART HEALTH: Scientists at the University of California, Davis, the University of Maine, Orono, and the School of Medicine at the University of Louisville, Kentucky, found that blueberries may help protect against cardiovascular disease. According to researchers at the University of Prince Edward Island in Atlantic Canada, rats fed diets containing wild blueberries for six weeks experienced decreased stroke-induced brain damage.

Tips on Using Blueberries

SELECTION AND STORAGE:
- Fresh blueberries should be deep blue and covered with a chalky white "bloom."
- Check for damp, moldy, or decayed berries.
- Frozen blueberries should move freely in the bag. If they are frozen in one clump, most likely they have been thawed and refrozen.

- Blueberries will last for seven to ten days if refrigerated.
- Do not wash the berries before storing.
- For freezing, spread unwashed berries on a cookie sheet and place it in the freezer until the berries are frozen, then transfer to a plastic freezer bag. They'll keep for up to a year.

PREPARATION AND SERVING SUGGESTIONS:
- Rinse fresh blueberries and pat dry.
- Frozen berries don't need to be washed before eating. Let thaw at room temperature before adding them to uncooked dishes.
- When adding fresh berries to batter, dust them first with flour, to keep them from settling.
- Toss some in a salad or on cereal, eat as a snack, or make a blueberry pie!

Bursting Blueberry Bread Pudding
by Chef Cheryl Bell
Servings: 12 • Prep and cooking time: 90 minutes

This recipe contains six powerhouse foods.

INGREDIENTS:

3 cups nonfat milk

3 large eggs

5 to 6 cups day-old torn whole wheat French bread or whole wheat bread

½ cup granulated sugar

¼ cup honey

¼ teaspoon almond extract

1 teaspoon vanilla extract

½ teaspoon lemon or orange zest (optional)

2 cups fresh blueberries (may also use frozen)

3 tablespoons whole wheat flour

DIRECTIONS:
Heat oven to 350 degrees. Spray an 11 × 7 baking dish. Whisk together milk, eggs, sugar, flavorings, and zest. Add bread and let stand for 10 to 15 minutes. In a separate bowl, "dust" blueberries with flour and discard excess flour when done. Add blueberries to bread mixture. Pour into the prepared baking dish. Set baking dish in a larger pan and add about 4 cups of hot water to make a steam bath for the pudding. Bake for 1 hour or until bread pudding is set

and is lightly browned on top. Serve warm with traditional rum
raisin, caramel, or lemon sauce. It's also great topped with fresh
fruit or served straight up!

LEMON SAUCE (optional)

¼ cup granulated sugar   *1 cup boiling water*
¼ cup honey   *1 teaspoon butter*
1 tablespoon cornstarch   *1 teaspoon lemon zest*
⅛ teaspoon salt   *1 lemon, juiced*
¼ teaspoon nutmeg

DIRECTIONS:
In a large saucepan, add sugar, honey, cornstarch, salt, and nutmeg. Gradually stir in boiling water. Simmer over low heat, gradually stirring until sauce thickens. Remove from heat; stir in butter,
lemon zest, and lemon juice. Serve drizzled over bread pudding.

BREAK IT DOWN . . .
Calories: 230; Total fat: 3g; Saturated fat: 0mg; Cholesterol: 45mg;
Sodium: 170mg; Total carbs: 46g; Fiber: 2g; Sugar: 30g; Protein: 6g.
with lemon sauce

Broccoli *(Brassica oleracea Italica)*

THE REAL DEAL
**Did you know . . . broccoli rabe, or turnip broccoli, is not really
broccoli but rather comes from the turnip family?**

What's the Story?

Broccoli is a member of the cruciferous family *Brassica oleracea,* specifically from the *Italica* cultivar, and is closely related to cabbage, cauliflower,
kale, collard greens, and brussels sprouts. There are two main types of
broccoli, heading and sprouting. Heading broccoli is by far the most com-

mon. You'll recognize the sprouting type by its stalk with many florets growing from it.

A Serving of Food Lore . . .

Broccoli has been around for at least 2,000 years and was first seen in the region of Asia Minor now known as Turkey. From Asia Minor it spread to Italy and Greece and eventually made its way throughout the rest of Europe. In the early nineteenth century, Italian immigrants carried the vegetable with them to North America. It was not popular with non–Italian Americans and took another century to catch on and be grown commercially. The first commercial harvest was celebrated in the borough of Brooklyn, New York, in 1920.

Where Is Broccoli Grown?

Canada, Japan, Hong Kong, Mexico, and the United States are the top contributors to broccoli production. Ninety percent of the broccoli grown in the United States comes from California's Salinas Valley and Santa Maria. In the winter months, the vegetable becomes available from Arizona, Texas, Florida, and Washington.

Why Should I Eat Broccoli?

Broccoli is an excellent source of vitamin C and a good source of vitamin A, mainly in the form of beta-carotene. Broccoli also contains folic acid, calcium, and chromium. Broccoli is rich in many plant compounds such as indoles and isothiocynates, which have been shown to have cancer-fighting properties. Broccoli sprouts are one of the most concentrated sources of an antioxidant called sulforaphane glucosinolate. Scientists discovered that a handful of three-day-old broccoli sprouts contained as much as twenty to fifty times as much sulforaphane glucosinolate as 114 pounds of regular broccoli!

Home Remedies

Getting vitamin C from fresh foods in the treatment of sinus infections is a plus, and broccoli, rich in C, along with other foods (like berries and citrus fruits), is eaten to both treat and prevent sinus problems. Used as a base of various juice blends, broccoli has long been advocated for relieving symptoms of herpes outbreaks. Now some scientists believe they may have found out why. Researchers at Northeastern Ohio University College of Medicine in Rootstown, Ohio, tested human and monkey cells and found that a naturally occurring compound present in broccoli (and other vegetables like cabbage and brussels sprouts), called indole-3-carbinol (I3C), may inhibit the herpes virus from reproducing.

Eating foods rich in calcium, such as broccoli, can also help prevent headaches and cramps from the menstrual cycle.

Throw Me a Lifesaver!

HEART HEALTH: Human studies have shown that people with mild to moderate LDL ("bad") cholesterol levels (and potentially at risk for heart problems) who consumed a beverage containing broccoli and cauliflower juice showed a decrease in LDL levels.

CANCER: There are over three hundred studies investigating the health benefits of sulphur-containing compounds such as sulforaphane glucosinolates, found in broccoli and, to a much greater extent, broccoli sprouts, in fighting breast and prostate cancers. Studies have shown that sulforaphane stopped the growth of breast and prostate cancer cells.

The growth of thyroid and goiter cancer cells slowed when they were treated with sulphur-containing substances in broccoli called indole-3-carbinol and diindolylmethane (DIM).

ULCERS: Sulforaphane in broccoli may prevent the growth of *H. pylori* bacteria, often attributed to causing stomach ulcers and other ailments. Even strains of bacteria that have been found resistant to antibiotics were effectively reduced in the presence of broccoli.

Tips on Using Broccoli

SELECTION AND STORAGE:
- Look for firm stalks and compact heads that are dark green in color.
- Place unwashed broccoli in an open bag in the refrigerator or in the crisper drawer.
- For best taste, use the broccoli within one to two days of buying.

PREPARATION AND SERVING SUGGESTIONS:

- Cut off the thick stalk. If you don't care for the fibrous outside layer you may use a vegetable peeler to remove it up to the florets. Cut the florets and stems into spears.
- Cooking broccoli may increase its cancer-killing properties. Researchers at the University of Illinois found that when broccoli was heated, the number of sulphoraphanes that fight cancer was enhanced.
- Steam broccoli until it is fork-tender but still crisp. It should be bright green in color.
- Stir-fry broccoli with carrots, snow peas, chicken (or any animal protein or vegetable protein such as tofu), and soy sauce.
- Eat raw with your favorite dip or in a salad for added flavor.

Family Favorite Broccoli Frittata
by Nicki Anderson

Servings: 8 • Prep and cooking time: 75 minutes

This recipe contains six powerhouse foods. If your kids aren't too keen on broccoli, this dish will certainly turn them around. Loaded with flavor, this is a dish even the pickiest of eaters will love!

INGREDIENTS:

1 tablespoon extra-virgin olive oil
½ cup onion, chopped
3 large egg whites
1 large egg
1 cup skim milk
½ teaspoon garlic salt (to taste)
½ teaspoon garlic, minced

¼ teaspoon black pepper
1 16-ounce package frozen
 broccoli, thawed and drained
½ cup whole grain bread crumbs
¾ cup low-fat sharp cheddar
 cheese, grated

DIRECTIONS:

Preheat oven to 350 degrees. Sauté onion and garlic in oil until onion is tender; set aside. Combine egg whites, egg, milk, salt, and pepper in large bowl. Stir in thawed broccoli, bread crumbs, cheese, and onion with egg mixture and mix thoroughly. Add all but ¼ cup of cheese and again, mix well. Carefully pour entire mixture into a 9 × 5 glass loaf pan. Sprinkle with leftover cheese and bake for one hour or until knife inserted in center comes out clean. Let cool for 5 or 10 minutes, slice in 1" slices, and serve.

BREAK IT DOWN . . .
Calories: 200; Total fat: 12g; Saturated fat: 6g; Cholesterol: 60mg; Sodium: 398mg; Total carbs: 13g; Fiber: 3g; Sugar: 5g; Protein: 11g.

Buckwheat *(Fagopyrum esculentum Moench)*

THE "BUCK" BEGAN HERE!

Did you know . . . Thomas Jefferson and George Washington were among the first Americans to grow buckwheat?

What's the Story?

Contrary to popular belief, buckwheat is not a cereal grain but rather a fruit. It is a seed that is closely related to the rhubarb plant. The Dutch named it after the beechnut, which it resembles. There are several varieties of buckwheat but the most popular comes unroasted or roasted and is also known as "kasha." Buckwheat also produces flowers from which bees make a dark, rich-flavored honey.

A Serving of Food Lore . . .

Buckwheat originated in central and western China and it was cultivated there in the tenth to the thirteenth centuries. The Crusaders brought it to Russia and Europe by the fourteenth and fifteenth centuries. It was first introduced to the United States by the Dutch in the seventeenth century, and has been used for human and animal consumption ever since. Buckwheat hulls are also used as filling in specialty pillows for the head, body, and eyes.

Where Is Buckwheat Grown?

Japan is the main producer of buckwheat, followed by Russia, Poland, Canada, France, and the United States. The three largest growers in the United States are Missouri, New York, and Pennsylvania.

Why Should I Eat Buckwheat?

Buckwheat is high in fiber, magnesium, B vitamins, and manganese. It contains flavonoids such as rutin, which helps lower bad cholesterol levels and maintain proper blood flow. Buckwheat has lignans, such as enterolactone, which may protect against breast cancer and heart disease. It contains the beneficial antioxidants vitamin E, tocotrienols, selenium, phenolic acids, and phytic acid.

Home Remedies

The Chinese Army feeds buckwheat to its soldiers because they believe it gives them more strength and stamina. The Hopi Indians gave their women an infusion of the whole buckwheat plant to stop bleeding after giving birth.

Throw Me a Lifesaver!

Rats and mice who were fed buckwheat flour had lower cholesterol levels, less body fat, and fewer gallstones than mice that were not fed buckwheat flour. Prematurely aging rats that were fed buckwheat flour had improved immune cell function compared to those who didn't consume it. A study done on diabetic rats found that buckwheat concentrate added to rat chow decreased their glucose levels by twelve to nineteen percent after eating. And buckwheat studies with humans also are showing promise—for appetite control. A study in 2005 found that people felt fuller after consuming buckwheat compared to other grains.

Tips on Using Buckwheat

SELECTION AND STORAGE:
- Bulk buckwheat should be free from condensation, clumping, or "webbing," a sure indication of pest infestation.
- When buying prepackaged buckwheat, check the expiration date and make sure the bag is free of moisture.
- Buckwheat can be stored up to a year in an airtight container if kept in a cool, dry place.
- Buckwheat flour should be kept in the refrigerator, where it will last a few months.

PREPARATION AND SERVING SUGGESTIONS:
- Buckwheat should first be rinsed under cold running water to get rid of dirt.
- To prepare, use one part buckwheat to two parts water. Bring buckwheat and water to a boil. Cover it and allow it to simmer for 20 minutes.
- Use buckwheat flour in combination with wheat or all-purpose flour to make bread, muffins, cookies, and pancakes.
- Use cooked buckwheat as a hot cereal. Add berries, brown sugar, or cinnamon for extra flavor. Add cooked buckwheat to salads and soups for added health benefits and flavor.

Buckwheat Banana Bread
from *Gluten-Free 101* by Carol Fenster
Servings: 12 (2 slices each) • *Prep time: 15 minutes*
Cooking time: 40 minutes

This recipe contains seven powerhouse foods.

INGREDIENTS:

2 large eggs

¾ cup skim milk

⅓ cup canola oil

1 teaspoon vanilla extract

2 medium bananas, mashed ripe

1½ cups Bob's Red Mill gluten-free
   all-purpose flour blend

½ cup cream of buckwheat cereal
   (Pocono brand by Birkett Mills)

¾ cup packed brown sugar

1½ teaspoons xanthan gum

2 teaspoons baking powder

1 teaspoon salt

1 teaspoon cinnamon, ground

¼ teaspoon nutmeg, ground

¼ cup walnuts, chopped

¼ cup raisins

DIRECTIONS:

Preheat oven to 375 degrees. Generously grease 3 mini 5 × 3-inch nonstick pans. In a medium bowl, beat eggs, milk, canola oil, vanilla, and bananas with electric mixer on medium speed until thoroughly blended. Add dry ingredients (flour through nutmeg) and blend thoroughly on low-medium speed. Gently stir in nuts and raisins. Transfer batter to prepared pans. Bake 35 to 40 minutes or until loaves are nicely browned. Remove from oven. Cool pans on wire rack for 10 minutes. Remove bread from pans and finish cooling on wire rack. Cut each loaf into 8 slices.

BREAK IT DOWN . . .
Calories: 250; Total fat: 10g; Saturated fat: 1g; Cholesterol: 35mg; Sodium: 300mg; Total carbs: 39g; Fiber: 3g; Sugar: 21g; Protein: 5g.

Cabbage *(Brassica oleracea capitata)*

CABBAGE PATCHIN'
Did you know . . . in some cultures, a bowl of cabbage soup is given to newlyweds the morning after their wedding as part of a fertility ritual? Perhaps that's where the concept for "cabbage patch kids" came from!

What's the Story?

Cabbage belongs to the *Brassicaceae* (mustard) family, which includes other vegetables such as brussels sprouts, broccoli, cauliflower, and kale. The leafy head is the only edible part. It is eaten raw, cooked, and preserved. There are over four hundred different varieties of cabbage to choose from. Popular varieties include green, red, and savoy, and Chinese varieties like Chinese cabbage, bok choy, and napa cabbage.

A Serving of Food Lore . . .

Cabbage has been cultivated for more than 4,000 years and domesticated for over 2,500 years. The first pickled version was cabbage preserved in brine, created by soldiers in China and Mongolia. The builders of the Great Wall of China also were known to exist on cabbage for energy and stamina. Fermented and pickled cabbage made its way into Europe from the East, carried by Hun and Mongol warriors. Cultivation of cabbage spread across northern Europe into Germany, Poland, and Russia, where it became a very popular vegetable in local food cultures. The savoy

cabbage variety found its first admirers in Italy. During extended explo-
ration voyages, Dutch sailors practically subsisted on sauerkraut, a dish
made from fermented cabbage. Sauerkraut's high vitamin C content
helped prevent scurvy. Cabbage and the traditional sauerkraut recipe
were introduced into the United States by early German settlers.

Where Is Cabbage Grown?

China, India, Russia, South Korea, Japan, and the United States are the
leaders in cabbage production, in that order. New York is the top producer
within the United States.

Why Should I Eat Cabbage?

Cabbage is a good source of vitamin C and fiber. Red cabbage also contains anthocyanins, a phytochemical also found in blueberries, beets, and
Bermuda onions. Sauerkraut is an excellent source of vitamin K and vitamin C, and a good source of folate, potassium, iron, and fiber. Sauerkraut
is equally rich in the friendly bacteria *lactobacillus acidophilus*. However, it
is also high in sodium whereas cabbage is not.

Home Remedies

Ancient Greek and Roman civilizations held cabbage in high regard as
they felt it was capable of treating a host of health conditions. Romans developed an ointment made from lard and ashes of burnt cabbages for use
in disinfecting wounds. Cabbage juice is often sold in health food stores as
a popular home remedy for ulcers.

Throw Me a Lifesaver!

CANCERS: Foods found in the crucifer family are rich in phytochemicals called glucosinolates, which may protect against cancer. Cabbage, especially raw sauerkraut (cooking cabbage appears to reduce these helpful
plant chemicals), is rich in the anti-cancer compounds indole-3-carbinole
(I3C), isothiocyanates (a type of beneficial compound found in *Brassica*
vegetables), and sulforaphane. These compounds help activate and stabi-

lize the body's antioxidant and detoxification mechanisms, which, in turn, eliminate cancer-producing substances. Cabbage intake has been linked to a lower incidence of colon, lung, cervical, and breast cancer.

BREAST CANCER: The Polish Women's Health Study included hundreds of Polish and Polish-born women in the United States. The study revealed that women who ate three or more servings of raw, lightly cooked, or fermented (sauerkraut) cabbage were seventy-two percent less likely to develop breast cancer as opposed to those women who only ate one and a half servings per week.

VIRUS: Scientists at Seoul National University in South Korea fed an extract of kimchi, a spicy Korean version of sauerkraut, to thirteen chickens infected with avian flu. A week later, eleven of the birds started to recover.

ULCERS: In a small study, participants who had stomach ulcers drank a liter of fresh cabbage juice daily for ten days. All ulcers had healed by the end of the ten days!

Tips on Using Cabbage and Sauerkraut

SELECTION AND STORAGE:
- Cabbage heads should be large and compact without discolored veins.
- Look for stems that are healthy-looking, closely trimmed, and are not dry or split.
- Buying precut cabbage may not be worth it as the leaves may have already lost their vitamin C content.
- Store the whole head of cabbage in a plastic bag in the refrigerator. Try to use any remaining cabbage in the next two days.

PREPARATION AND SERVING SUGGESTIONS:
- Cabbage can be prepared any number of ways including steaming, frying, boiling, braising, and baking.
- Cabbage can be used cooked or raw in dishes from corned beef and cabbage, soups and stews, to cold dishes such as coleslaw.

- Eating sauerkraut on a hot dog may reduce some of the harmful effects of nitrates and nitrites found in processed meats. Try it on a turkey sandwich with mustard or in a pasta salad.

SAUERKRAUT:

- The sodium content is pretty intense but can be easily lowered by rinsing in a colander under cold water.
- Look for fresh sauerkraut. The friendly bacteria content is much higher than what you would find in pasteurized jars. Once opened, sauerkraut should be used within three days.

Vegetarian Polish Cabbage Rolls
by Ma Tomich
Servings: 6 • Prep and cooking time: 90 minutes

This recipe contains eight powerhouse foods.

FILLING INGREDIENTS:

2 cups brown rice, cooked

1 large head of cabbage

*1 pound Boca crumbles or lean
    ground turkey*

½ cup yellow onion, finely chopped

1 clove garlic, minced

1 teaspoon black pepper

2 omega-3 eggs

½ cup vegetable broth

2 tablespoons olive oil

SAUCE INGREDIENTS:

1 can diced tomatoes

1 can tomato soup

DIRECTIONS:

Preheat oven to 375 degrees. Core cabbage, place in pot, and cover with water. Bring to boil. Lower heat to medium and cover with lid and cook until slightly softened. Remove cabbage and place on a dish to cool. Meanwhile, in a large pot, sauté onions and garlic in olive oil until transparent. Add crumbles, rice, egg, vegetable broth, and pepper. Mix well. When cabbage is warm to the touch, peel leaves and place on a cutting board. Divide mixture into six equal parts. Fill cabbage leaves and roll. Place rolls with folded end down into 9 × 13 baking dish. Combine soup and tomatoes in a separate bowl. Ladle over rolls. Cover rolls in aluminum foil and bake for 45 minutes or until cabbage is easily pierced with fork.

BREAK IT DOWN . . .
Calories: 360; Total fat: 11g; Saturated fat: 2g; Cholesterol: 60mg; Sodium: 760mg; Total carbs: 46g; Fiber: 11g; Sugar: 14g; Protein: 23g.

Cardamom *(Elettaria, Amomum, Aframomum)*

CHEW AFTER EVERY MEAL

Did you know . . . long before toothbrushes, ancient Egyptians chewed cardamom seeds to clean their teeth?

What's the Story?

The name cardamom, also seen as cardamon, refers to three varieties from the ginger family: *Elettaria,* commonly known as green cardamom or true cardamom; *Amomum,* known as black cardamom; and *Aframomum,* found and used mainly in Africa and Madagascar. All cardamom species have been used in cooking and for healing purposes. Cardamom has a strong, unique taste, with an intensely aromatic fragrance. It is often used in baked goods but can be found in such dishes as masala, meat loaf, sausages, curries, and in beverages such as chai, coffee, and tea throughout the world. Cardamom is especially popular across the Arab world.

A Serving of Food Lore . . .

Cardamom is thought to be native to India and southeastern Asia. It may have been brought to Europe around eight hundred years ago, and, by means of trade, introduced throughout the rest of the world.

Where Is Cardamom Grown?

Cardamom is cultivated mainly in India, but only a small share of its production is exported due to the large domestic demand. Guatemala, Nepal,

Sri Lanka, Mexico, Thailand, and Central America are the main exporters of cardamom.

Why Should I Eat Cardamom?

Cardamom is loaded with essential oils that have high antioxidant properties.

Home Remedies

In India, green cardamom is used to treat a range of maladies such as periodontal infections, sore throats, lung congestion, tuberculosis, inflammation, and digestive disorders. It is also reportedly used as an antidote for both snake and scorpion venom.

The *Amomum* species is used extensively in traditional Indian medicine. Traditional Chinese medicine uses cardamom for treating stomachaches, constipation, diarrhea, and other digestive difficulties. Cardomon has been traditionally used as an antispasmotic.

Throw Me a Lifesaver!

DIGESTIVE HEALTH: Cardamom possesses the ability to kill harmful *H. pylori* bacteria associated with ulcers. It also exerts a calming effect on the rest of the digestive tract and has been used to treat dyspepsia and gastritis.

ANTI-INFLAMMATORY: An animal study found that Swiss Albino mice who received cardamom extract daily for eight weeks had significant reductions in many markers of inflammation. Increased death of colon cancer cells was also observed in the group that received cardamom extract.

Tips for Using Cardamom

SELECTION AND STORAGE:
- Cardamom is sold in two ways: a high-quality ground and fresh in its pod, typically in the green and black varieties.
- Cardamom is best stored in pod form, because once the seeds are exposed or ground, they quickly lose their flavor.

- Keep ground cardamom in a cool, dry place in a tightly sealed container.

PREPARATION AND SERVING SUGGESTIONS:
- For recipes requiring whole cardamom pods, a generally accepted equivalent is 10 pods equals 1½ teaspoons of ground cardamom.
- Green cardamom is traditionally mixed together with roasted coffee beans to make the Arabian coffee beverage called *Gahwa*.
- Add ground cardamom to flan, rice pudding, or hot breakfast cereals. Add whole cardamom to tea with milk or chai beverages.
- Cardamom is traditionally offered after dinner in Indian restaurants as a breath-freshener.

Fried Tofu in Curry Sauce
by Dave Grotto
Serves: 8 • Prep and cooking time: 25 minutes

You can substitute chicken or fish for the tofu, if you like. This recipe contains an amazing 10 powerhouse foods.

INGREDIENTS:

2 pounds firm tofu cut into ½" slices

1 tablespoon olive oil

2 large onions, peeled and quartered

1 large green pepper, sliced into 2" strips

1 teaspoon crushed garlic

1 teaspoon fresh grated ginger

3 teaspoons curry powder

1 (15-ounce) can tomato sauce

1 (10-ounce) can coconut milk

1 tablespoon whole cloves

1 teaspoon ground cardamom

1 cinnamon stick

Salt and pepper

DIRECTIONS:

Heat olive oil in a large skillet over medium-high heat, sauté tofu pieces until crispy and browned. Remove tofu from skillet and set aside. Sauté onion and green pepper in skillet until onion is translucent; add ginger and garlic and cook for 2 to 3 minutes until fragrant, then stir in curry powder. Return tofu to skillet and add tomato sauce, coconut milk, cloves, cardamom, and cinnamon stick. Season

with salt and pepper to taste and stir all together. Reduce heat to low
and simmer for about 15 minutes.

BREAK IT DOWN . . .
*Calories: 210; Total fat: 12g; Saturated fat: 7g; Cholesterol: 0mg; Sodium:
430mg; Total carbs: 17g; Fiber: 3g; Sugar: 11g; Protein: 11g.*

Carob *(Ceratonia siliqua)*

HIS DAILY BREAD

**Did you know . . . carob is also known as "locust" or "St. John's
bread" because the "locusts" that John the Baptist fed upon in the
Bible in actuality were carob pods?**

What's the Story?

Carob is a member of the pea family. The fruit of the carob tree lies inside a
long reddish-colored pod that grows up to a foot in length. Clifford, Santa
Fe, Tylliria, Amele, and Casuda are among the most popular varieties.
Locust bean gum is an extract from carob seeds which is used as a stabilizer
in many commonly found foods. This is the most popular use for carob.

A Serving of Food Lore . . .

Carob most likely originated in the Middle East, where it has been cultivated for the past 4,000 years. It became popular in the Mediterranean region and from there spread throughout Europe. The Spaniards brought
carob to Mexico and South America, while the British brought it to South
Africa, India, and Australia. In 1854 carob arrived in North America and
in 1873 the first seeds were planted in California.

Where Is Carob Grown?

Most carob is still grown in the Mediterranean region. Sicily, Cyprus,
Malta, Spain, and Sardinia are the main producers in this area. California
is the main grower of carob in the United States.

Why Should I Eat Carob?

Carob is a good source of fiber and protein; the minerals magnesium, calcium, iron, and potassium; and the vitamins A, D, and B. It contains the polyphenols catechin, gallic acid, and quercetin—all powerful antioxidants. Carob also contains tannins that work as antioxidants that aid the digestive tract.

Home Remedies

A popular remedy for digestive difficulties (diarrhea, nausea, vomiting) is a drink made with one tablespoon carob powder mixed with one cup of liquid, such as water, oat, almond, or rice milk. Ground leaves and bark of the carob tree have been used to treat or reduce the symptoms of syphilis and other venereal diseases. Chemicals called tannins that are found in carob can bind to and inhibit the growth of bad bacteria.

Throw Me a Lifesaver!

HEART HEALTH: Subjects with high cholesterol showed that those who consumed carob pulp—rich in insoluble fiber—had lower LDL cholesterol and triglycerides, and improved LDL/HDL ratio.

WEIGHT MANAGEMENT: Another study on the benefits of carob pulp pointed to fat-burning properties of the fruit.

DIABETES: A study done on rats fed locust bean gum with a meal slowed the rate of food digestion, improved insulin response, and prevented rebound hypoglycemia, an abnormal lowering of blood glucose.

Tips for Using Carob

SELECTION AND STORAGE:
- Carob is available in powder, chips, and syrup. It comes prepackaged or in bulk at many health food stores.
- Once carob is brought home from the store you want to keep it in a cool, dry place, where it can be kept for up to twelve months. If you buy carob powder and lumps form, sift the powder in a flour sifter or strainer.

PREPARATION AND SERVING SUGGESTIONS:
- If you are using carob powder as a substitute for cocoa powder, re-place one part cocoa with 1½ to 2 parts carob. You must keep in mind that carob powder is similar in taste to—but not as flavorful as—chocolate.
- Powder: Use in cakes, cookies, candy, or pancakes.
- Chips: Substitute for chocolate chips in muffins and cookies.
- Add carob syrup or powder to warm milk for a hot chocolate substitute.

Carob Walnut Cake
by Chef J. Hugh McEvoy
Servings: 32 • Prep and baking time: 60 minutes

This recipe contains five powerhouse foods.

INGREDIENTS:

1 12-ounce bag carob chips	4 medium omega-3 eggs
1 stick margarine	¼ cup cocoa powder,
1 cup brown sugar	unsweetened
½ cup whole wheat flour	2 teaspoons vanilla extract
½ cup unbleached white flour	½ teaspoon baking powder
8 ounces dried English walnut	1 teaspoon sea salt
halves	½ cup powdered sugar

DIRECTIONS:

Preheat oven to 350 degrees. Melt carob chips in a double boiler and set aside. Cream brown sugar and 1 stick margarine in large bowl. Slowly beat in eggs. Add melted carob chips and vanilla, mixing well. Sift in cocoa powder, flour, salt, and baking powder. Blend just until smooth. Fold in walnuts. Place batter in a greased and paper-lined 9 × 12-inch cake pan. Bake until done—approximately 35 to 40 minutes. Let cool on rack and dust with powdered sugar.

BREAK IT DOWN . . .

Calories: 160; Total fat: 8g; Saturated fat: 1g; Cholesterol: 25mg; Sodium: 120mg; Total carbs: 22g; Fiber: 2g; Sugar: 8g; Protein: 8g.

Carrots

SUCH A BABY!

Did you know . . . most "baby" carrots were once longer carrots that have been trimmed to size? True baby carrots are removed from the ground early.

What's the Story?

Carrots belong to a diverse group of vegetables called "taproots." They are unique as they grow downward into the soil rather than upward toward the sun. Carrots come in many different shapes and sizes but the most popular color is orange and the most popular size is seven to nine inches in length. Over forty different pigmented varieties are available that vary in the types of phytochemicals they contain. But the majority of cultivated carrots are usually orange, purple, yellow, or white. They all fall within the two basic categories: eastern (Asiatic) carrots or western (carotene).

A Serving of Food Lore . . .

The cultivation of carrots dates back thousands of years. Native to central Asia and the Middle East, they soon spread throughout the Mediterranean region. India, China, and Japan had established carrots as a food crop by the thirteenth century. In Europe, however, carrots did not gain favor until the Renaissance. During the seventeenth century, farmers started cultivating different varieties of carrots including the orange-colored variety we know today.

Where Are Carrots Grown?

China is the largest producer of carrots, followed by the United States, Russia, France, England, Poland, and Japan.

Why Should I Eat Carrots?

Carrots are an excellent source of carotenes, particularly beta-carotene. One cup of diced carrots provides roughly 686.3 percent of the RDA for vitamin A. Carrots are also a good source of fiber, manganese, niacin, potassium, vitamin B6, and vitamin C.

Home Remedies

Long ago, Greeks used carrots to cure stomach ailments and Romans ate carrots to improve their love life. Carrots also have other traditional "roots": During Rosh Hashanah, the Jewish New Year, for example, carrots are served in the shape of coins, as a symbol of future prosperity.

Throw Me a Lifesaver!

HEART DISEASE: Multiple studies examined the association between high-carotenoid diets and reduced risk of heart disease. One of those studies, reported over ten years ago in a leading journal, followed 1,300 elderly persons who ate at least one serving of carrots and/or squash each day. The results showed that those who were on the carotenoid-rich diet had a sixty percent reduction in their risk of heart attacks compared to those who ate less than one serving.

CANCER: High carotenoid intake has been linked with a twenty percent decrease in postmenopausal breast cancer and up to a fifty percent decrease in the incidence of cancers of the bladder, cervix, prostate, colon, larynx, and esophagus. Extensive human studies suggest that a diet including as little as one carrot per day could conceivably cut the rate of lung cancer in half. Precancerous colon lesions in animals given diets containing carrots or falcarinol (a natural phytochemical in carrots) were much smaller than those in the control animals, and far fewer lesions had progressed to become tumors.

Though a large population study called CAROT showed that smokers who ingest beta-carotene supplements were more prone to lung cancer, a study from the National Cancer Institute found that lung cancer occurrence was higher in men whose diets did not supply a healthy intake of alpha-carotene.

DIABETES: Human research suggests that eating foods rich in carotenoids, like carrots, may aid in making insulin more effective, thus improving blood-glucose control.

EMPHYSEMA: Animal research conducted at Kansas State University showed that diets rich in vitamin A reduced lung inflammation and the occurrence of emphysema.

VISION: Beta-carotene helps to protect vision, especially night vision. Beta-carotene's powerful antioxidant actions help provide protection against macular degeneration and the development of cataracts, the leading cause of blindness in the elderly.

Tips on Using Carrots

SELECTION AND STORAGE:
- Carrots that are deep orange in color contain the most beta-carotene.
- Avoid carrots that are cracked, shriveled, soft, or wilted.
- Carrots are best kept refrigerated in the crisper section, but don't store them with fruits. Fruits produce ethylene gas as they ripen. This gas will decrease the storage life of the carrots.

PREPARATION AND SERVING SUGGESTIONS:
- Peeling carrots may make them look pretty but generally it is unnecessary. Besides, peeled carrots lose some of their vitamins.
- Steaming, braising, roasting, and grilling are the preferred methods of preparing carrots. There is more nutrient loss when carrots are boiled. And though cooking carrots in a microwave may be a time-saver, there is a reduction in beta-carotene content when you do so.
- Season raw or cooked carrots with dill, tarragon, ginger, honey, brown sugar, parsley, lemon, or orange juice.

Roasted Carrot Butternut Soup
by Chef J. Hugh McEvoy
Servings: 12 • Prep and cooking time: 60 minutes

This recipe contains seven powerhouse foods.

INGREDIENTS:

1 pound fresh baby carrots
1 pound fresh butternut squash,
   cubed
1½ cups Vidalia onions, chopped
4 cups low-sodium chicken broth
3 tablespoons olive oil
1 fresh garlic clove

12 cinnamon sticks
½ teaspoon fresh thyme
¼ teaspoon nutmeg, whole
   grated
12 fresh peppermint leaves
1 teaspoon dried whole bay leaves

DIRECTIONS:

Preheat oven to 375 degrees. Roast carrots and squash until tender, approximately 20 minutes. In a large stock pot, sauté onions and garlic in olive oil until translucent. Add squash, carrots, chicken stock, bay leaf, and thyme. Bring to boil, reduce heat, and simmer 15 minutes. Remove bay leaf and thyme. Using a food processor, blend until very smooth. Season to taste with salt and pepper. Serve in wide bowls. Garnish with single cinnamon stick, fresh grated nutmeg, and floating mint leaf.

BREAK IT DOWN . . .
Calories: 80; Total fat: 3g; Saturated fat: 2g; Cholesterol: 8mg; Sodium: 56mg; Total carbs: 12g; Fiber: 2g; Sugar: 4g; Protein: 3g.

Cauliflower *(Brassica oleracea)*

ONE SMART HEAD

"Cauliflower is nothing but a cabbage with a college education."

—MARK TWAIN

What's the Story?

Cauliflower is a member of the *Brassicaceae* family that includes brussels sprouts, cabbage, and broccoli. It is a crucifer: a sulfur-containing vegetable that forms a compact head referred to as a "curd." Cauliflower comes in several colors and varieties ranging from white to light green to purple. The three main varieties are white cauliflower, broccoflower (a mix between cauliflower and broccoli), and romanesco, which grows in a yellow-green color. White is the most common variety found in the United States, while the purple and green varieties are most appreciated in Italy.

A Serving of Food Lore . . .

Cauliflower originated in Asia Minor, where it has been cultivated since 600 B.C. From Asia Minor it moved to Italy, and around the sixteenth century it was brought to France and elsewhere in Europe, and across the channel to England. In the early 1600s, the English introduced it to North America, where it has been grown since.

Where Is Cauliflower Grown?

Cauliflower is grown in the United States, France, Italy, India, China, Canada, and Mexico. In the United States, California is the leading supplier.

Why Should I Eat Cauliflower?

Cauliflower is an excellent source of fiber and vitamin C, as well as a good source of the B vitamins biotin and folate. Cauliflower contains a phytochemical called sulforaphane, which helps the liver produce enzymes that block cancer-causing chemicals from damaging the body.

Home Remedies

Biotin, a water-soluble vitamin found in cauliflower, has been shown to control dandruff. Biotin also helps thicken nails and reduce splitting and cracking. Munching of crunchy foods such as cauliflower before bed may help stop jaw-clenching while sleeping.

Throw Me a Lifesaver!

CANCER PREVENTION: In a study published in the *British Journal of Cancer,* researchers reported on the cancer-fighting properties of indole-3-carinol (I3C). This study showed that what we eat can influence cancer genes. Several other studies support this direction for further investigation into breast cancer. Researchers have seen that the chemical sulforaphane, found in cruciferous vegetables like cauliflower, stopped lung cancer cells in an animal trial, and helped kill off and stop the growth of prostate cancer cells in a test tube study on human cells.

RHEUMATOID ARTHRITIS: Researchers who followed a group of older women for over ten years found that those who consumed more cruciferous vegetables had a decreased risk of rheumatoid arthritis.

Tips on Using Cauliflower

SELECTION AND STORAGE:
- Look for white or creamy-colored heads. They should be firm, compact, and heavy when lifted.
- Keep cauliflower refrigerated, stem side up, to avoid moisture buildup and rapid spoiling, preferably in the crisper drawer, for up to five days.

PREPARATION AND SERVING SUGGESTIONS:
- Remove the outer leaves and cut the florets where they meet the stem base. Rinse the florets in a colander under cold running water.
- To minimize the smell and nutrient loss, steam the florets for a short amount of time, no longer than three to five minutes.

- Cooking cauliflower in an aluminum pan causes the vegetable to yellow; cooking it in an iron pan causes it to turn blue-green.
- Eat cauliflower raw with veggie dip or salad dressing.
- Add raw cauliflower to green or mixed vegetable salads, and cooked cauliflower to soup, casseroles, or quiche.
- Mash cauliflower in with mashed potatoes.

Creamy Cauliflower Soup

from *Lean Mom, Fit Family: The 6-Week Plan for a Slimmer You and a Healthier Family* by Michael Sena and Kirsten Straughan
Servings: 6 • Prep and cooking time: 60 minutes

This recipe contains six powerhouse foods.

INGREDIENTS:

1 pound cauliflower flowerets, fresh

4 medium potatoes, peeled and cubed

1 large onion, chopped

1 tablespoon extra-virgin olive oil

3 cups reduced-sodium chicken broth

2 cups skim milk or low-fat soy milk

½ teaspoon ground black pepper

½ teaspoon cayenne pepper hot sauce

2 teaspoons fresh thyme leaves (or 1 teaspoon dried)

Salt to taste

DIRECTIONS:

Sauté the onion in olive oil until translucent. Place cauliflower in a separate large saucepan, cover with water, and bring to boil. Reduce heat and simmer until slightly tender. Drain off water. Add potatoes, sautéed onion, chicken broth, milk, pepper, and hot sauce, and return to simmer. Cook for about 40 minutes until all vegetables are fully cooked. Remove from heat. Place 1 to 2 cups of hot soup mixture into a blender and mix at low speed until smooth. Pour into separate container. Repeat with remaining soup mixture. Add salt to taste.

BREAK IT DOWN . . .

Calories: 190; Total fat: 7g; Saturated fat: 1.5g; Cholesterol: 5mg; Sodium: 115mg; Total carbs: 27g; Fiber: 4g; Sugar: 8g; Protein: 7g.

Celery *(Apium graveolens)*

CHEWING THE FAT?
Did you know . . . some believe that it takes more calories to digest
celery than those provided by eating it? This remains to be proven,
but one thing is clear—celery is a great part of anyone's diet!

What's the Story?

Celery's name is derived from the Celtic word meaning "water." Celery belongs to the same family that includes carrots, fennel, parsley, and dill.
There are three main types of cultivated celery: Chinese celery, which is
closest to wild celery; celeriac, known for its mild, sweet taste and most
popular in Europe; and *var dulce* (meaning "sweet"), a variety most commonly found in North America. The tender stalks in the center are called
the heart.

A Serving of Food Lore . . .

Celery was first cultivated in the Mediterranean region about 3,000 years
ago. It was presented to the winners of athletic games in Greece, much like
we give bouquets of flowers today. The first use of celery as a culinary ingredient was as a flavoring and the earliest printed record of its use as a
food is from France, dating to 1623. The Chinese also cultivated celery as
early as the fifth century.

Where Is Celery Grown?

Celeriac variety is grown widely throughout Europe. France, Germany,
Holland, and Begium are the main producers, with fifty percent of the
harvest going to the pickling industry. The *var dulce* variety of celery is
grown year-round in the United States, primarily in California, Michigan,
Texas, and Ohio. The largest harvest each year in the United States is called
the "Thanksgiving Pull," for the traditional preparation of stuffing for the
turkey.

Why Should I Eat Celery?

Celery is a good source of vitamin A—the darker the green, the higher the level of vitamin A. Celery also contains vitamins C, B1, and B2; calcium; iron; magnesium; phosphorus; and potassium. The leaves contain many of these nutrients and can work well as a replacement for parsley. Celery contains phalides, which may help lower cholesterol, and coumarins, possibly useful in cancer prevention.

Home Remedies

Wild celery was used as a medicinal plant throughout the Middle Ages. People used it to "treat" conditions such as anxiety, insomnia, rheumatism, gout, and arthritis. Wild celery was also thought to provide strength and purify the blood. The Romans wore wreaths of celery leaves as an antidote against the intoxicating effects of wine and the ensuing headache. In Vietnam, celery has been used as a remedy for lowering high blood pressure. Celery also has a reputation as an aphrodisiac. Celeriac oil has a calming effect, is useful as a diuretic, and is a traditional remedy for skin complaints and rheumatism.

Throw Me a Lifesaver!

CHOLESTEROL: In an animal study, celery juice significantly lowered total cholesterol by increasing bile acid secretion.

CANCER PREVENTION: Perillyl alcohol, present in the essential oil of celery seeds, has been shown to have anticancer properties. The National Cancer Institute is conducting human clinical trials with perillyl alcohol to investigate its effectiveness in halting breast cancer. Animal studies have demonstrated positive results in regressing pancreatic, mammary, and liver tumors and may hold hope for preventing and treating many other types of cancer.

ANTIBACTERIA AND FUNGI (MOLD): Celery contains polyacetylenes, substances highly toxic against fungi and bacteria. This compound also has anti-inflammatory effects and makes blood more slippery.

Tips on Using Celery

SELECTION AND STORAGE:

- The leaves of the celery stalk should be bright green and not wilted. Gently squeeze the middle of the stalk. If you hear a squeaky sound, the celery is fresh.
- Celeriac (celery root) comes in two varieties: a smaller knob version sold earlier in the fall and a larger knob version sold later.
- Rinse celery and place in a plastic bag. Sprinkle or add water to the plastic bag to maintain the freshness of the celery. Keep in the refrigerator's vegetable bin, where it should last about two weeks.

PREPARATION AND SERVING SUGGESTIONS:

- If you didn't rinse the celery for storage, be sure to rinse it thoroughly to remove sand and dirt from its stalks before use.
- Cut the stalks just prior to serving them. If you need to prepare them well in advance, put the cut celery stalks in ice water for up to an hour before serving.
- Fill celery with peanut butter or low-fat cream cheese, or use as a healthy dip-scooper instead of chips.
- Sauté celery and add to your favorite soup or casserole. Add fresh to any salad.

Celery Slaw

from *Charting a Course to Wellness: Creative Ways of Living with Heart Disease and Diabetes* by Treena and Graham Kerr

Servings: 4 • Prep time: 10 minutes

This recipe has six powerhouse foods.

INGREDIENTS:

4 cups chopped celery

1 cup grated carrots

½ cup chopped yellow onion

½ cup chopped red bell pepper

½ cup raisins

¼ cup canola oil mayonnaise

¼ cup plain, nonfat yogurt

2 tablespoons apple cider
   vinegar

1 tablespoon Dijon mustard

DIRECTIONS:
Combine celery, carrots, onions, red pepper, and raisins together in a large bowl. In a separate small bowl, combine mayonnaise, yogurt, vinegar, and mustard, and whisk until smooth. Add dressing to vegetables and mix well.

BREAK IT DOWN . . .
Calories: 163; Total fat: 5g; Saturated fat: 1g; Cholesterol: 6mg; Sodium: 342mg; Total carbs: 27g; Fiber: 4g; Sugar: 19g; Protein: 3g.

Chard *(Beta vulgaris)*

A SWISS MISSED
Did you know . . . Swiss chard is not native to Switzerland but rather Sicily? A botanist named it after his Swiss homeland.

What's the Story?

Swiss chard is a member of the beet family but does not produce an edible bulb. There are many varieties of chard such as Fordhook Giant, Ruby Chard, Argenta, and Bright Lights. Fordhook is the most popular variety grown in the United States; other common varieties are bunched together under the label "Rainbow chard." Chard's taste is somewhere between spinach and beets.

A Serving of Food Lore . . .

The origins of chard can be traced back to ancient Babylonia. Aristotle wrote about chard in the fourth century B.C. During the Middle Ages, travelers from Italy brought it to North and Central Europe. From there chard traveled to the Far East and China. Today, chard is especially popular in Southern France, Catalonia, Spain, and Sicily, Italy.

Where Is Chard Grown?

Chard is grown in Italy, France, Spain, Holland, Switzerland, and the United States. California, Texas, and Arizona are the primary growers in the U.S.

Why Should I Eat Chard?

Chard is a good source of fiber and is an excellent source of vitamins A, C, and K. It is a good source of vitamin E, magnesium, potassium, iron, and mangenese. Chard contains the carotenoids zeaxanthin and lutein, which benefit vision.

Home Remedies

Chard has been used for the treatment of ulcers, tumors, leukemia, and other cancers. In South Africa, the drinking of chard juice is supposed to ease the discomfort of hemorrhoids. Chard juice has also been used as a decongestant and to neutralize stomach acidity.

Throw Me a Lifesaver!

CANCER: Components in chard were found to inhibit cell proliferation of human cancer cells. A study performed on human breast cancer cells found that the flavonoids present in chard stopped the growth and DNA reproduction of the cells.

DIABETES AND HEART HEALTH: Several studies performed on diabetic rats found that feeding them chard controlled blood glucose and either reversed, stabilized, or prevented the negative effects of diabetes such as nerve damage and heart disease.

Tips on Using Chard

SELECTION AND STORAGE:
- Select chard leaves that are a bright green color with a crisp stalk. Avoid buying chard that is browning or yellowing or has small holes.
- Unwashed chard can be kept in plastic in the crisper drawer of your refrigerator for up to three days.

PREPARATION AND SERVING SUGGESTIONS:
- Chard should be washed well under cold water to remove any dirt or sand. Next, trim the end of the stalk and cut the leaves into one-inch pieces.
- Avoid cooking chard in an aluminum pot because the oxalates it contains will cause the pot to change color.
- Use chard in place of spinach in lasagna or salads. The stem of chard can be used as a broccoli substitute.
- Add chard to eggs and pasta dishes for added nutritional benefits.

Swiss Chard Tacos with Carmelized Onion, Fresh Cheese, and Red Chile
from *Mexican Everyday* by Rick Bayless
Servings: 6 (2 tacos each) • Prep and cooking time: 30 minutes

This unlikely taco filling is fantastic! Don't worry about the huge volume of chard called for in the recipe; it cooks down considerably. This recipe contains seven powerhouse foods.

INGREDIENTS:

12-ounce bunch of Swiss chard (other greens can be substituted)

1½ tablespoons of olive oil

1 large white or red onion sliced ¼-inch thick

3 garlic cloves, peeled and chopped or crushed through a garlic press

1 teaspoon red pepper flakes

½ cup reduced-sodium chicken broth or water

½ teaspoon salt

12 warm corn tortillas

1 cup crumbled queso fresco, feta, or goat cheese, for serving

¾ cup Frontera Guajillo Chile or Chipotle Salsa

DIRECTIONS:
Cut the chard crosswise into ½-inch slices. In a large skillet, heat the oil over medium heat. Add onion and cook, stirring frequently, until golden brown but still crunchy, about 4 to 5 minutes. Add the garlic and red pepper flakes and stir for a few seconds, until aromatic, then add the broth or water, ½ teaspoon salt, and the greens. Reduce the heat to medium-low, cover the pan (if you don't have a lid, a cookie sheet works well), and cook until the greens are almost

tender—about 5 minutes. Uncover the pan, raise the heat to medium-high, and cook, stirring continually, until the mixture is nearly dry. Taste chard and then season with additional salt, if you think it necessary. Serve with the warm tortillas, crumbled cheese, and salsa for making soft tacos.

BREAK IT DOWN . . .
Calories: 240; Total fat: 9g; Saturated fat: 3g; Cholesterol: 15mg; Sodium: 610mg; Total carbs: 35g; Fiber: 5g; Sugar: 3g; Protein: 10g.

Cherries *(Prunus cerasus L. and Prunus avium L.)*

FEELIN' CHERRY GOOD!

Did you know . . . cherries are a natural pain reliever? The University of Michigan identified two plant pigments in cherries that block an enzyme (COX-2) believed to cause pain.

What's the Story?

The cherry is a member of the rose family. It falls within the classification of a drupe, meaning that it is a fruit that contains a pit covered with edible flesh. The two main types of cherries are sweet and sour (also known as pie or tart). The sweet cherry includes many varieties such as Bing, Ranier, Lambert, Royal Anne, and Van. The Bing is the most popular type of eating cherry in the United States. The Montmorency cherry is the sour cherry most often used in pies. One cherry tree can produce enough cherries to make about twenty-eight pies.

A Serving of Food Lore . . .

Sweet cherries originated in two places: the Caucasus Mountains and Turkey. The sour cherry originated in Eastern and Central Europe. During the Norman invasion in 1066, the cherry was brought to England. In the seventeenth century, British and French settlers brought cherries with them to North America. Wild cherries (also known as chokecherries) are indigenous to North America and were spread across the country by the Native Americans. Cherry trees adorned French gardens in Midwestern settlements.

Where Are Cherries Grown?

Sweet cherries are grown throughout Europe and North America. Spain, Switzerland, France, Italy, Russia, and Germany are big producers in Europe. Sour cherries are grown in the United States, Russia, Germany, and Eastern Europe. Germany tops the world in cherry production, followed by the United States. In the United States, sweet cherries are grown in Idaho, Oregon, Washington, and California. Sour cherries are grown in Michigan, New York, and Wisconsin.

Why Should I Eat Cherries?

Cherries contain vitamins A, C, and the Bs; the minerals calcium, iron, and potassium; and fiber. Cherries are an important source for a variety of phytochemicals. Beta-sitosterol, a plant sterol that has been linked to lower blood-cholesterol levels, and anthocyanins give the cherry its red color and may also reduce inflammation and pain. Quercetin may help prevent heart disease. Amygdalin may reduce tumor growth and size. Ellagic acid may help fight bacterial infections and also cancer. Perillyl alcohol is an antioxidant that may have antitumor activity. Sour cherries have more phenolic compounds than sweet cherries and are also a natural source of free radical scavengers called superoxide dismutase (SOD).

Home Remedies

Native Americans used wild cherries (chokecherries) as a cough suppressant. Hot cherry pits have been used to heat beds on cold nights. Tart cherries have been used for tooth decay, prevention of varicose veins, and headaches. Cherries have been known to have laxative effects and can relieve constipation.

Throw Me a Lifesaver!

CANCER: Studies with tart cherries suggest that they contain substances that substantially reduce the formation of heterocyclic aromatic amines (HCAAs), the carcinogenic chemicals that occur from the charring of meat. A mouse study found that anthocyanins, a phytochemical in tart cherries, reduced colon cancer cell growth.

HEADACHE: Eating around twenty cherries a day may help with reducing headaches, according to researchers from Michigan State University.

EXERCISE-INDUCED MUSCLE PAIN: Men who drank tart cherry juice after performing weight-training exercises had less muscle pain and strength loss. (Women may also benefit but this particular study looked exclusively at men.)

GOUT, ARTHRITIS, INFLAMMATORY PAIN: Black or Bing cherries have both antioxidant and anti-inflammatory properties, specifically a substance called cyanidin, which may shut down the pain caused by uric acid crystals. In one study, healthy men and women ate Bing cherries for twenty-eight days. Inflammation markers were reduced and remained low for days even after discontinuation of cherry intake. The inclusion of cherries in the diet may be a powerful tool for preventing inflammatory disease before it becomes painfully apparent!

HEART HEALTH: A study done on men and women found that eating Bing cherries decreased certain blood markers of heart disease.

DIABETES: Anthocyanins in tart cherries were found to increase insulin production in animal pancreatic cells by fifty percent.

SLEEP: Tart Montmorency cherries are rich in the antioxidant melatonin, which may help in promoting sleep.

Tips on Using Cherries

SELECTION AND STORAGE:
- Cherries should be free from any dents or discoloration. One bad cherry can cause the entire batch to deteriorate quickly.
- Be sure the cherries you select are as ripe as you wish them to be. They will not ripen after they are picked.
- Place unwashed cherries in the refrigerator for up to one week.

PREPARATION AND SERVING SUGGESTIONS:
- To freeze cherries, take the stems off and freeze on a cookie sheet. You can keep them in the freezer for up to 10 months.
- To pit a cherry, cut the cherry in half with a paring knife and pick out the pit.
- For cherry-stained hands, squeeze fresh lemon juice all over hands and rinse with warm water.
- Eat cherries by themselves or on top of ice cream, salads, and cereal. Mix into cookie and muffin batter, or even in a sauce on meat and fish.
- Use frozen cherries to make a cherry pie.

Cherry Oatmeal Bake
Adapted from the Cherry Marketing Institute
Servings: 4 • Prep and cooking time: 50 minutes

This recipe contains five powerhouse foods.

INGREDIENTS:

½ cup dried tart cherries　　　*2 cups skim or soy milk*
½ cup quick oats, uncooked　　*¼ cup egg substitute*
¼ cup agave syrup　　　　　　*½ teaspoon almond extract*
½ teaspoon salt

DIRECTIONS:
Combine cherries, oats, agave syrup, and salt in a medium bowl. Stir in milk, egg substitute, and almond extract. Spray four 10-ounce custard cups with a nonstick cooking spray. Divide mixture evenly between the cups. Place filled cups on baking sheet. Bake in preheated 350-degree oven for 30 to 40 minutes or until the centers are slightly soft. Serve warm.

BREAK IT DOWN . . .
Calories: 210; Total fat: 3.5g; Saturated fat: 0g; Cholesterol: 0mg; Sodium: 330mg; Total carbs: 39g; Fiber: 3g; Sugar: 27g; Protein: 7g.

Chocolate (*Theobroma cacao*)

A "DOG-GONE" SHAME!

Did you know . . . chocolate may be healthy for humans but the antioxidant theobromine found in chocolate can be toxic to dogs, cats, parrots, and horses?

What's the Story?

Chocolate comes from fruit pods of the cacao tree. (*Cacao* is the Aztec word for "chocolate.") The pods contain seeds that are turned into a paste called chocolate liquor. Many chocolate products are made from the liquor. There are three varieties of cocoa available today: Criollo, Forastero, and Trinitario. Forastero accounts for nearly eighty percent of world chocolate production.

A Serving of Food Lore . . .

According to the Mayan and Aztec legends, cacao was discovered by the gods in a mountain in South America. The cacao tree is believed to have originated in the foothills of the Andes in the Amazon, and in South America. From there, the Mayans brought the cocoa tree to Central America. The first documented commercial shipment of cocoa beans occurred in 1585 between Veracruz, Mexico, and Seville, Spain. The first cocoa beverage outside of South and Central America was served in Italy in 1606. Soon after, cocoa spread throughout Europe. The Spaniards introduced the cacao tree to the Philippines, and finally, to the West Indies and the United States.

Where Is Cocoa Grown?

The largest producing countries are Côte d'Ivoire, Ghana, and Indonesia. The Criollo variety is found in Ecuador, Nicaragua, Guatemala, and Sri Lanka. *Forastero*, which means "foreigner" in Spanish, is now the predominant variety cultivated in Africa. Trinitario is grown mainly in Trinidad.

Why Should I Eat Cocoa?

Cocoa beans contain minerals such as magnesium, calcium, iron, zinc, copper, potassium, and manganese. They also contain vitamins A, B1, B2, B3, C, E, and pantothenic acid. Cocoa has more phenolic phytochemicals and a higher antioxidant capacity possibly than any other food, including green tea, black tea, red wine, and blueberries. Flavonoids found in chocolate include the flavonols, notably epicatechin, catechin, and proanthocyanidins. It is also a rich source of the antioxidant theobromine. Many dark chocolate products with a high percentage (seventy percent) of cocoa contain more of these type of antioxidants, but that is not always a guarantee. Processing of cocoa can cause substantial losses so look for cocoa products that boast of its flavonol content. Cocoa also contains some caffeine. An eight-ounce serving of cocoa provides not more than 5 to 10 mg of caffeine, less than the amount found in coffee, black tea, and cola, which typically ranges anywhere from 20 to 120 mg.

Home Remedies

Cocoa butter is an old-time favorite to reduce the appearance of stretch marks. Aztecs were the first to use cocoa medicinally for stomach and intestinal complaints. Native Indians used cacao to cool fevers. In 1672 it was noted that chocolate could cure "pustules or swellings" of sailors who did not eat a "fresh diet."

Throw Me a Lifesaver!

HEALTHIER SKIN: Though chocolate is often blamed for contributing to skin breakouts, a study found that women who regularly consumed a high-flavonol cocoa beverage showed increased hydration, and decreased roughness and scaling.

DIARRHEA: A study conducted by researchers at Children's Hospital & Research Center in Oakland, California, discovered that flavonoids in cocoa beans can combat diarrhea.

HEART HEALTH: Several human studies have shown that flavonoid-rich dark chocolate improves endothelial function and reduces LDL ("bad") cholesterol, lowering the risk for heart disease. Studies have shown that adding chocolate to one's diet lowers blood pressure as compared to people who do not eat chocolate.

DIABETES: A human study found that the flavonols in dark chocolate increased nitric oxide in the subjects tested, which improved insulin sensitivity and blood flow and lowered blood pressure.

COUGHS: A team of researchers discovered that theobromine, a derivative found in cocoa, is nearly a third more effective in stopping persistent coughs when compared with codeine, currently considered the best cough medicine. The use of theobromine as a cough suppressant is still being investigated.

COLON CANCER: Researchers from the University of Barcelona in Spain found that antioxidants in cocoa may be effective in suppressing genes that trigger colon cancer cell growth.

COGNITIVE FUNCTION: Dr. Bryan Raudenbush, a researcher from Wheeling Jesuit University in West Virginia, discovered that verbal and visual memory were significantly higher in those subjects who consumed milk chocolate as opposed to dark chocolate.

Tips on Using Chocolate: (Do you really need any? Ha!)

SELECTION AND STORAGE:
- Chocolate comes in a variety of forms such as cocoa powder; dark chocolate, also known as "bittersweet"; milk chocolate; and baking chocolate. White chocolate is *not* chocolate.
- Avoid purchasing chocolate that has a grayish tone, white spots on the surface, or small holes.
- Chocolate will keep for several months at room temperature or refrigerated or frozen.

PREPARATION AND SERVING SUGGESTIONS:
- When melting chocolate, be careful to keep its temperature under 120° F (49° C), because overheating will alter its flavor.

- Make a chocolate fondue and dip strawberries, cake, mango, watermelon, or just about any fruit you can think of.
- In Spanish and Mexican cuisine, chocolate is used to flavor sauces for seafood and poultry.

Giselle's Dairy-Free Birthday Cupcakes
by Giselle Ruecking

Servings: 24 cupcakes • Prep and cooking time: 25 minutes

My goddaughter, Giselle, has battled severe asthma all of her life. Dairy products, for her, were a powerful trigger for attacks, which meant that she couldn't eat many items we take for granted, like regular birthday cake. So, her parents came up with this delicious recipe that Giselle and her family have now enjoyed for the past fourteen years. This recipe contains three powerhouse foods and is a "lifesaver" for those with dairy allergies.

INGREDIENTS:

1½ cups whole wheat flour
1½ cups all-purpose white flour
¾ cup sugar
2 teaspoons baking soda
½ cup cocoa powder
2 teaspoons white vinegar

¾ cup canola oil
½ teaspoon salt
2 teaspoons vanilla extract
1 cup vanilla soy milk
1 cup cold water

DIRECTIONS:
Place all ingredients in a large bowl and mix for three minutes. Pour mixture into cupcake baking cups until two-thirds filled. Bake at 350 degrees for 12 to 15 minutes. Poke with toothpick to test if done.

BREAK IT DOWN . . .
Calories: 150; Total fat: 8g; Saturated fat: .5g; Cholesterol: 0g; Sodium: 160mg; Total carbs: 19g; Fiber: 2g; Sugar: 6g; Protein: 2g.

Cilantro/Coriander
(Coriandrum sativum)

A REAL STINKER!

Did you know . . . the name "coriander" is derived from the Greek word *koris*, which means "bug." It may have earned this name because of the "buggy," offensive smell that it has when unripe.

What's the Story?

Coriander is considered both an herb and a spice since both its leaves and its seeds are used as a seasoning condiment. Fresh coriander leaves, more commonly known as cilantro, resemble Italian flat-leaf parsley, a close family member. The seeds have a flavor that is similar to citrus peel and sage. Ground coriander is a major ingredient in curry powder, certain Belgian-style beers, and other aromatic dishes. Coriander is often used commercially as an ingredient to make medications more palatable. It is also used as a flavoring in gin, pickles, and sausages, and as a component of makeup and perfumes.

A Serving of Food Lore . . .

The use of coriander can be traced back over seven thousand years, making it one of the world's oldest known spices. It is native to the Mediterranean and Middle Eastern regions and has been in Asia for thousands of years. Coriander was cultivated in ancient Egypt and is mentioned in the Old Testament. (*"And the house of Israel called the name there of Manna: and it was like coriander seed, white; and the taste of it was like wafers made with honey."* Exodus 16:31.)

It was used as a spice in both Greek and Roman cultures, the latter using it to preserve meats and flavor breads. Coriander seed and leaf were widely used in medieval Europe for their ability to mask the taste and smell of rotten meat. In 1670, coriander was brought to the British colonies in North America. It was one of the first spices cultivated by early settlers.

Where Is Coriander Grown?

Most coriander is produced in Morocco, Romania, and Egypt. China and India also offer limited supplies. Fresh coriander production can be found throughout Central and South America and in the United States.

Why Should I Eat Coriander?

Coriander's volatile oil is rich in a variety of phytonutrients including carvone, geraniol, limonene, borneol, camphor, elemol, and linalool. Coriander contains flavonoids including quercetin, kaempferol, rhamnetin, and epigenin and also contains active phenolic acid compounds, including caffeic and chlorogenic acid, which have been found helpful in fighting cancer, diabetes, and heart disease. Coriander is a source of iron, magnesium, and manganese.

Home Remedies

Coriander is promoted as an aphrodisiac in *The Tales of the Arabian Nights*. It is thought to increase the appetite and is still widely used in tonic and cough medicine in India. Coriander has been used for the relief of anxiety and insomnia in Iranian folk medicine. Recent experiments in mice may provide the secret to its enduring usage for anxiety.

Throw Me a Lifesaver!

DIABETES: When coriander was added to the diet of diabetic mice, it helped stimulate their secretion of insulin and lowered their blood sugar.

HEART HEALTH: Coriander was given to rats that had been fed a high-fat and -cholesterol diet. The spice lowered total cholesterol and triglycerides significantly.

ANTIBACTERIAL: Researchers isolated a compound in coriander called dodecenal, which in laboratory tests was twice as effective as the commonly used antibiotic drug gentamicin at killing salmonella.

DIGESTIVE HEALTH: Researchers examined the effects of coriander combined with other spices on digestion and found the spice mix enhanced the activities of pancreatic digestive enzymes and also stimulated bile flow and secretion.

Tips on Using Coriander

SELECTION AND STORAGE:

- Fresh leaves should look vibrantly fresh and be deep green in color. They should be firm, crisp, and free from yellow or brown spots.
- Buy whole coriander seeds instead of coriander powder since the latter loses its flavor more quickly.
- Both seeds and powder should be kept in an opaque, tightly sealed glass container in a cool, dark, and dry place. Ground coriander will keep for about four to six months, while the whole seeds will stay fresh for about one year.
- Fresh coriander should always be stored in the refrigerator with its roots in a glass of water and its leaves covered with a loosely fitting plastic bag. Fresh leaves will last about three days.

PREPARATION AND SERVING SUGGESTIONS:

- Clean coriander by placing it in a bowl of cold water and swishing it around with your hands. Empty the bowl, refill it with clean water, and repeat this process.
- Coriander seeds can be easily ground with a mortar and pestle or an electric spice grinder.
- Over low heat, combine vanilla soy milk, honey, coriander, and cinnamon in a saucepan for a delicious beverage.
- Add coriander seeds to soups, broths, and fish.
- Adding ground coriander to pancake and waffle mixes will give them a Middle Eastern flavor.

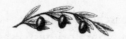

Lime-Cilantro Dressing

Adapted from *Mexican Everyday* by Rick Bayless

Servings: makes 1½ cups (12 servings) • Prep time: 15 minutes

Don't skimp here: Use fresh lime juice—it's worth it. Add one-quarter cup of honey for a sweeter option. This recipe contains six powerhouse foods.

INGREDIENTS:

½ cup canola oil

¼ cup olive oil

¼ cup honey (optional)

⅓ cup fresh lime juice

½ teaspoon lime zest, grated

½ cup (packed) cilantro, roughly chopped

1 serrano or 1 jalapeño, stemmed and roughly chopped (optional)

1 teaspoon (or less) salt

DIRECTIONS:

Combine oils, lime juice, honey, lime zest, cilantro, salt, and chiles in a blender jar and blend until smooth. You may want to start off with ½ teaspoon of salt and add more if needed. Store in the refrigerator until ready for use. Shake well immediately before pouring on tender greens, raw or cooked vegetables, or any dish that warrants that fresh lime-cilantro flavor!

BREAK IT DOWN . . .

Calories: 150; Total fat: 14g; Saturated fat: 1.5g; Cholesterol: 0mg; Sodium: 100mg; Total carbs: 7g; Fiber: 0g; Sugar: 6g; Protein: 0g.

Cinnamon
(*Cinnamomum zeylanicum* and *Cinnamomum cassia*)

MUMMY LIKES IT!

Did you know . . . cinnamon was used in ancient Egypt to embalm the dead?

What's the Story?

There are actually four types of cinnamon. *Cinnamomum zeylanicum,* more commonly known as "Ceylon," is considered "true cinnamon." The others are relatives with the most popular being *cinnamomum cassia,* also known as Chinese cassia or Indonesian cinnamon. Both come from the bark of an Asian evergreen tree. The bark is peeled off, dried, and allowed to form a roll—the common "cinnamon stick" that we know today. Though close in taste, Ceylon has a slightly richer and sweeter taste. Most of the cinnamon bought in the United States is the less expensive cassia variety.

A Serving of Food Lore . . .

Cinnamon has a long history. Ceylon cinnamon originated from the island of Sri Lanka. Chinese writings have documented use of cinnamon since 2700 B.C. Around 1000 B.C., West Asia, Europe, and Africa imported cinnamon from India and this began the spread of the spice. Cinnamon became really popular in Europe during the Crusades and its popularity grew throughout the world.

Where Is Cinnamon Grown?

The main countries that produce Ceylon cinnamon are India, Sri Lanka, Madagascar, and Brazil. Chinese cinnamon (cassia) is mainly grown in China, Vietnam, and Indonesia.

Why Should I Eat Cinnamon?

Cinnamon is a source of manganese, iron, calcium, and fiber and contains cinnamaldehyde, cinnamyl acetate, and cinnamyl alcohol, substances that work as antioxidants in the body. Cinnamaldehyde reduces stickiness of platelets.

Home Remedies

The Chinese have believed that consuming cinnamon will improve your complexion and give you a youthful appearance. The people of India believe that chewing on a cinnamon stick will help to regulate the menstrual cycle, and their midwives and physicians use the spice for pain relief during childbirth. Gargling with a mixture of one teaspoon each of cinnamon and honey mixed into hot water has been used to battle bad breath.

Throw Me a Lifesaver!

ARTHRITIS: Researchers from Nanjing University in China evaluated 122 Chinese herbs for their effectiveness in reducing uric acid, the trigger for gout and arthritis flare-ups. Cinnamon cassia extract proved the most effective of them all for inhibiting the enzyme responsible for producing uric acid.

HEART HEALTH: Cinnamon has been shown to reduce lipids and have anti-inflammatory and platelet-adhesion properties. The results of a study demonstrated that intake of small amounts of cinnamon per day (no more than six grams or one-fifth of an ounce) reduced serum glucose, triglyceride, LDL cholesterol, and total cholesterol in people with type 2 diabetes.

TYPE 2 DIABETES: In an animal study, male rats who were given an extract of cinnamon had lower blood glucose levels. A human study found that giving cinnamon extract to type 2 diabetics significantly reduced their blood sugar levels.

BLOOD PRESSURE: In one study, rats were given a sugar solution to increase their blood pressure. Then they were given ground cinnamon, cinnamon extract, or a placebo. The rats that were given the ground cinnamon and cinnamon extract had reduced blood pressure.

Tips for Using Cinnamon

SELECTION AND STORAGE:
- Cinnamon is available in ground and in stick form.
- To check for freshness, smell the cinnamon. Fresh cinnamon has a sweet odor.
- When buying cinnamon you need to be careful because Ceylon and Chinese cinnamon are often labeled the same. If you want the "true" Ceylon cinnamon, try buying it at a spice store or at an ethnic food mart.
- Cinnamon should be kept in an airtight container in a dark place. Ground cinnamon will start to lose flavor after six months. Stick cinnamon will last for one year.
- Though it may be tempting to buy the jumbo economy-size container of cinnamon, the optimal strategy is to buy small amounts to preserve freshness, taste, and phytochemical content.

PREPARATION AND SERVING SUGGESTIONS:
- Cinnamon sticks can be ground by using a coffee grinder or a cheese grater.
- Use cinnamon in desserts such as rice pudding, pies, and cakes.
- Use the spice to flavor meats. Cinnamon, along with cumin, turmeric, and ginger are a classic combination for flavoring Middle Eastern and North African meat and poultry dishes.
- Mix cinnamon with coffee and drink as a hot beverage.
- Top whole grain toast with a little bit of butter, cinnamon, and sugar on top. Yum!

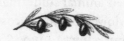

Banana–Cinnamon French Toast
by Sharon Grotto
Servings: 4 • Prep and cooking time: 15 minutes

This recipe contains four powerhouse foods.

INGREDIENTS:

2 large bananas

8 slices whole wheat Italian
  bread

2 eggs

2 egg whites

1 cup vanilla soy milk

1 cup skim milk

1 teaspoon cinnamon

1 teaspoon vanilla extract

1 pinch nutmeg (fresh-ground)

DIRECTIONS:

Place all ingredients, except bread, in food processor and blend well. Transfer into a shallow mixing bowl. Take one slice of bread at a time and soak in mixture for one minute. Coat a nonstick skillet with vegetable oil spray and heat over medium-high heat. Place bread on skillet and cook each side for 3 minutes or until golden brown. Remove from frying pan and top with your choice of maple syrup, honey, fresh fruit, or preserves.

BREAK IT DOWN . . .

Calories: 310; Total fat: 19g; Saturated fat: 3g; Cholesterol: 80mg; Sodium: 380mg; Total carbs: 9g; Fiber: 2g; Sugar: 2g; Protein: 25g.

Cloves *(Eugenia caryophyllus)*

SPEAK IN CLOVED TONGUE

Did you know . . . during the Han dynasty, people were required to put a piece of clove in their mouths to hide bad breath before they were allowed to talk to the Emperor?

What's the Story?

Cloves are dried flower buds that come from the Evergreen clove tree. The English word "clove" stems from the Latin word *clavus* which translates to "nail." Cloves have a sweet, warm flavor and smell. Cloves and clove oil are used in cooking, perfumes, and artificial flavorings.

A Serving of Food Lore . . .

Cloves originated in the Molucca Islands of Indonesia. The spice was first mentioned in Chinese writings during the Han dynasty over two thousand years ago. Arab traders brought cloves to the Venetians in Europe four hundred years later.

Where Are Cloves Grown?

The principle producer of cloves is Zanzibar in East Africa. Indonesia, Sumatra, Jamaica, West Indies, and Brazil are the world's other top producers.

Why Should I Eat Clove?

Cloves contain manganese, vitamins C and K, magnesium, calcium, and fiber. Cloves also contain eugenol, a substance helpful for relieving pain, killing bacteria, and reducing inflammation.

Home Remedies

Make a paste from one-quarter teaspoon clove powder and one teaspoon cinnamon oil. Apply this to the forehead for headaches or to any other painful area. To relieve a toothache, chew on a clove or dip cotton in clove oil and apply it to the painful area.

Throw Me a Lifesaver!

HEART HEALTH: A few grams of cloves per day boosted insulin function while lowering cholesterol, according to two reports presented at the 2006 Experimental Biology meeting in San Francisco. The clove study found that all participants who ingested cloves, regardless of the amount, showed a drop in glucose, triglycerides, and LDL ("bad") cholesterol levels. Blood levels of HDL ("good") cholesterol remained unaffected. Clove oil was found to inhibit lipid peroxidation, which can lead to heart disease.

INFLAMMATION: Eugenol, a component in cloves, has been found to inhibit enzymes and pathways that lead to inflammatory conditions in human cell studies.

YEAST INFECTION: An animal study found a reduction in yeast infections when clove oil was applied to the infected area.

LUNG CANCER: One study found that when mice with induced lung cancer were given an IV clove infusion, cancer growth was reduced.

PAIN: A human study found that clove oil may be helpful in dentistry before a needle is injected into the gums. The subjects in the study reported feeling less pain.

PREMATURE EJACULATION: One study found when a cream containing clove was applied to the penis, men were able to increase the length of time before ejaculation.

Tips on Using Cloves

SELECTION AND STORAGE:
- Choose whole cloves whenever possible. The powder form loses its flavor quickly.
- Fresh cloves release an oil when squeezed. Also, if a clove is fresh, it will float vertically.
- Whole and ground cloves should be stored in an airtight container in a cool, dark, dry place. Whole cloves can be kept for one year; ground cloves can be kept for six months.

PREPARATION AND SERVING SUGGESTIONS:
- Use a coffee grinder to grind whole cloves. Grind just before use.
- Use cloves in combination with other herbs to flavor meats.
- Add cloves when making pickles, stews, marinades, or wines.
- Add ground cloves to your favorite cake, cookie, or pie.

Clove Tequila Shrimp
by Chef J. Hugh McEvoy

Servings: 22 • Prep and cooking time: 30 minutes (but must be marinated overnight)

This recipe contains eight powerhouse foods.

INGREDIENTS FOR SHRIMP BOIL:

⅛ teaspoon ground cloves	2 green onions, chopped
1 pound large shrimp, raw	1 teaspoon sea salt
⅛ cup tequila	1 teaspoon black pepper
6 cups water	1 teaspoon dried ground chipotle
1 lemon, sliced	chili pepper
1 lime, sliced	

MARINADE INGREDIENTS:

⅛ cup lime juice	1 tablespoon green onion
⅛ cup lemon juice	1 tablespoon chopped cilantro
1 tablespoon tequila	leaves
½ cup extra-virgin olive oil	¼ teaspoon ground cloves
1 cup Pinot Grigio white wine	1 clove crushed garlic

GARNISH INGREDIENTS:

¼ pound thinly sliced prosciutto or   1 bag crostini
    smoked French ham

DIRECTIONS:

Add water, tequila, cloves, lemon, lime, green onion, salt, pepper, and dried chipotle peppers to a large sauce pot. Bring ingredients to a rolling boil. Add shrimp and cook just until shrimp turns pink (less than 5 minutes). Do not fully cook. Drain shrimp and run under very cold water. Peel and devein shrimp. Set aside for next step.

In a large bowl, blend together all ingredients for marinade. Place peeled shrimp into a large Ziploc bag. Add marinade to bag. Close tightly. Refrigerate marinating shrimp bag overnight or a minimum of twelve hours. Toast ¼" sliced French bread or use crostini. Brush toasted bread lightly with marinade. Place thinly sliced prosciutto or French smoked ham on toast. Remove shrimp from marinade and place over toast with ham. Garnish each tapas with cilantro.

BREAK IT DOWN . . .

Calories: 43; Total fat: 3g; Saturated fat: 0g; Cholesterol: 17mg; Sodium: 47mg; Total carbs: 1g; Fiber: 0g; Sugar: 0g; Protein: 3g.

Coffee (*Coffea arabica, C. robusta*)

COUNTIN' BEANS

Did you know . . . coffee is the second most traded commodity in the world, right after oil?

What's the Story?

Coffee comes from an evergreen tree that produces red coffee "cherries." The process starts by removing the skin of the cherry to reveal a green coffee "bean." The coffee beans are then dried and roasted to make a brown bean.

Most coffee consumed comes from either arabica or robusta varieties of beans. Arabica coffee accounts for seventy percent of the world's coffee production. It has a mild flavor and is aromatic. Robusta coffee comes from Southeast Asia and Brazil. It has a somewhat bitter taste and contains about fifty percent more caffeine than Arabica.

A Serving of Food Lore . . .

Coffee is thought to have originated in central Ethiopia in 850 A.D. and was brought to Yemen, where it has been cultivated since 1000 A.D. Coffee was mainly used for medicinal purposes until around one thousand years ago, when people began drinking it as a hot beverage. Coffee was always popular among Middle Eastern people but it took time for the beverage's popularity to grow in Europe. Christians first thought that coffee was evil until the Pope tried some and thought it was delicious and blessed it. This began the start of the coffeehouse culture, which soon spread from Italy to France, England, and the Americas.

Where Is Coffee Grown?

Coffee is grown in over fifty-three countries worldwide. These countries have in common their southern latitude; they all lie along the equator between the tropics of Cancer and Capricorn, otherwise known as the "Bean Belt." Brazil is the largest producer of coffee, followed by Colombia, Mexico, Guatemala, Costa Rica, Kenya, Indonesia, Yemen, and Vietnam. Hawaii and Puerto Rico also grow and produce coffee.

Why Should I Drink Coffee?

> Did you know . . . moderate intake (three six-ounce cups per day) of coffee provides the same amount of hydration as an equal amount of water? This is especially true for "seasoned" coffee drinkers.

Coffee doesn't contain significant amounts of vitamins or minerals, yet its antioxidant properties are off the charts. It is one of the top antioxidant beverages consumed worldwide. Coffee contains phytochemicals such as chlorogenic acids, with similar antioxidant benefits to those found in fruits and vegetables that may improve glucose (sugar) metabolism. An average cup of regular coffee contains anywhere between 60 and 130 mg of caffeine. Caffeine is a stimulant that can help with alertness and may improve athletic performance; however, too much can cause jitteriness and irritability.

Home Remedies

Concoctions from the leaves and roots of the coffee tree have been used for fevers, colds, and pneumonia. Many people believe that administering a coffee enema detoxifies the liver while cleaning the colon. Coffee does have a laxative effect on many people.

Throw Me a Lifesaver!

PARKINSON'S DISEASE: In a study of over one million people, caffeine consumption was associated with a reduced risk of Parkinson's disease in men (but not in women).

HEART HEALTH: Though coffee consumption has been associated with hypertension and elevated homocysteine, one study that followed 41,836 postmenopausal women for fifteen years showed that coffee consumption reduced the risk of cardiovascular disease and other inflammatory conditions.

LIVER PROTECTOR: In a study of more than 125,000 people, one cup of coffee per day cut the risk of alcoholic cirrhosis by twenty percent. Four cups per day reduced the risk by eighty percent!

MEMORY LOSS: A study done on elderly men showed that those who drank three cups of coffee per day had less memory loss than those who did not. In another study observing an elderly population, University of Arizona researchers found that decaffeinated-coffee drinkers had a decline in memory performance as the day wore on but this was not the case with caffeinated coffee drinkers.

TYPE 2 DIABETES: An eleven-year study with women found that those who consumed coffee (especially decaffeinated) had less risk of developing type 2 diabetes. A review of fifteen studies on coffee and type 2 diabetes, published in *The Journal of the American Medical Association,* found that people who regularly drank coffee were at lower risk.

BREAST CANCER: Human breast cancer cells responded positively to a treatment with caffeic acid and chlorogenic acid from coffee.

Tips on Using Coffee

SELECTION AND STORAGE:
- To select the best-tasting coffee beans, make sure they are freshly roasted and ground. The beans should be fragrant and free of any cracks.
- The darker the roast, the stronger and more bitter the flavor.
- Troubled by stomach pain when drinking coffee? Phenols, not phenolic acids, may be responsible. Reduced-acid coffees are now available.
- Keep coffee in an airtight container in a cool, dry place. Refrigerate ground coffee for storage of longer than a week but don't freeze coffee as it causes moisture to accumulate and unwanted odors can be absorbed.

PREPARATION AND SERVING SUGGESTIONS:
- Grind coffee beans just before using. Finer grinds brew faster.
- For strong coffee, use two tablespoons of coffee for every six ounces of water.
- Using cold water will help maximize the flavor of the ground coffee beans.
- Run your coffee maker with a mixture of one part vinegar and one part water a few times each month. This eliminates buildup of oils that have become oxidized and can produce a bitter taste in your coffee.
- Use strong black coffee as an ingredient in cakes and other desserts for extra flavor.
- Leftover coffee grinds can be used in a marinade for meats.

Banana Mocha Swirls
Courtesy of Folgers
Servings: 2 • Prep time: 10 minutes

This recipe can be made with any prepared coffee; however, Simply Smooth is a nonacidic coffee that's gentler on the stomach. This recipe contains five powerhouse foods.

INGREDIENTS:

1 cup Folgers Simply Smooth
   coffee, cooled
1 cup nonfat milk
5 heaping teaspoons dark cocoa
   powder

2 tablespoons agave syrup
1 large banana, sliced
½ cup ice cubes

DIRECTIONS:

Combine all ingredients in a blender until frothy. Pour into glasses and serve right away.

BREAK IT DOWN . . .
Calories: 190; Total fat: 1g; Saturated fat: .5g; Cholesterol: 0mg; Sodium: 70mg; Total carbs: 70mg; Fiber: 3g; Sugar: 36g; Protein: 6g.

Corn *(Zea mays)*

LITTLE CORNY
Baby corn is just sweet corn picked in its "infancy."

What's the Story?

There are five principal classes of corn: dent or field corn, flint corn, pop or Indian corn, flour corn, and sweet corn. Dent is the predominant type grown throughout the world. Sweet corn is the common "corn on the cob" that we eat today.

A Serving of Food Lore . . .

Archaeological studies indicate that corn was cultivated in the Americas at least 5,600 years ago. Corn, also known as maize, was domesticated in Mesoamerica, which in pre-Columbian cultures included southern Mexico, Guatemala, Belize, El Salvador, western Honduras, and parts of Nicaragua and Costa Rica. Corn spread to the rest of the world after Spaniards came to the Americas in the late fifteenth century and early sixteenth century. Today, there are over six hundred food and nonfood products made from corn.

Where Is Corn Grown?

The United States is by far the largest producer of corn, accounting for forty percent of world production, followed by Canada, China, Brazil, and many other nations. The "Corn Belt" includes the states of Iowa, Illinois, Nebraska, Minnesota, Indiana, Ohio, Wisconsin, South Dakota, Michigan, Missouri, Kansas, and Kentucky, with the first four states accounting for over fifty percent of corn production in the United States. About seventy-five percent of corn produced in the United States is fed to livestock.

Why Should I Eat Corn?

Corn is a good source of fiber, vitamin B1, folate, vitamin C, and pantothenic acid. Corn contains the phytochemicals beta-cryptoxanthin, lutein, saponins, alkaloids, sitosterol, stigmasterol, malic acid, palmitic acid, tartaric acid, oxalic acid, and maizenic acid, which have heart health and cancer-fighting properties.

Home Remedies

The entire corn plant has long been used in Native American cultures for medicinal purposes. Cornsilk is a well-studied tea that has diuretic properties, and, accordingly, has been used for difficult, painful, or frequent urination. Cornmeal boiled with milk has been applied to burns, inflammations, and swellings. Cornstarch, applied as a powder, may soothe chafing. Cornmeal mixed with castor or corn oil has been used to relieve skin irritations. In Chinese traditional medicine, corn has been used for gallstones, jaundice, hepatitis, and cirrhosis. The cobs stripped of the fruit have been used to treat nosebleeds and unusual uterine bleeding. The hulls have been used to treat diarrhea in children.

Throw Me a Lifesaver!

HEART HEALTH: Corn is high in folate, a vitamin known to reduce homocysteine, an inflammatory marker attributed to heart disease.

LUNG CANCER: Corn is rich in beta-cryptoxanthin, an orange-red carotenoid that may significantly lower the risk of developing lung cancer. One study evaluated the diet of 63,257 adults in Shanghai, China, finding that those who ate the most crytpoxanthin-rich foods had a twenty-seven percent reduction in lung cancer risk. Smokers who ate the crytopoxanthin-rich foods were found to have a thirty-seven percent reduction in risk compared to those who didn't eat them.

COLON CANCER: Corn is very high in phenolic compounds that may help in preventing colon cancer and other digestive cancers. Corn is also high in resistant starch that helps promote butyrate, a short-chain fatty acid found in the colon that may be beneficial in fighting colon cancer.

DIABETES: Cornstarch, a component of corn, was shown to improve glucose metabolism in normal and overweight women.

Tips on Using Corn

SELECTION AND STORAGE:
- Corn kernels come fresh, frozen, canned, and canned creamed.
- Avoid ears of corn with shriveled husks that look burned or have a dark-colored slime in the tassel.
- Leave the husks on and place corn, uncovered, in the refrigerator. Use within a few days for best quality.

PREPARATION AND SERVING SUGGESTIONS:
- Fresh corn can be boiled, steamed, microwaved, or roasted on the grill or in the oven.
- Enjoy cold in salads.

- Use polenta (the Italian word for cornmeal) as a pizza crust for a healthy pizza.
- Use resistant cornstarch to replace up to twenty-five percent of flour to increase fiber content of your baked goods.

Corn Chowder
Adapted from *The Gathering Place* by Graham Kerr
Servings: 6 • Prep and cooking time: 60 minutes

This recipe contains five powerhouse foods.

INGREDIENTS:

1 teaspoon extra-virgin olive oil
2 cups yellow onion, finely chopped
6 ears of corn, kernels shaved off
    of the cob (substitute frozen
    corn if unavailable)
½ teaspoon thyme
1 teaspoon parsley stalks,
    finely diced

¼ teaspoon table salt
⅛ teaspoon black pepper
12 ounces evaporated skim milk
2 cups soy milk
2 tablespoons cornstarch
4 tablespoons dry white wine

GARNISH:

⅓ cup Canadian or veggie bacon,
    chopped

⅓ cup red bell pepper, finely diced
1 tablespoon parsley, chopped

DIRECTIONS:

Heat oil in a large saucepan over medium heat. Sauté the onion and ½ cup of the corn kernels until very soft, 12 to 15 minutes. Stir occasionally. Add thyme, parsley, salt, and pepper. Transfer onion mixture to blender and add ½ cup evaporated milk. Puree mixture for two minutes. Add remaining evaporated milk and blend for another three minutes or until smooth. Return to saucepan along with remaining corn. Rinse the blender with soy milk to pick up any ingredients left behind. Add to saucepan with corn. Bring to a boil. Reduce heat and simmer for 10 minutes. Combine cornstarch with wine to make a slurry. Remove soup from heat and stir in slurry until thickened. Sauté bacon, pepper, and parsley over medium heat for three minutes. Set aside. Serve chowder in warmed bowls and top with 1 tablespoon of garnish.

BREAK IT DOWN . . .

Calories: 240; Total fat: 5g; Saturated fat: 1g; Cholesterol: 10mg; Sodium: 550mg; Total carbs: 39g; Fiber: 3g; Sugar: 13g; Protein: 12g.

Cranberries *(Vaccinium macrocarpon)*

BIRD IN THE BUSH

Did you know . . . "craneberry," as it was called by American Pilgrims, was given that name because the spring bush blossom resembled a crane. It was then shortened to "cranberry" sometime later.

What's the Story?

Cranberries are one of three fruits native to the United States and Canada. They grow in fruit beds called bogs. The most common way of harvesting cranberries is to flood the fruit beds and "beat" the fruit loose using a specialized harvester. The floating fruit is then gathered and loaded onto trucks for delivery to a receiving station.

A Serving of Food Lore . . .

Historically used as both a culinary ingredient and as medicine by Native Americans, cranberries first became popular in our culture during the Revolutionary War. Henry Hall, a war veteran, planted the first commercial cranberry beds in Dennis, Massachusetts, in 1816. Today, cranberries account for nearly 40,000 acres across the northern United States and Canada, and over 300 million pounds of the berries were sold in 2004 to become fresh, frozen, juiced, dried, jellied, sauced, and even "pilled" products.

Where Are Cranberries Grown?

They are mainly grown commercially in Wisconsin, Massachusetts, New Jersey, Oregon, Washington, and also in the Canadian provinces of British Columbia and Quebec.

Why Should I Eat Cranberries?

Cranberries are rich in fiber and are an excellent source of vitamin C and phytonutrients, such as flavonoids and proanthocyanidins (PAC). They contain more phenolic antioxidants than nineteen of the most popular consumed fruits according to a study published in the *Journal of Agriculture and Food Chemistry.*

Home Remedies

A lot of the initial work with cranberries, especially with its role in fighting urinary tract infections (UTIs), was anecdotal. It was mom's advice and she knew it worked. Now research is finding that mothers were right all along! The National Institutes of Health has twelve studies underway focusing primarily on further defining cranberries' activity against UTIs.

According to Martin Starr, PhD, scientific advisor to the Cranberry Institute, cranberries are not only nutritious but have unique antiadhesion and antibacterial properties not found in other fruit:

> There have been multiple clinical studies done using cranberry juice and it turns out that cranberry has unique antiadhesion properties that prevent certain harmful bacteria from sticking to cells in our body. This newer concept of antiadhesion is not just limited to UTIs [urinary tract infections] but potentially other harmful bacteria as well, including those responsible for stomach ulcers and gum disease.

Throw Me a Lifesaver!

CANCER: Multiple studies have found that flavonoid compounds including anthocyanins, flavonols, and proanthocyanidins, found naturally in cranberries, may be able to fight leukemia, breast, lung, colon, and potentially many other types of cancer.

HEART DISEASE: Flavonoids may also reduce the risk of atherosclerosis. The flavonoid and phenolic compounds in cranberries have been shown to reduce LDL ("bad") cholesterol, a known risk factor for atherosclerosis, while potentially raising protective HDL ("good") cholesterol.

Amazingly, cranberry juice may be as effective in fighting heart disease as using the whole cranberry!

DIGESTIVE HEALTH: Cranberry juice has been shown to inhibit the bacteria associated with peptic ulcers, *H. pylori*. Though most ulcers are not life-threatening, *H. pylori* bacteria has been associated with stomach cancer, acid reflux disease, and gastritis. Cranberries' properties have also been shown to help reduce diarrhea.

PERIODONTAL DISEASE: In a study that appeared in the *Journal of the American Dental Association*, a component of cranberry juice was demonstrated to have the ability to stop bacteria from adhering to teeth and gums, thus reducing dental plaque and periodontal disease.

Tips on Using Cranberries

SELECTION AND STORAGE:
- Purchase prepackaged in plastic bags. Look for plump, firm, and bright berries.
- Besides raw cranberries, you can also purchase dried (usually sweetened), juice (sweetened and unsweetened), sauce, jelly, and even cranberry supplements.
- Store cranberries in the crisper section of the refrigerator, in their original bag, for up to four weeks, or in the freezer section for up to six months.

PREPARATION AND SERVING SUGGESTIONS:
- Unsweetened juice can be rather bitter tasting by itself, so it's best mixed with equal parts of apple juice or any other sweet juice of choice. It also comes in the "cocktail" form, sweetened or artificially sweetened.
- Topping a bowl of cereal with a small handful of dried cranberries, tossing in a salad, or including as a focal point to almost any side dish (such as a cranberry pilaf) adds that "sweet-tart" taste that's delightful.

Kamut-Cranberry Salad
by Chef J. Hugh McEvoy
Servings: 6 • Prep and cooking time: 60 minutes

This makes a great breakfast cereal alternative. Serve with maple syrup and cinnamon. This recipe contains six powerhouse foods.

INGREDIENTS:

12 ounces organic kamut berries
4 ounces Vidalia onions, chopped
2 teaspoons butter, unsalted
2 teaspoons extra-virgin olive oil
1 teaspoon garlic cloves, chopped fine

1 ounce dried sweetened cranberries
2 ounces dry roasted pecans, unsalted
Kosher salt and black pepper to taste

DIRECTIONS:

Using a heavy sauce pot, cook kamut berries in one gallon of boiling salted water until tender, approximately 45 to 50 minutes. Drain cooked grain and reserve for next steps.

Using the pot the grain was cooked in, sauté chopped onion in extra-virgin olive oil and butter until lightly browned. Add garlic, sauté until just soft, then add cooked grain, nuts, and cranberries. Bring mixture up to a simmer. Season with salt and black pepper to taste. Remove from heat and serve immediately.

BREAK IT DOWN . . .

Calories: 261; Total fat: 10g; Saturated fat: 2g; Cholesterol: 3mg; Sodium: 60mg; Total carbs: 42g; Fiber: 7g; Sugar: 15g; Protein: 8g.

Cumin *(Cuminum cyminum)*

MUMMY'S LITTLE HELPER

Did you know . . . cumin was used for both culinary and medicinal purposes in ancient Egypt? Egyptians not only seasoned their meats with it but also mummified their dead with cumin.

What's the Story?

Cumin is related to coriander and is a member of the parsley family. Some countries consider caraway to be a foreign form of cumin and vice versa. That is why you may see cumin referred to as Roman caraway, Eastern caraway, Egyptian caraway, and Turkish caraway as you globe-trot in search of culinary adventure.

The seed component of the plant is what is mainly used as a spice and it is a key ingredient in both chili powder and curry powder. Cumin has a strong and sharp taste and is ubiquitous in the cuisines of Mexico, Thailand, and Vietnam. It is an inseparable part of the Indian curry *masala* and is also one of several spices for meat and poultry marinades in North African, Middle Eastern, and Mediterranean cooking.

A Serving of Food Lore . . .

Cumin's origins are thought to range from the eastern Mediterranean region to India. Its use dates back to biblical times. The Romans and the Greeks used it medicinally—and cosmetically to induce a pale complexion. Cumin also symbolized greed at one time, particularly in the lore of the Roman emperor Marcus Aurelius, who came to be known privately as "Cuminus." Much later, in Europe, cumin symbolized faithfulness. In Germany, guests of a wedding carried cumin, dill, and salt in their pockets during the ceremony to prevent the bride or groom from straying.

Where Is Cumin Grown?

Historically, Iran had been the principal supplier of cumin, but today the major producers are India, Syria, Pakistan, Turkey, and China.

Why Should I Eat Cumin?

Cumin is a source of iron. Rich in essential oils such as cuminaldehyde and pyrazines, cumin is associated with blood glucose–lowering effects.

Home Remedies

Some Middle Eastern countries consider the combination of cumin, black pepper, and honey a natural sexual aid. Cumin seeds mixed with milk and honey have been used during pregnancy to ease childbirth, reduce nausea, and increase lactation. In traditional medicine, cumin helps aid digestion. Cumin has antibacterial properties and has been known to protect against hookworm infection. In traditional Indian medicine, cumin seeds are smoked in a pipe with ghee (clarified butter) to relieve the hiccups.

Throw Me a Lifesaver!

ARTHRITIS: One study showed that rats that were given an extract of black cumin had reduced inflammation attributed to arthritis.

DIABETES: Rats who consumed cumin for six weeks had marked reduction in blood glucose, hemoglobin A1c, cholesterol, and triglycerides. Researchers also found cumin supplementation to be more effective than glibenclamide (an oral hypoglycemic medication to help control blood glucose) in the treatment of diabetes mellitus.

COLON CANCER: Cumin added to the diets of rats slowed down the formation of colon cancer cells.

ULCERS: Cumin was found to be highly effective at killing *H. pylori,* a bacteria associated with stomach ulcers.

Tips on Using Cumin

SELECTION AND STORAGE:
- Because cumin can lose its flavor quickly, fresh-ground seeds are preferable to cumin powder.
- Cumin seeds and cumin powder should be kept in a tightly sealed glass container in a cool, dark, and dry place. Ground cumin will

keep for about six months, while the whole seeds will stay fresh for about one year.

PREPARATION AND SERVING SUGGESTIONS:

- Lightly roast whole cumin seeds to bring out the flavor before using them in a recipe.
- Cumin goes well with chicken.
- Add to legumes such as lentils, garbanzo beans, and black beans.
- Sprinkle on plain brown rice along with dried apricots and almonds for a tasty side dish.

Roasted Fish with Cumin Sweet Potatoes
by Nicki Anderson

Servings: 4 • Prep and cooking time: 1 hour, 10 minutes.

This delectable dish contains six powerhouse foods.

INGREDIENTS:

1 pound sweet potatoes, sliced ¼" thick

½ teaspoon ground cumin

1 tablespoon olive oil

4 catfish or other fish fillets (4–6 ounces each)

1 teaspoon chili powder

1 cup chopped yellow/green zucchini

¾ cup diagonally sliced scallions

1 tablespoon fresh cilantro

DIRECTIONS:

Preheat oven to 400 degrees. In a 13 × 9 baking dish, sprinkle potatoes with cumin and toss with oil to coat. Spread in even layer and roast until potatoes are browned, about 45 minutes. Remove from oven. Increase oven temperature to 450 degrees. Use wide spatula to gently turn potato slices. Arrange fish on top of potatoes. Sprinkle with chili powder and scallions. Return to oven and roast until fish is opaque in center, 8 to 10 minutes per inch of thickness. With wide spatula, lift a portion of potatoes with fish on top onto serving plates. Garnish with fresh cilantro.

BREAK IT DOWN . . .

Calories: 300; Total fat: 9g; Saturated fat: 2g; Cholesterol: 100mg; Sodium: 95mg; Total carbs: 25g; Fiber: 3g; Sugar: 11g; Protein: 30g.

Currants *(Ribes)*

ARE YOU KEEPING CURRANT?

"Zante currants" are not really currants at all. They are actually dried grapes and are often found in scones.

What's the Story?

Currants are related to gooseberries and are not smaller versions of raisins. The English word "currant" has been used for this fruit only since 1550, taken from the fruit's resemblance to the dried currants of Greece, which, in fact, *are* raisins made from a small seedless grape. The main varieties available are: red, black, white, green, and pink. Red and black are the most common type and are used for culinary purposes. White currants are an albino form of the red, and pink currants are a mix between the white and red.

A Serving of Food Lore . . .

Currants are native to Europe, Asia, and North America. Cultivation began in Europe in the 1500s and the first American colonists began cultivating them in the late 1700s. The black currant has been known in the United States as a "forbidden fruit" since 1911, when a ban was placed on the fruit because it caused disease to the white pine tree. Although the ban was lifted in 1966, several states still prohibit growing black currants.

Where Are Currants Grown?

Russia is the number one producer of currants. Poland, Germany, Ukraine, and Austria also grow currants commercially. There is very little commercial production in the United States; however, Oregon, Washington, and New York grow them at modest levels.

Why Should I Eat Currants?

Currants are an excellent source of vitamin C and fiber, and a good source of calcium, iron, potassium, and vitamins A and B. Currants are rich in the phytochemical ellagic acid, a phenolic compound that may reduce some cancers and cholesterol, and anthocyanins, which have shown anti-inflammatory and antioxidant properties.

Home Remedies

BLACK CURRANTS: Boiled black currant juice has been used for sore throats. The leaves have been used to reduce fevers and increase urination. Extract from the bark of the black currant tree has been used for hemorrhoids. Black currant jelly mixed with hot water has been helpful for colds.

RED CURRANTS: The leaves have been used to relieve pain from arthritic symptoms, sprains, and dislocated bones. The fruit has been used as a laxative. It has also been used to prevent scurvy. Red currants have also been made into facial masks for firm skin.

Throw Me a Lifesaver!

CANCER: One study found that black currant juice stopped the growth of tumors in mice.

BLOOD PRESSURE: Currant seed oil was given to a group with mildly high blood pressure. Scientists attribute their significant decline in blood pressure to the gamma-linoleic acid found in the berry.

Tips on Using Currants

SELECTION AND STORAGE:
- Currants come fresh, dried, juiced, and in jams and jellies.
- Choose berries with the darkest colors. Currants can also be bought frozen.
- Keep currants refrigerated and use them within two days. Wash just before use. Fresh currants can be frozen.

PREPARATION AND SERVING SUGGESTIONS:
- Wash the berries in cold running water. Remove stems or leaves. Drain and pat dry.
- Use currants as a garnish for any dish.
- Add dried currants to brown rice.
- Top ice cream with fresh currants or a currant sauce.

Red Currant Grill Sauce
by Chef J. Hugh McEvoy
Servings: 38 • Prep and cooking time: 40 minutes

This recipe contains five powerhouse foods.

INGREDIENTS:

FIRST STAGE:

½ cup fresh red currants
8 ounces red currant preserves
¼ cup fresh lemon juice
1 ounce fresh lemon zest
½ teaspoon ground cinnamon

⅛ teaspoon ground cloves
⅛ teaspoon black pepper
⅛ teaspoon chili powder
2 cups fat-free beef broth, unsalted

SECOND STAGE:

¼ cup Worcestershire sauce
¼ cup Burgundy red wine

4 ounces blackstrap molasses
¼ cup organic tomato ketchup

DIRECTIONS:

Combine first nine ingredients in a heavy saucepan. Mix until evenly blended. Bring mixture to a boil. Reduce heat to a low simmer. Simmer mixture until it has reduced by one half. In a separate bowl, whisk together the remaining four ingredients. Add the second group of ingredients [the second stage] into the simmering sauce. Mix thoroughly until color is even. Simmer until sauce comes back to a boil. Reduce heat to very low. Serve sauce hot with grilled lamb, pork, or flavorful fish such as salmon or bluefish. Serve with a robust red wine such as Burgundy or Cabernet Sauvignon.

BREAK IT DOWN . . .

Calories: 30; Total fat: 0g; Saturated fat: 0g; Cholesterol: 0mg; Sodium: 54mg; Total carbs: 8g; Fiber: 0g; Sugar: 6g; Protein: 0g.

Eggplant *(Solanum melongena L.)*

CRAZY LOVE

Did you know . . . the Spanish called eggplant *berengenas*, "the apples of love"; whereas other Europeans called it *mala insana*, "mad apple," because they thought it caused insanity.

What's the Story?

Eggplant, along with potatoes, tomatoes, and peppers, is a member of the nightshade family. Eggplant hangs from vines on a plant very much like tomatoes and comes in several widely available varieties such as classic (oval shape with purple color), Italian (small and mauve with white streaks), Japanese (white with purple streaks), pink, and green. Eggplant can be egg-shaped, oval-shaped, or balloon-shaped with a pear-shaped end, and has a somewhat bitter taste and spongy texture.

A Serving of Food Lore . . .

Eggplant is thought to have originated in southeast India around Assam and the adjoining area then known as Burma. From Southeast Asia it was brought by traders from the Middle East to the Mediterranean in the early Middle Ages. The Moors introduced eggplant to Spain in the twelfth century and it soon made its way throughout the rest of Europe. Four hundred years later, Spanish traders brought it to the Americas.

It was not until fifty years ago that eggplant was even considered acceptable to eat in the United States because many believed eating it caused insanity, leprosy, and cancer.

Where Is Eggplant Grown?

Most of the world's eggplant is grown in China. Italy, Turkey, Egypt, and Japan also produce significant harvests of the vegetable. Florida is the largest U.S. producer of eggplant, accounting for more than thirty percent of the crop. New Jersey is the second largest, followed by California. Mexico exports eggplant to the U.S. during the winter.

Why Should I Eat Eggplant?

Eggplant is high in potassium, copper, folate, magnesium, and fiber. It contains flavonoids and phenols such as caffeic acid and chlorogenic acid, which may fight cancer, viruses, and harmful bacteria, and protect against damage to cells.

Home Remedies

In Asia, the roots are often used for coughs, phlegm, and sore throats. It is believed that crushing a baked, blackened eggplant and applying it to teeth and gums will promote a healthy mouth. This concoction is also said to stop bleeding gums and nosebleeds. Eggplant has been used as an antidote for poisonous mushrooms, to reduce hemorrhoids, soothe burns, and relieve cold sores.

Throw Me a Lifesaver!

HEART HEALTH: An animal study in Japan found that an anthocyanin unique to eggplant peels had anti–heart disease attributes. Rabbits with high cholesterol that were fed eggplant had decreased weight, total cholesterol, LDL cholesterol, and triglycerides.

DETOXIFIER: A cell study found that eggplant triggered enzymes that detoxify and remove drugs and other harmful chemical substances in the human body.

LIVER CANCER: A cell study found that a component of eggplant called glycoalkaloids killed human liver cancer cells.

Tips for Using Eggplant

SELECTION AND STORAGE:
- Look for firm, shiny, smooth, deep purple skin. Avoid eggplant with cracked or shriveled skin, and stay away from brown, blue, or yellow eggplants.
- Eggplant is best used right away, but may be kept in the refrigerator's crisper drawer for up to one week.

PREPARATION AND SERVING SUGGESTIONS:
- The skin can be peeled with a potato peeler or it may be kept on.
- To tenderize the eggplant and remove some of the bitter flavor, sprinkle the eggplant with salt, let it sit for 30 minutes, and then wash the salt off.
- Eggplant can be baked, roasted, steamed, fried, or sautéed. The eggplant is done when a fork goes through easily.
- Scrape out some of the middle of the eggplant and stuff it with vegetables and cheese, then bake.
- Add eggplant to stir-fry, lasagna, or other pasta dishes.
- Puree eggplant with lemon juice, garlic, and olive oil for a bread spread or vegetable dip.

Elisa's Cheesy Spaghetti with Eggplant and Tomato
by Elisa Zied

Servings: 8 • Prep and cooking time: 50 minutes

This recipe contains six powerhouse foods.

INGREDIENTS:

1 box thin whole wheat spaghetti	1 tablespoon onion powder
4 tablespoons extra-virgin olive oil	1 tablespoon garlic powder
1 eggplant cut into ½-inch cubes	8 ounces fresh mozzarella
1 pint (2 cups) grape tomatoes, cut in half	¾ cup Parmesan cheese, grated

DIRECTIONS:
Make spaghetti as directed and set aside. In a large, nonstick skillet, add two tablespoons of olive oil to the pan, and set on medium heat.

Wash eggplant and cut into cubes. Set aside. Wash grape tomatoes and cut in half. Place eggplant and tomatoes into a large plastic baggie. Add onion powder and garlic powder to the eggplant and tomatoes. Add two tablespoons olive oil to the baggie. Seal the bag and shake vigorously until all ingredients are well mixed. Add eggplant and tomato mixture to the pan and lower heat to low-medium. Every few minutes, stir eggplant and tomato so they cook evenly. Cook for about 20 minutes or until eggplant is tender. Meanwhile, make sure to drain cooked pasta and put it back into the pot in which it was cooked. When eggplant and tomato mixture is thoroughly cooked, place in a large bowl lined with paper towels. Blot with more paper towels to remove excess oil. Add eggplant and tomato in with spaghetti. Cut up mozzarella cheese into cubes and add to pasta mixture. Set on low heat. Stir mixture for about 5 minutes until cheese is melted. Mix in grated Parmesan cheese and serve.

BREAK IT DOWN . . .
Calories: 370; Total fat: 15g; Saturated fat: 6g; Cholesterol: 20mg; Sodium: 300mg; Total carbs: 43g; Fiber: 8g; Sugar: 4g; Protein: 13g.

Eggs

EGG HER ON!
Did you know . . . a hen can produce an egg every day?

What's the Story?

Any way you crack them, all eggs contain a yellow yolk surrounded by a clear egg white (also known as albumin), all encased in a shell. Chicken eggs are the most widely consumed type of egg but other kinds such as duck, quail, and turkey are also eaten throughout the world.

When it comes to chicken eggs, there are basically two kinds to choose from: white and brown. White eggs come from hens with white feathers and white earlobes whereas brown eggs come from hens with red feathers and red earlobes. White and brown eggs have the same nutritional quality; notwithstanding many claims to the contrary, neither is better than the other. Fresh eggs are graded and sized by the United States Department of Agriculture (USDA). AA is the highest grade, followed by A and B. Size ranges from jumbo to extra large, large, medium, small, and peewee.

A Serving of Food Lore . . .

What came first? We may never know, but what is for sure is that eggs have been around a long, long time. Throughout history, the egg has been used to symbolize everything from fertility to nobility. Domesticated chickens can be traced back to 3200 B.C. in India. Full-blown egg production in the Middle East and Asia began as early as 3,500 years ago. Eggs were brought to the Western world in the fifth century A.D. Several hundred years later eggs were added to the list of foods not eaten during Lent because they were seen as luxurious. On Easter, people were allowed to begin eating eggs again, which explains their importance and popularity on that holiday.

Where Do Eggs Come From?

As with so many food essentials, China is the world's largest producer of eggs, meeting its own needs and also supplying eggs to some neighboring markets. Other big suppliers are India, Mexico, the European Union, and the United States. Iowa, Ohio, Indiana, Pennsylvania, California, and Texas are, in that order, the United States' leading producers.

Why Should I Eat Eggs?

The quality of egg protein is the highest of any whole food product, second only to human breast milk. Eggs are also a good source of the amino acid tryptophan, selenium, vitamin B2, and vitamin B12, and are one of the rare sources of natural vitamin D. Eggs are a good source of choline, which is important for brain function, gene regulation, and heart health. Eggs also contain lutein and zeaxanthin, two phytochemicals that may reduce the risk of cataracts and macular degeneration.

Home Remedies

Eggs have been used in a variety of ways for medicinal purposes. One popular remedy for colic consists of beating four to five egg whites and putting them on a piece of leather, sprinkling the mixture with pepper and ginger, and then placing the mixture over the child's belly button. The age-old remedy of mixing one egg, a teaspoon of Worcestershire sauce, a dash of vinegar, a dash of Tabasco sauce, and a little salt and pepper reportedly has helped many in getting over a hangover. Be aware that from a food-safety standpoint, eating raw eggs is not a good idea!

Throw Me a Lifesaver!

CATARACTS AND MACULAR DEGENERATION: According to one study, people who ate foods high in lutein and zeaxanthin, such as eggs, had a twenty percent reduction in developing cataracts and a forty percent reduction in developing macular degeneration.

OBESITY: A report in the *Journal of the American College of Nutrition* presented promising research on the possible "hunger-fighting power" of eggs. An egg first thing in the morning may lead to reduced calorie consumption for the rest of the day.

Tips on Eggs

SELECTION AND STORAGE:
- Check for cracks before purchasing.
- Look for an expiration date on the side of the carton and only buy eggs that are refrigerated.
- There are varieties of eggs that are rich in omega-3 fats and are actually lower in cholesterol than regular eggs (180mg versus 215mg in a large egg).
- Store your eggs in the refrigerator and they will stay good for about one month.
- Do not put them in the refrigerator door as they will be exposed to warmer temperatures when the door is opened. Keep them in their original carton.
- Egg whites freeze fairly well for several months.

PREPARATION AND SERVING SUGGESTIONS:
- Wash your hands, utensils, and work surfaces with hot, soapy water before and after handling eggs to prevent cross-contamination of salmonella.
- Cook until yolks are firm.
- Don't keep eggs and egg products out of the refrigerator for more than two hours.
- Eggs are used in French toast, pancakes, quiche, soufflés, salads, and a variety of other dishes.

Cheesy Asparagus and Mushroom Scramble
by Elisa Zied
Servings: 4 • Prep and cooking time: 20 minutes

If you don't like your veggies crunchy, sauté the asparagus and mushrooms first. This recipe contains three powerhouse foods.

INGREDIENTS:

8 large egg whites, raw
4 egg yolks, raw
1 cup asparagus, chopped
1 cup white mushrooms,
　chopped

4 slices low-sodium, light
　Swiss cheese, cut into
　small slivers
Salt and pepper to taste
Nonstick cooking spray

DIRECTIONS:

On medium heat, coat the bottom of a nonstick large frying pan with nonstick cooking spray. Put 4 whole eggs into a medium bowl. Remove egg yolks from 4 other eggs and add the remaining whites to the bowl with the whole eggs. Mix eggs and pour into the pan when heated. Let the eggs set for 1 minute. Slide the pan gently and bring eggs to center. Add asparagus, mushrooms, and Swiss cheese and stir gently for a few minutes until all ingredients are scrambled. Serve.

BREAK IT DOWN . . .

Calories: 190; Total fat: 11g; Saturated fat: 6g; Cholesterol: 233mg; Sodium: 270mg; Total carbs: 4g; Fiber: 1g; Sugar: 2g; Protein: 19g.

Elderberry *(Sambucus nigra)*

ELDER STATESMAN

Did you know . . . the elder tree has been called "the medicine chest of the common people"?

What's the Story?

There are over twenty species of elder trees in existence today. Formerly thought to be in the honeysuckle family *Caprifoliaceae,* elder is now classified in the Moschatel family *Adoxaceae.* The flowers, leaves, berries, bark, and roots have all been used in traditional folk medicine for centuries. The fruit goes into elderberry wine, brandy, and the popular drink Sambuca, which is made by infusing elderberries and anise into alcohol. When cooked, elderberry can be used to make pies and jam. Raw berries contain hydrocyanic acid (cyanide) and sambucine alkaloids, which can cause diarrhea and nausea. Their harmful effects can be deactivated simply by cooking the berries.

A Serving of Food Lore . . .

Elderberry gets its name from the Anglo-Saxon word "aeld" meaning "fire," perhaps referring to its fiery red branches that hold the berries. Interestingly, Egyptians used elder flowers for healing burns. Many Native American tribes used elderberry, and its variants, in teas and other beverages. In the Middle Ages, legend held that its tree was home to witches and that cutting one down would bring on the wrath of those residing in the branches. As early as the seventeenth century, the British became known for homemade wine and cordials that were consumed for various health challenges including fighting the common cold. For the past several centuries, reference to the medicinal benefits of elderberry can be found in a variety of pharmacopoeias throughout greater Europe.

Where Are Elderberries Grown?

Elderberries are grown commercially in the Russian Federation and throughout Europe, particularly in Poland, Hungary, Portugal, and Bulgaria. They are also grown, on a smaller scale, in North America, in Nova Scotia, New York, Ohio, and Oregon.

Why Should I Eat Elderberries?

The berries contain more vitamin C than any other fruit except rose hips and black currants. Elderberries also contain vitamin A and carotenoids, flavonoids, tannins, polyphenols, and anthocynanins. Many of these phytochemicals have been shown to be powerful antioxidants with anti-inflammatory, antiulcerative, antiviral, and anticancer properties.

Home Remedies

Hippocrates and other healers have used elderberry as an anti-inflammatory, anti-rheumatic, diuretic, and laxative agent, as well as for the treatment of dysentery, stomach ailments, scurvy, and urinary tract problems. Warm elderberry wine is a remedy for sore throat and influenza, and induces perspiration to reverse the effects of a chill. The juice from the berries is an old-fashioned cure for colds, and is also said to relieve asthma and bronchitis. Infusions of the fruit are beneficial for nerve disorders and back pain, and have been used to reduce inflammation of the urinary tract and bladder.

Throw Me a Lifesaver!

INFLUENZA: Several studies have shown the effectiveness of elderberry in killing influenza strains A and B. In one study, sixty patients who had influenza-like symptoms for less than two days were randomized in a double-blind, placebo-controlled study. In those receiving elderberry extract, less medication was required and symptoms were relieved an average of four days earlier compared to those who had received the placebo. In another study with an elderberry-treated group, over ninety-three percent of participants experienced significant relief, including the absence of fever, within two days.

COLITIS: Rats with colitis received an extract of elderberry for one month. Compared to the control group, the elderberry-fed group had a fifty percent reduction in damage to the colon.

Tips on Using Elderberry

SELECTION AND STORAGE:
- Avoid picking berries that have become overripe. Wash well and strip from the stalks using a dining fork.
- Elderberries can be stored in the refrigerator for up to one week.

PREPARATION AND SERVING SUGGESTIONS:
- They can be frozen, canned, and made into pie filling.
- Elderberries can be added to apple pie or blackberry jam.

Fourth of July Elderberry Ice Cream Pie
by Sharon, Chloe, Katie, and Madison Grotto

Servings: 8 • Prep and cooking time: 30 minutes.
Freeze until firm: 3 to 4 hours

This recipe contains two powerhouse foods.

INGREDIENTS:
FOR THE CRUST:

1½ cups graham cracker crumbs
2 tablespoons honey

2 tablespoons butter, melted

FOR THE FILLING:

12 ounces elderberries
¼ cup honey
1 teaspoon vanilla extract
⅓ cup water
1 tablespoon cornstarch

2 cups low-fat strawberry ice cream or frozen yogurt
2 cups low-fat vanilla ice cream or frozen yogurt

DIRECTIONS (CRUST):
Place graham cracker crumbs, honey, and butter in a 9-inch pie plate. Mix and firmly press mixture to form pie crust. Place in freezer for thirty minutes.

DIRECTIONS (FILLING):

While crust is freezing, dissolve cornstarch in water and mix with elderberries, honey, and vanilla extract in a medium saucepan, bring to a boil, cook until thickened (about two minutes). Let sauce cool completely.

Place softened strawberry ice cream on top of frozen pie crust. Layer ½ of berry sauce over ice cream. Layer vanilla ice cream over berry sauce. Layer top of vanilla ice cream with remaining berry sauce. Wrap with plastic wrap and freeze 3 to 4 hours or until firm.

BREAK IT DOWN . . .

Calories: 260; Total fat: 8g; Saturated fat: 3.5g; Cholesterol: 15mg; Sodium: 160mg; Total carbs: 48g; Fiber: 3; Sugar: 30g; Protein: 4g.

Fennel *(Foeniculum vulgare)*

CHEW ON THIS!

Did you know . . . Puritans referred to fennel as the "meeting seed" as they would chew it during their long church services?

What's the Story?

Fennel is composed of a white or pale green bulb with stalks that are topped with feathery green leaves and flowers that produce fennel seeds. All parts of the fennel plant are edible. Fennel has a sweet aromatic flavor and aroma. Varieties include Cantino, Fino (Zefa Fino), Herald, Perfection, Sirio, Sweet Florence, and Tardo (Zefa Tardo). Fennel is popular in southern European cooking.

A Serving of Food Lore . . .

Fennel is native to southern Europe and southwestern Asia. It was known to the ancient Greeks and spread throughout Europe by Imperial Rome. Legend has it that the Battle of Marathon, the town for which the famous race is named, was fought in a field of fennel. Greek mythology reveals that fennel was favored by Dionysus, the Greek god of food and wine, and that knowledge of the gods was passed on to man via a fennel stalk.

Where Is Fennel Grown?

Wild fennel is the form mainly cultivated in central and eastern Europe, while sweet fennel is grown mainly in France, Italy, Greece, and Turkey. Much of the seed of European commerce comes from India. In the U.S., California and Arizona are the top producers.

Why Should I Eat Fennel?

Fennel is a source of fiber, folate, and potassium. It contains a significant amount of vitamin C. Fennel also contains the phytochemicals anethole and other terpenoids that have been shown to have anticancer, anti-inflammatory, and digestive properties.

Home Remedies

Chinese and Hindus used it as a snakebite remedy. The seeds are utilized in many herbal medicines to reduce gas and intestinal colic, allay hunger, and diminish indigestion. In the first century, it was noted that after snakes had shed their skins, they ate fennel to restore their sight. It has since been used as a wash for eyestrain and irritations. Fennel seed is widely used in India as an after-dinner breath freshener and also to help in digestion.

Fennel has also been used as a diuretic, to stimulate lactation, and to help with yellow jaundice, gout, and occasional cramps. Chinese medicine prescribes fennel for gastroenteritis, hernia, indigestion, and abdominal pain, to resolve phlegm, and to stimulate milk production.

Throw Me a Lifesaver!

COLIC: About forty percent of infants who received fennel seed oil showed relief of colic symptoms, as compared to only fourteen percent in the placebo group.

CANCER: The phytonutrient anethole, which occurs naturally in fennel, has been shown to reduce the gene-altering and inflammation-triggering molecule called NF-kappa B. It also helps reduce tumor necrosis factor (TNF), a cancer-signaling molecule, thus enhancing cancer cell death.

STOMACH RELIEF: Anethole and other terpenoids have been known to inhibit spasms in the intestinal tract, acting as a gas-relieving and cramp-relieving agent.

Tips on Using Fennel

SELECTION AND STORAGE:
- Select fennel bulbs that are whitish or pale green in color and firm without signs of damage.
- Store fresh fennel in the refrigerator crisper for up to four days.

PREPARATION AND SERVING SUGGESTIONS:
- The three different parts of fennel—the base, stalks, and leaves—can all be used in cooking.
- Use it for meats and poultry, but even more for fish and seafood.
- Toasting fennel seeds accentuates their flavor. They can be added to meat dishes for an authentic Italian flavor. Sauté fennel seeds with sliced peppers, onion, and sausage for a quick pasta sauce.
- Fennel is often combined together with thyme and oregano in olive oil–based marinades for vegetables and seafood.

Baked Stuffed Garlic Fennel
by Chef Cheryl Bell
Servings: 4 • Prep and cooking time: 60 minutes

This recipe contains three powerhouse foods.

INGREDIENTS:

2 fennel bulbs
1 cup chicken or vegetable broth
¼ cup minced garlic
2 tablespoons grated Parmesan
   cheese

2 tablespoons seasoned whole
   wheat breadcrumbs
Kosher salt and black pepper to
   taste

DIRECTIONS:

Heat oven to 375 degrees. Spray an 11 × 9-inch baking dish with nonstick cooking spray. Trim the frilly tops off of the fennel bulbs. Remove outer skin that may be thick and tough. Cut fennel bulbs vertically into ¼-inch-thick slices. Lay slices flat in the baking pan, keeping slices intact. Add the chicken broth to the baking dish. Place 1 teaspoon of minced garlic on top of each fennel slice. Sprinkle with salt and pepper, if desired. Cover pan tightly with aluminum foil and bake for 45 to 50 minutes, or until fennel can be pierced through with a fork without any resistance. In a small bowl, combine the Parmesan, breadcrumbs, and pepper. Remove fennel from oven and sprinkle Parmesan mixture over fennel slices. Bake uncovered for 10 to 15 minutes, or until the crumbs are lightly browned. Serve right away with pan juices.

BREAK IT DOWN . . .
Calories: 80; Total fat: 1g; Saturated fat: .5g; Cholesterol: 0mg; Sodium: 380; Total carbs: 16g; Fiber: 4g; Sugar: 2g; Protein: 4g.

Figs *(Ficus carica L.)*

GO "FIG-URE"

Did you know . . . according to the Bible, the first known fashion statement was made with fig leaves?

> *"Then the eyes of both [Adam and Eve] were opened and they realized that they were naked; so they sewed fig leaves together and made coverings for themselves."*

Genesis 3:7

What's the Story?

Figs are commonly thought of as a fruit but they are actually inverted flowers with the seeds being the actual fruit. There are hundreds of different varieties of figs but the most popular are the Celeste, Brown Turkey, Brunswick, and Marseilles. In the United States, the Calimyrna and Black Mission are most common.

A Serving of Food Lore . . .

The fig is a symbolic fruit that dates back to ancient and biblical times and is the most frequently mentioned fruit in the Bible. Figs were revered by Cleopatra for their health benefits, and Greek Olympians not only ate figs but wore them as medals for their accomplishments. Figs were introduced to the United States in 1669. Spanish missionaries were the first to bring figs to California, planting them in a mission in San Diego in the mid-1700s. They became known as "Black Mission" figs. The golden-brown Calimyrna (formally known as "smyrna") variety arrived from Turkey and was brought to California in 1882.

Where Are Figs Grown?

Turkey and Greece are the leading producers of figs in the world. The United States comes in third place with figs grown in California, Texas, Utah, Oregon, and Washington. However, one hundred percent of all harvested dried figs and ninety-eight percent of all fresh figs in the United States are grown in California's San Joaquin Valley, primarily in Fresno, Madera, and Merced counties.

Why Should I Eat Figs?

Figs are higher in fiber than any other fresh or dried fruit per serving, containing about five to six grams per ¼ cup (about three figs). They are rich in potassium, calcium, magnesium, and iron, and are also an excellent source of polyphenols, plant-based chemicals thought to play a role in fighting disease. Research reports that figs are one of the healthiest dried fruits, with "superior quality" antioxidants.

Throw Me a Lifesaver!

SKIN DISORDERS: Figs contain a substance called Psoralens that, when combined with exposure to ultraviolet light, has shown success in treating several skin diseases and certain forms of lymphoma in some studies.

DIGESTION: Figs are naturally high in fiber and contain digestive enzymes that promote regularity and can aid in digestion.

WEIGHT MANAGEMENT: Fiber may play a role in making people feel full faster and slowing absorption of calories.

HEART HEALTH: Antioxidants called phenols, found specifically in dried figs, decrease damage and mutations to individual cells in the body, possibly offering a protective effect against heart disease and cancer.

DIABETES: The type of fiber found in figs may reduce the risk of developing adult-onset diabetes (type 2) by slowing down the digestion and absorption of sugars in foods.

Tips on Using Figs

SELECTION AND STORAGE:
- Fresh figs: Choose figs that are slightly soft and bent at the neck. They can only be refrigerated for approximately 2 to 3 days after harvest.
- Dried figs: The white "frost" that occurs on figs is called "sugaring" and it is a natural occurrence when sugars from the fig rise to the surface. Keep refrigerated to reduce "frost."
- Figs also come in juice concentrate and pastes.
- Figs are one of the first recorded fruits to be dried and stored for food. Dried figs can be stored for six to eight months without loss of quality. Unopened, they will last for up to two years!

PREPARATION AND SERVING SUGGESTIONS:
- For baking and cooking, just snip off the stem and slice, chop, or puree as the recipe suggests.
- Dipping the blade of your knife in hot water helps prevent sticking when cutting.
- Fresh and dried figs can be processed and used in baked products, jams, jellies, and preserves.
- Diced figs are a great topping for salads.
- Mix in chopped figs with oatmeal or on top of any cold cereal.
- Soak figs for thirty minutes, puree, and add to tomato sauce to sweeten it.

Moroccan Chicken with Figs
by Chef Kyle Shadix

Servings: 8 • Prep and cooking time: 60 minutes

For a vegetarian version, substitute the chicken with seitan (wheat gluten—I've fooled many a nonvegetarian with it!). This recipe contains ten powerhouse foods.

INGREDIENTS FOR SAUCE:

1½ cups coarsely chopped yellow onions

2 tablespoons freshly ground ginger

2 tablespoons extra-virgin olive oil

½ teaspoon ground coriander

½ teaspoon ground cumin

1½ cups tomato sauce

2 cups peeled and cubed white potatoes

1½ cups fresh or dried figs cut into halves

INGREDIENTS TO ACCOMPANY CHICKEN/SEITAN:

2 pounds seitan or other chicken substitute, cut into 1–2" square pieces

¼ cup extra-virgin olive oil

½ cup fresh cilantro, chopped

Salt and pepper to taste

DIRECTIONS:

Heat 2 tablespoons olive oil in saucepan and sauté onions and fresh ginger until tender. Add cumin and coriander to onions and ginger mixture and stir until spices are cooked. Add all other sauce ingredients in the saucepan and set aside. Heat ¼ cup olive oil in a large pot over medium-high heat. Add the chicken, seitan, or other chicken substitute and brown, cooking for 2 to 3 minutes on each side. Pour the sauce over the seitan or other chicken substitute and simmer, covered, over medium heat until cooked through, 30 to 45 minutes. Serve over rice. Garnish with chopped cilantro.

BREAK IT DOWN . . .

Calories: 370; Total fat: 13g; Saturated fat: 2g; Cholesterol: 65mg; Sodium: 360mg; Total carbs: 37g; Fiber: 7g; Sugar: 24g; Protein: 29g.

Flax *(Linum usitatissimum)*

**Did you know . . . oil from flax is also known as "linseed" oil when it
is used to make paints, varnishes, lacquer, and ink?**

What's the Story?

Flax is a plant that is native to southwest Asia and southeastern Europe. Its
Latin name means "most useful," as all parts of the flax plant have been
used historically for a variety of purposes. The seed of flax is small and full
of oil. It has a nutty flavor and can be used in many different culinary
dishes. Flax is mostly grown for its nutritional value but it also is widely
used for various commercial nonfood products such as in paints, ink, and
linoleum.

A Serving of Food Lore . . .

Flax cultivation can be traced back to 3000 B.C. in Babylon. In fact, linen
made from flax fiber was used to wrap Egyptian mummies. About six
hundred years ago, Hildegard von Bingen used flax meal in hot com-
presses for the treatment of both external and internal ailments. In the
United States, early colonists grew small amounts of flax for home use,
but it wasn't until 1753 that commercial production began. Following the
invention of the cotton gin, forty years later, flax production declined to a
minimum.

Where Is Flax Grown?

Canada is the leading producer and exporter of flax, followed by China,
the United States, India, the European Union, and Argentina. States with
the greatest flax production in the U.S. include North Dakota, South
Dakota, Minnesota, and Wisconsin.

Why Should I Eat Flax?

Flaxseeds are a rich source of omega-3 fats. They are an excellent source of soluble and insoluble fiber, beneficial for regulating cholesterol, blood glucose, and digestion. Flax is a superb source of lignans, plant compounds that act like a weak form of estrogen. Some scientists believe that lignans may protect against certain kinds of cancer, particularly breast and colon cancer.

Home Remedies

Flax is known as a "blessed plant" that can bring good fortune, restore health, and protect against witchcraft. Historically, flax has been used to relieve abdominal pains, coughs, boils, skin abscesses, and constipation.

Throw Me a Lifesaver!

HEART DISEASE: Women who added fifty grams of ground flaxseed each day for four weeks to their daily diet lowered their total cholesterol by nine percent and LDL ("bad") cholesterol by eighteen percent. Flaxseed also reduces inflammatory markers associated with increased risk for heart disease.

PROSTATE CANCER: Lignans, a fiber compound found in flax, slowed tumor growth in prostate and breast cancer patients.

BREAST CANCER: A mouse study showed that flaxseed may enhance the effectiveness of the cancer drug tamoxifen in halting the growth of breast cancer. Women with high levels of enterolactone (a weak phyto-estrogen), linked to high lignan intake from foods like flax, have been shown to experience a fifty-eight percent reduction of breast cancer risk.

COLON CANCER: An animal study found supplementation of flaxseed oil to be effective in preventing colon tumor development whereas corn oil, mostly omega-6 fats, promoted tumor growth.

DIABETES: The addition of flax or components of flax in animal studies slowed the onset of type 2 diabetes and protected kidneys from the typical damage caused by diabetes.

ATTENTION DEFICIT HYPERACTIVITY DISORDER (ADHD): A pilot study conducted in India evaluated the effect of flax oil on behavior in children with ADHD. There was significant improvement in their symptoms, reflected by reduction in total hyperactivity scores.

Tips on Using Flax

SELECTION AND STORAGE:
- Whole flaxseed is available either in bulk or packaged and can be found at health food stores, some supermarkets, or direct from manufacturers.
- The color of flax makes little difference when it comes to taste or nutritional value.
- Flax oil is sold in liquid and gelatin capsules. Your greatest health benefit is from ground flaxseeds.
- Look for flax-enriched breads and cereals.
- Flax oil should be kept refrigerated. Milled flax may be refrigerated in an airtight container for up to 90 days, and whole flaxseed may be stored at room temperature for up to one year.

PREPARATION AND SERVING SUGGESTIONS:
- Grind flaxseeds fresh in a coffee grinder whenever possible.
- Do not cook with flax oil as it burns easily. Flaxseed oil works best in cold foods.
- You can sprinkle milled flax on cereal, salads, soups, casseroles, baked breads, and other cooked foods.
- Replace high-saturated-fat ingredients like butter with milled flax. Three tablespoons milled flax equals 1 tablespoon butter, margarine, shortening, or vegetable oil.
- Replace eggs, too! For every egg, mix 1 tablespoon milled flax with three tablespoons water in a small bowl and let sit for one or two minutes.

Cinnamon-Walnut Granola

From *The Amazing Flax Cookbook* by Jane Reinhardt-Martin

Servings: 25 (½ cup) • Prep and cooking time: 40 minutes

This recipe contains five powerhouse foods.

INGREDIENTS:

7½ cups old-fashioned oatmeal

1 cup walnuts, chopped

1 cup coconut, shredded

½ cup flaxseed, ground

½ cup brown sugar

½ cup canola oil

½ cup honey

½ tablespoon cinnamon

1 tablespoon vanilla extract

DIRECTIONS:

Preheat oven to 275 degrees. In a mixer bowl, combine oats, coconut, walnuts, and ground flaxseed. In another bowl (microwavable), combine brown sugar, oil, honey, cinnamon, and vanilla. Cook on high in microwave until mixture starts bubbling. Pour mixture over oat mixture and mix well. Spray cookie sheet with nonstick spray. Spread mixture thinly onto cookie sheet. Bake for 15 minutes. Stir and bake for an additional 15 minutes or until oats are toasted. Cool and store in an airtight container.

BREAK IT DOWN . . .

Calories: 233; Total fat: 11g; Saturated fat: 2.5g; Cholesterol: 0mg; Sodium: 14mg; Total carbs: 29g; Fiber: 4g; Sugar: 10g; Protein: 5g.

Garlic (*Allium sativum*)

YOU'RE "ODOR-ABLE"

Did you know . . . garlic is known universally as "the stinking rose"?

What's the Story?

Garlic is a member of the lily family and is closely related to the onion, shallot, and leek. There are two common classifications of garlic: hardneck and softneck. Wild garlic is of the hardneck variety; domestic garlic may be either hardneck or softneck. Popular hardneck varieties include Roja, German Red, and Valencia. Silverskin, artichoke, and Italian are the most popular "softneck" varieties.

A Serving of Food Lore . . .

Although there isn't a lot of information about garlic's history of domestication, inscriptions on the Cheops pyramid in Egypt told of the wonders of garlic. Indians referred to garlic some 5,000 years ago and Babylonians used it 4,500 years ago. Ancient writings tell of garlic's use in China as far back as 4,000 years ago. The center of origin for garlic is thought to be a region that stretches from China to India.

Where Is Garlic Grown?

China and the United States lead in domestic production. Garlic grows wild in central Asia, predominantly in Kyrgyzstan, Tajikistan, Turkmenistan, and Uzbekistan. Gilroy, California, is often referred to as the garlic capital of the world and every year it celebrates by hosting an annual garlic festival.

Why Should I Eat Garlic?

Though garlic contains many nutrients, you'd have to eat quite a bit to achieve an appreciable level of nutrition. But what garlic lacks in nutritional value, it more than makes up with phytochemicals attributed to protecting your body from harm, such as allicin, a bacteria killer; saponin, a cholesterol soaker-upper; and coumaric acid, a cancer-fighter, to name a few.

Home Remedies

Garlic is the original crime fighter! It battles villains inside and outside the body from vampires to the dreaded "evil eye" (*malocchio* in Italian) to the common cold.

Egyptian slaves were fed garlic to keep their strength up. Roman soldiers ate garlic to inspire them and give them courage.

Throw Me a Lifesaver!

ANTIMICROBIAL/ANTIFUNGAL AGENT: Louis Pasteur demonstrated how, under laboratory conditions, garlic killed bacteria and acted as an effective antibacterial. The amount of allicin produced in one clove of garlic after chopping was found to be effective against killing vancomycin-resistant *Enterococci* and methicillin-resistant *Staphylococcus aureus* in two recent studies.

HEART HEALTH: A randomized, double-blind human study found that after 12 weeks of garlic supplementation, low-density lipoprotein cholesterol (LDL-C) was reduced by eleven percent. In another study involving 261 patients, those taking garlic extract for sixteen weeks had lowered their cholesterol levels by twelve percent and their triglycerides by seventeen percent. A ten-month study evaluated the effect of aged garlic extract (AGE) on the lipid profiles of men with moderately high cholesterol. Platelet adhesion and fibrinogen (makes blood sticky, increasing risk of clotting) was reduced by approximately thirty percent in subjects taking AGE.

REDUCED RISK OF PREECLAMPSIA DURING PREGNANCY: Researchers in London found that garlic may help to boost the birth weight of babies and decrease preeclampsia complications at birth.

CANCER: Nearly thirty studies have shown that garlic has some cancer-preventive effect. The evidence is particularly strong for a link between garlic and prevention of prostate and stomach cancers.

Tips on Using Garlic

SELECTION AND STORAGE:
- A "bulb" usually contains between ten and twenty individual cloves of garlic. Fresh garlic should be plump and firm with tight skin.
- Garlic is also available in powder, flakes, and oil form, as well as chopped and pureed versions.
- Store in a cool, dark place—do not refrigerate!
- Frozen: Garlic can be peeled, pureed, and frozen for longer storage.

PREPARATION AND SERVING SUGGESTIONS:
- Peeling, crushing, and cutting garlic increases the number and variety of active compounds including an enzyme called allinase that produces diallyl disulfide (DADS). Don't cook with it right away! Scientists recommend waiting 15 minutes between peeling and cooking garlic to allow the allinase reaction to occur.
- Garlic can burn easily, so brown it carefully.
- Make peeling easy: Press a clove with the broad side of a large knife until the skin splits and then it can be pulled off.
- Roasted: Simply put unpeeled heads of garlic in a roasting pan, sprinkle with olive oil and rosemary, and roast at 350 degrees for 30 to 40 minutes. Elephant garlic is delicious prepared this way.
- Garlic and salads: Rub the salad bowl with a cut clove of garlic before putting in the salad greens.

Sicilian Spread
by Mary Corlett
Servings: 8 • Prep time: 15 minutes

This recipe contains five powerhouse foods.

INGREDIENTS:

16 ounces sun-dried tomatoes in oil, drained and rinsed, coarsely chopped

1 anchovy fillet, pureed with some of the tomato

½ cup kalamata olives, coarsely chopped

4 cloves garlic, minced

¼ cup capers, coarsely chopped

DIRECTIONS:

Blend ingredients, serve with crackers. Also makes a great sandwich spread. You won't even know the anchovy is there!

BREAK IT DOWN . . .

Calories: 80; Total fat: 5g; Saturated fat: 0.5g; Cholesterol: 0mg; Sodium: 330mg; Total carbs: 8g; Fiber: 2g; Sugar: 0g; Protein: 2g.

Ginger *(Zingiber officinale)*

WHAT'S "ALE-ING" YOU?

Did you know . . . at one time, it was popular to sprinkle fresh ginger in steins of beer at English pubs, hence the name and origin of "ginger ale"?

What's the Story?

Though often referred to as a root, ginger is actually a reedlike herb that has rough, knotty rhizomes (underground stems). There are several different varieties to choose from, including the most popular kind, called Jamaican, African/Indian that features a darker skin, and Kenyan varieties that come in white, red, and yellow.

A Serving of Food Lore . . .

The origins of ginger can be traced back to southeastern Asia, China, and India, where its use as a culinary spice dates back at least 4,400 years. Romans brought ginger from China nearly 2,000 years ago and its popularity spread throughout Europe. In the 1850s, many English and Irish pubs and restaurants featured fresh ginger on every table, much like salt and pepper today. Spaniards brought ginger to the Western Hemisphere, introducing it throughout South America and Mexico.

Where Is Ginger Grown?

India, China, Indonesia, Nigeria, the Philippines, and Thailand currently are the main ginger producers. In the United States, ginger is grown mostly in California, Hawaii, and Florida.

Why Should I Eat Ginger?

Ginger is a rich source of powerful antioxidants such as gingerols, shogaols, and zingerones.

Home Remedies

Ginger has been used as a home remedy through many generations for treating a variety of conditions. It has been taken internally for loss of appetite, stomach upset, diarrhea, stomachache, colic, dyspepsia, flatulence, post-surgical pain, motion and morning sickness, general and chemotherapy-induced nausea, rheumatoid arthritis, osteoarthritis, migraine headache, upper respiratory tract infections, cough, and bronchitis. Topically, it has been used for treating thermal burns and as an analgesic.

Throw Me a Lifesaver!

MORNING SICKNESS: A double-blind, randomized, placebo-controlled trial found that 125mg of ginger extract consumed four times per day for four days significantly reduced morning sickness in women less than 20 weeks pregnant. A trial investigated the effect of 1.05 grams of ginger on nausea and vomiting among women less than 16 weeks pregnant. Fifty-three percent of women consuming the ginger capsule reported a reduction in both nausea and vomiting associated with pregnancy.

MOTION SICKNESS: Two double-blind studies showed that ginger had a significant effect on preventing and treating motion sickness.

OSTEOARTHRITIS: In a randomized, double-blind study, researchers found that those participants with osteoarthritis who had consumed ginger extract experienced much greater reduction in knee pain than those in the control group.

CANCER: A mouse study found that the antioxidant 6-gingerol, which gives ginger its flavor, resulted in fewer tumors and their size was considerably smaller than those of mice who did not receive gingerol.

OVARIAN CANCER: Ginger induced apoptosis (programmed cell death) and autophagy (cells digesting themselves) in ovarian cancer cells. Ginger was also effective at controlling inflammation, thus stopping the cancer cells from growing.

COLON CANCER: Ginger was found to protect against the formation of colon cancer in mice injected with cancer cells.

Don't Throw Me an Anvil!

Ginger has blood-thinning qualities and may be contraindicated if you are on blood thinners. Check with your doctor or a registered dietitian for advice on the inclusion of ginger.

Tips on Using Ginger

SELECTION AND STORAGE:
- Ginger can be found fresh, pickled, dried, or in powdered form.
- Choose fresh ginger that is free from bruises, and light brown to cream in color.
- Fresh ginger should be stored at room temperature.

PREPARATION AND SERVING SUGGESTIONS:
- Fresh ginger provides the freshest taste and can be shredded, finely minced, sliced, or grated, and does not have to be peeled.
- Fresh ginger can be successfully substituted for ground ginger and should be done at a six-to-one ratio, fresh to ground ginger respectively.
- The center of the root is more fibrous and contains the most powerful flavors.
- When shredding, be sure to shred in the direction of the fibers.
- Slice fresh ginger and enjoy on top of a bed of lettuce or boil to make a soothing tea.
- Use dried or powdered ginger to spice up any main dish or to make a delicious marinade.
- Use pickled ginger as an accompaniment to main Asian dishes or to beautifully garnish a meal.

Strawberry Ginger Sauce (or Dressing)
by Cynthia Sass

Servings: 6 · Prep time: 10 minutes

Every ingredient in this recipe is a powerhouse food.

INGREDIENTS:

1½ cups strawberries (stems removed)

1½ tablespoons honey

2 tablespoons fresh lime juice

2 teaspoons fresh grated ginger

DIRECTIONS:

In a blender or food processor, combine all ingredients and blend until smooth. Refrigerate and use as a dressing (great on spinach salad), dip, or topping.

BREAK IT DOWN . . .

Calories: 20; Total fat: 0g; Saturated fat: 0g; Cholesterol: 0mg; Sodium: 0mg; Total carbs: 6g; Fiber: 1g; Sugar: 5g; Protein: 0g.

Goji Berries (*Lycium, Wolfberries*)

WILL THE REAL GOJI PLEASE STAND UP!

Did you know . . . the term "goji" refers only to the Tibetan variety of Lycium berry that is indigenous to the Tibetan and Mongolian regions?

What's the Story?

There are more than forty species of the goji berry, also known as "wolf-berry." The more commonly consumed variety of goji berry is *Lycium barbarum*. The berries, small and orange to light red in color, are filled with seeds. The taste is somewhat like a cross between a cranberry and a cherry. They are shade-dried before packaging. Goji can be eaten raw, cooked, consumed as juice or wine, brewed into a tea, or prepared as a tincture.

A Serving of Food Lore . . .

The goji plant hails from Tibet and Inner Mongolia and has a 3,000-year history in Chinese and Eastern medical traditions. The use of goji was first described in the Chinese *Materia Medica,* published nearly 2,000 years ago.

Where Is Goji Grown?

The Chinese have been growing goji for thousands of years and the plant continues to be cultivated throughout China and Tibet. Ningxia, located in northwest China along the Yellow River, is often referred to as the goji capital of the world. There is even an annual two-week festival to honor the goji berry. It is also grown as a cultivated plant throughout Asia, the Middle East, Great Britain, and North America.

Why Should I Eat Goji Berries?

Although goji contains a wide variety of nutrients and trace minerals, this berry is not especially rich in any one vitamin or mineral. However, its concentration of the plant chemicals beta-carotene and zeaxanthin more than makes up for any shortfall in nutrient density.

Home Remedies

Whatever ails you! Goji has been used to treat inflammations, skin irritations, nosebleeds, and aches and pains. In Chinese medicine, goji is recommended for long life, sharp eyesight, and healthy liver function, to boost sperm production, and to improve circulation, among other benefits.

Throw Me a Lifesaver!

HEART HEALTH: Goji fruit extracts significantly reduced blood glucose, total cholesterol, and triglycerides, and at same time markedly increased high-density lipoprotein ("good") cholesterol levels after rabbits consumed them for ten days.

INSULIN RESISTANCE: Diabetic rats who were treated with goji for three weeks had significant decreases in triglycerides, weight, and cholesterol, and had improved insulin sensitivity.

CANCER: An extract of goji stopped the spread and encouraged death of liver cancer cells in a cell study. Another cell study showed that goji inhibited leukemia cancer cells, and a mouse study showed that goji enhanced the killing effect of radiation therapy.

Tips on Using Goji Berries

SELECTION AND STORAGE:
- Goji can be purchased at Chinese supermarkets and herb shops and health food stores.
- Goji berries are processed into a variety of other forms including juice, powdered, and dried.
- Store in a cool, dry place.

PREPARATION AND SERVING SUGGESTIONS:
- Goji berries can be eaten right off of the vine!
- Wash and then soak dried goji berries for fifteen minutes before eating.
- Dried goji berries can be eaten alone as a snack food or as a great addition to a trail mix.
- Throw a handful of berries into a smoothie.
- Top off hot or cold cereals, stews, or baked goods and cereal bars with some berries.

Goji Berry Rice Pudding
by Chef J. Hugh McEvoy

Servings: 6 • Prep and cooking time: 90 minutes (but chill at least two hours)

This recipe contains seven powerhouse foods.

INGREDIENTS:

3 ounces dried goji berries

3 ounces seedless golden raisins

½ cup quick-cooking long-grain brown rice

1 cup water

3 cups 2% milk or soy milk

¾ cup agave syrup or honey

3 omega-3 eggs

1 teaspoon vanilla extract

1 teaspoon sea salt

⅛ teaspoon ground cinnamon

DIRECTIONS:

Using a large, heavy sauce pot bring water to a rolling boil. Add salt and rice. Cover, reduce heat, and cook rice until done, approximately 15 to 20 minutes. Stir in milk and sugar. Cover and cook over very low heat for approximately 1 hour. The mixture should look like thin oatmeal. Whip eggs to a froth. Add vanilla and cinnamon. Slowly add about 6 ounces of hot mixture to beaten egg mixture to temper the egg. Blend until smooth. Then add egg mixture to hot rice, stirring constantly. Blend until smooth. At very low heat, cook until mixture thickens, about 2 minutes. Add goji berries and raisins. Mix until even. Remove from heat immediately. Portion into six Pyrex or ceramic dessert dishes. Chill in refrigerator at least two hours or overnight. Serve garnished with fresh mint leaves and powdered cinnamon.

BREAK IT DOWN . . .
Calories: 217; Total fat: 4g; Saturated fat: 2g; Cholesterol: 77mg; Sodium: 174mg; Total carbs: 39g; Fiber: 1g; Sugar: 28g; Protein: 6g.

Grapefruit *(Citrus paradisi)*

YOU SMELL BEAUTIFUL

Did you know . . . if men want women to look younger, they should smell some grapefruit? While wearing masks that were infused with various aromas, men and women were asked to estimate the age of models who appeared in photos. When women wore the mask infused with grapefruit, their guesstimate was closer to the real age. But when men smelled the grapefruit, they guessed the models were six years younger than they actually were!

What's the Story?

Grapefruit is thought to be a cross between an orange and a pummelo that was brought to Barbados from Indonesia in the seventeenth century. Some of the most popular grapefruit varieties include Duncan, Foster, Marsh,

Oroblanco, Paradise Navel, Redblush, Star Ruby, Sweetie, Thompson, and Triumph. The two most common Western varieties include the Marsh and Ruby Red.

A Serving of Food Lore . . .

The grapefruit was first discovered in Barbados in 1750 and was later found in Jamaica in 1789. When introduced to Florida in the nineteenth century, the grapefruit tree was grown only for novelty, as the actual fruit was rarely consumed. In 1874, New York imported 78,000 grapefruits from the West Indies to meet a growing popularity and demand. In 1962, an American horticulturist proposed to change the name of grapefruit to "pomelo" in an attempt to increase sales; however, this was unsuccessful.

Where Is Grapefruit Grown?

The United States is one of the largest growers of grapefruits. Florida is the country's main grower, with help from California, Arizona, and Texas. Other countries with commercial production include Israel, South Africa, Brazil, Mexico, and Cuba.

Why Should I Eat Grapefruit?

Grapefruit is an excellent source of vitamin C. The pink and red varieties are fifty times higher than white grapefruit in carotenoids that act as powerful antioxidants. It is also a good source of potassium, calcium, and, in the case of red grapefruit, vitamin A. One half of a grapefruit contains more than 150 phytonutrients, mostly flavonoids, believed to help the body fight against aging, allergies, infection, cancer, ulcers, and heart disease.

Home Remedies

Most of the home remedies utilize the grapefruit seed versus the fruit. Grapefruit seed extract is thought to be useful in treating external skin conditions, especially fungal-related conditions such as athlete's foot, jock itch, and dandruff.

Throw Me a Lifesaver!

PERIODONTAL DISEASE: A study found that bleeding associated with periodontitis was significantly reduced after drinking grapefruit juice. The researchers attribute the amazing results to the vitamin C content of grapefruit juice, known to help wound and tissue repair.

HEART HEALTH: Researchers studied the effect of eating one grapefruit a day on fifty-seven patients who had bypass surgery. Those who consumed one red grapefruit a day for thirty days showed decreases in total cholesterol, LDL ("bad") cholesterol, and triglycerides.

WEIGHT LOSS: One study found that obese individuals who consumed one half of a fresh grapefruit before meals for twelve weeks lost a significant amount of weight and had improvements in insulin resistance associated with metabolic syndrome. A fad diet based on eating grapefruits was developed in Hollywood, California, and first became popular in the 1930s, making a later resurgence in the 1970s. Medical and nutritional experts found it to be nutritionally incomplete and unsound. But be assured—adding grapefruit to a healthy diet is sound advice and may be a valuable tool in achieving an optimal weight!

CANCER: A study found that a particular flavonoid found specifically in grapefruit helps to repair damaged DNA in human prostate cancer cells. A diet including grapefruit reduced inflammatory markers and increased apoptosis (programmed cell death) associated with colon cancer in a rat study.

Don't Throw Me an Anvil!

Grapefruit juice may interfere with the rate of absorption of many prescription medications. Check with your doctor, a pharmacist, or a registered dietitian to see if grapefruit juice is right for you.

Tips on Using Grapefruit

SELECTION AND STORAGE:
- There are two main varieties of grapefruit, white and pink/red, that can be found year-round.

- Choose firm and heavy grapefruits for their size. Avoid those that appear to have water-soaked areas or have an overly soft spot at the stem. Watch for signs of dehydration and skin collapse at the stem.
- Store grapefruits in the refrigerator crisper for up to two to three weeks, but keep in mind that they are juicier when served warm rather than cool.

PREPARATION AND SERVING SUGGESTIONS:
- Slice the fruit in half, separating the flesh from the membrane and scooping out each section with a spoon. A grapefruit spoon simplifies this process.
- If seeds are present, remove the seed before eating. A less labor-intensive way to consume a grapefruit is to peel and eat it like an orange.
- Serve chilled, cut in half and flesh precut from the membranes. Sweeten with honey, agave syrup, or sugar.
- Add grapefruit sections to green salads for added tang.

Roasted Grapefruit Salad
by Cynthia Sass
Servings: 1 • Prep and cooking time: 20 minutes

Make sure you use a ripe, sweet grapefruit for this recipe. Try brushing a little agave syrup on the surface if the grapefruit isn't as sweet as you would like. This recipe contains six powerhouse foods.

INGREDIENTS:

1 medium grapefruit, sectioned	1/4 cup red onion, sliced
1 cup baby spinach leaves	2 tablespoons fresh avocado, diced
1/4 cup yellow grape tomatoes, sliced in half	1 tablespoon walnuts, chopped
	2 tablespoons balsamic vinegar

DIRECTIONS:
Gently remove seeds from grapefruit sections. Lay on cookie sheet. Broil until bubbly; remove and set aside. Toss spinach with balsamic vinegar and place in salad bowl. Top with grapefruit, tomatoes, nuts, onion, and avocado, and serve.

BREAK IT DOWN . . .

Calories: 110; Total fat: 4.5g; Saturated fat: .5g; Cholesterol: 0mg; Sodium: 25mg; Total carbs: 17g; Fiber: 4g; Sugar: 11g; Protein: 2g.

Grapes *(Vitis)*

HEARD IT THROUGH THE GRAPEVINE

Did you know . . . more grapes are grown throughout the world than any other fruit?

What's the Story?

Grapes range in shape from oval to round, and from seeded to seedless. They may be green, red, amber, purple, or blue-black. The skin and seeds of grapes are edible too, although many people believe that chewing the seeds may be harmful—not so! But you should avoid chewing the seeds if you have a medical condition called diverticulitis (pouches in the intestine). Out of literally thousands of different kinds to choose from, only about twenty varieties make up the vast majority of what we consume today. European grapes, North American grapes, and French hybrid grapes dominate the market for everything from ready-to-eat table grapes to raisin grapes to wine grapes.

A Serving of Food Lore . . .

In 6000 B.C., grapes were first cultivated in Caucasia, in the region between the Black and Caspian Seas near northern Iran. Cultivation spread to Asia around 5000 B.C. and from there to Egypt and Phoenicia around two thousand years later. Grapes were used for winemaking during the Greek and Roman times and the fruit's many uses spread throughout Europe. In the seventeenth century, grapes were planted in the United States at a Spanish mission in New Mexico, and from there they spread to the central valley of California.

Where Are Grapes Grown?

The major producers of grapes today are Italy, Spain, France, Mexico, the United States, and Chile. Over ninety-nine percent of commercially available table grapes produced in the United States come from California.

Why Should I Eat Grapes?

Grapes contain vitamin C and potassium, and a small amount of fiber. Grape seeds contain an abundance of powerful antioxidants. Studies show that the predominant antioxidant, proanthocyanidin, has twenty times greater antioxidant power than vitamin E and fifty times greater than vitamin C. Resveratrol, a key phytonutrient found mainly in the skins of grapes, has anti-inflammatory and anticarcinogenic properties. Grapes are also high in flavonoids. Red grapes contain the carotenoid lycopene, which may help in fighting breast and prostate cancer.

Home Remedies

The juice of green grapes that is combined with water, alum, and salt has been reported to lessen the scars of acne when applied to the face. To overcome constipation, consume about a cup and a half of grapes daily.

Throw Me a Lifesaver!

HEART HEALTH: A study using mice fed freeze-dried grape powder found that LDL cholesterol was protected from being converted into the more dangerous type that can lead to heart disease. Researchers found that the flesh extract of grapes was just as protective for the heart as skin extract. Beyond the heart-health importance of resveratrol, found abundantly in grapes, significant concentrations of other antioxidants such as caffeic, caftaric, coumaric, and coutaric acids have been found in the skin and flesh of both red and white grape varieties. Drinking Concord grape juice significantly increased good cholesterol (HDL) and significantly lowered two markers of inflammation in people with stable coronary artery disease.

CANCER: A number of studies have shown a link between grapes and cancer prevention, including the ability to inhibit growth of cancer cells.

Specific cancer types that have been tested include breast, colon, stomach, and leukemia. A rat study found that consumption of Concord grape juice significantly inhibited breast cancer tumor growth.

A cell study using advanced human prostate cancer cells found that treatment with grape seed extract inhibited cell growth and caused them to die. Another study showed that drinking four or more glasses of red wine per week cut the risk of prostate cancer in half.

COGNITIVE FUNCTION: Concord grape juice significantly improved laboratory animals' short-term memory in a water maze test, as well as co-ordination, balance, and strength.

WEIGHT CONTROL: A study found that grape seed extract may be helpful in limiting absorption and accumulation of dietary fat in cells observed under a microscope.

Tips on Using Grapes

SELECTION AND STORAGE:
- Look for grapes that are intact, plump, and free of wrinkles.
- Red grapes should be mostly red, green grapes should have a slight yellowish hue, and blue-black and purple grapes should be deep in color.
- Wrap unwashed grapes in a paper towel, place in a plastic bag, and put in the refrigerator for longer storage.
- Grapes will keep fresh for several days at room temperature.

PREPARATION AND SUGGESTED USES:
- Wash with cold water right before use and pat dry.
- Use scissors to cut small clusters from the stem, which prevents the stem from drying out and keeps remaining grapes fresher.
- Add grapes to your fruit or mixed green, chicken, or tuna salad.
- Freeze grapes for a refreshing snack.

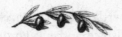

Grapes of Wrap
by Sharon Grotto
Servings: 6 • Prep Time: 10 minutes

This recipe contains eight powerhouse foods.

INGREDIENTS:

¾ cup red grapes, quartered
2 cans tuna or chicken, drained
½ cup celery, chopped coarse
⅓ cup red onion, chopped coarse
1 teaspoon dill, chopped fine
¼ cup canola oil mayonnaise
½ teaspoon black pepper

2 teaspoons honey
1 teaspoon fresh lemon juice
¼ teaspoon toasted sesame oil
   (optional)
½ teaspoon dry mustard powder
6 whole wheat tortillas

DIRECTIONS:

Combine all ingredients and mix well. Spread some of the salad in a whole wheat tortilla. Garnish with lettuce and tomato, hold together with a toothpick, and serve.

BREAK IT DOWN . . .
Calories: 190; Total fat: 4.5g; Saturated fat: 0g; Cholesterol: 20mg; Sodium: 460mg; Total carbs: 26g; Fiber: 2g; Sugar: 4g; Protein: 18g.

Guava *(Psidium guajava L.)*

TAKE ONE GUAVA AND CALL ME IN THE MORNING

Did you know . . . Amazon Indians used guava fruit to remedy sore throats, digestive challenges, and vertigo, and to regulate menstrual periods?

What's the Story?

The guava belongs to the myrtle family (*Myrtaceae*), which includes spices such as clove, cinnamon, allspice, and eucalyptus. Guava comes in a range of shape and sizes and, for the most part, is sweet and fragrant. The inside flesh is juicy and ranges in color from white to yellow to pink to red. Depending on the variety, the center may be filled with hard yellow seeds or no seeds at all. Tree-ripened fruit is optimal but guava usually falls prey to birds before it can make it to market. Therefore, the vast majority are picked early and artificially ripened for six days in straw at room temperature.

A Serving of Food Lore . . .

Guava's place of origin is most likely in southern Mexico down to Central America. Spanish and Portuguese explorers brought it from the Americas to the East Indies and Guam. From there, guava traveled throughout Asia, Africa, and the Middle East. Guava was first introduced to Hawaii during the reign of King Kamehameha I. By 1847, guava was commonly found in the Bahamas, Bermuda, and southern Florida. The first commercial guava-processing plant was established in Palm Sola, Florida, in 1912.

Where Is Guava Grown?

Guava grows in abundance in India, China, Mexico, and South America. In the United States, Hawaii, Florida, and California are the leading producers of guava.

Why Should I Eat Guava?

Pound for pound, guava is higher in vitamin C than citrus and contains appreciable amounts of vitamin A as well. Guava fruits are also a good source of pectin, a dietary fiber, and rich in potassium and phosphorus. Guava contains an amazing amount of phytochemicals including tannins, phenols, triterpenes, flavonoids, essential oils, saponins, carotenoids, and lectins. The leaves of guava are also rich in flavonoids, in particular quercetin, which has demonstrated antibacterial activity and is thought to contribute to the antidiarrheal effect of guava.

Home Remedies

Guava leaves have been used as a remedy for diarrhea for their supposed antimicrobial properties. Leaves were chewed to cure bleeding gums and bad breath too. Guava has been used as an antibacterial, antifungal, pain reliever, and antihypertensive, for controlling blood glucose, and for promoting menstruation.

Throw Me a Lifesaver!

DIABETES: Diabetic mice who received guava juice for four weeks experienced a reduction in glucose of nearly twenty-five percent as compared with the diabetic control group. Guava leaf has also been used successfully in experiments for controlling blood glucose.

HEART HEALTH: Participants who consumed guava experienced a marked reduction of total cholesterol, triglycerides, and LDL ("bad") cholesterol, along with improved HDL cholesterol. Their blood pressure improved as well.

ANTIBACTERIAL: Guava leaves have antibacterial properties and have been shown to have a highly lethal effect on salmonella and other harmful bacteria.

Tips on Using Guava

SELECTION AND STORAGE:
- Guavas come fresh, canned, in a paste, jelly, juice, and nectar. These are readily available in Latin supermarkets.
- Ripe guavas bruise easily, are highly perishable, and must be eaten within a few days.

PREPARATION AND SERVING SUGGESTIONS:
- Guavas need to be quite ripe before they are eaten.
- Cut it into quarters, remove the seeds, and peel away the skin.
- Raw guavas can be eaten out of one's hand or served sliced as dessert or in salads.
- A traditional dessert that is popular throughout Latin America is stewed guava shells (*cascos de guayaba*).
- Guava syrup is great over waffles, ice cream, and puddings, and in milkshakes.

Guava and Cheese Empanadas
Adapted from *Steven Raichlen's Healthy Latin Cooking*
Servings: 12 (1 serving = 3 empanadas) • *Prep and cooking time: 15 minutes*

Oprah called Steven Raichlen the "Gladiator of Grilling" and Howard Stern hailed him as the "Michael Jordan of Barbecue." For this recipe, I consider him the "Emperor of Empanadas"! This recipe contains two powerhouse foods.

INGREDIENTS:

36 (3-inch) wonton wrappers
    or round Chinese
    ravioli wrappers
1 egg white, lightly beaten

4 ounces guava paste, cut into
    36 small pieces
4 ounces low-fat cream cheese, cut
    into 36 small pieces

DIRECTIONS:

Preheat the oven to 400 degrees. Coat a nonstick baking sheet with nonstick spray. Arrange a few wonton wrappers on a work surface. Lightly brush the edge of each wrapper with egg white. (The egg white helps make a tight seal.) Place 1 piece of guava paste and 1 piece of cream cheese in the center and fold the wrapper in half to make a triangular pastry, or a half moon–shaped pastry if using round wrappers. Crimp the edges with a fork. Place the finished empanadas on the prepared baking sheet while you make the rest. Coat the tops of the empanadas with nonstick spray. Bake, turning occasionally, for 6 to 8 minutes, or until crisp and golden brown.

BREAK IT DOWN . . .

Calories: 110; Total fat: 0g; Saturated fat: 0g; Cholesterol: 5mg; Sodium: 21mg; Total carbs: 21g; Fiber: less than 1g; Sugar: 0g; Protein: 4g.

Hazelnuts *(Corylus avellana L.)*

GO NUTS!
Did you know . . . hazelnuts are one of the main ingredients in the famous Italian Nutella spread?

What's the Story?

Hazelnuts, also known as filberts, are a nut that grows on a bushy tree. A hazelnut is shaped like an acorn and has a fuzzy outer husk that will open as the nut matures, exposing a smooth, hard shell. Hazelnuts have a rich flavor and are often used in baking products and also used to make hazelnut butter, meal and flour, paste, and oil. They can also be purchased in their shell, chopped, ground, or roasted.

A Serving of Food Lore . . .

Hazelnut is one of the oldest agricultural food crops and is thought to have originated in Asia. Chinese manuscripts from 5,000 years ago refer to the hazelnut as a sacred food from heaven. The Romans and Greeks used hazelnuts for medicinal purposes.

Where Are Hazelnuts Grown?

The main producers of hazelnuts are Turkey, Italy, Spain, and France. In the United States they are mainly grown in Oregon and Washington.

Why Should I Eat Hazelnuts?

Not only are hazelnuts a high-quality source of protein and fiber, they also contain a variety of antioxidants such as vitamin E and a host of phytonutrients that benefit the immune system. Hazelnuts are a rich source of the amino acid arginine that relaxes blood vessels. Hazelnuts have the highest concentration of folate among all of the tree nuts. Folate reduces the risk of neural tube birth defects, and may help to reduce the risk of cardiovascular disease, certain cancers, Alzheimer's disease, and depression. Hazelnuts also contain the blood pressure–lowering minerals calcium, magnesium, and potassium. Hazelnuts are also a rich source of squalene, a plant chemical—also found in olive oil, wheat germ oil, rice bran oil, shark oil, and yeast—that has anticancer and cholesterol-lowering properties.

Home Remedies

Hazelnut oil has been used externally as a way to rid the skin of cellulite. The ancient Greek physician Dioscorides boasted of hazelnut's ability to quiet chronic coughs, fight the common cold, and even grow hair in bald areas of the head.

Throw Me a Lifesaver!

HEART HEALTH: A small human study showed that men with elevated cholesterol who were fed a diet containing hazelnuts for eight weeks had decreased plaque-promoting lipids and increased HDL ("good") cholesterol compared to the control group.

Tips on Using Hazelnuts

SELECTION AND STORAGE:
- If they're in the shell, choose nuts that are heavy and full. Unshelled nuts can be stored in a cool, dry place for about a month.
- Shelled nuts should have tight skins and nuts that are plump. They can be stored in the refrigerator or freezer, where they will keep fresh for about four months.

PREPARATION AND SERVING SUGGESTIONS:
- The skin can be removed by toasting the nuts and then rubbing them. Hazelnuts can be roasted using a conventional oven and a cookie sheet.
- You can grind them by placing them in a food processor.
- Try hazelnut butter as an alternative to peanut butter.
- Add hazelnuts to your favorite salad, cookies, stir-fry, or breakfast cereal.
- Add an exciting texture to your yogurt with diced hazelnuts.

Cranberry Pear Salad with Curried Hazelnuts
Courtesy of the Hazelnut Council
Servings: 8 • Prep and cooking time: 45 to 60 minutes

This recipe contains an amazing thirteen powerhouse foods!

INGREDIENTS:
DRESSING:

8 ounces yogurt, plain, fat-free

1 cup cucumber, peeled, seeded,
   and chopped

1 tablespoon honey

1 teaspoon lemon juice

1 teaspoon tarragon, dried

1 teaspoon chives, chopped

1/4 teaspoon garlic, minced

1/4 teaspoon salt

1/8 teaspoon white pepper, ground

HAZELNUTS:

1 3/4 cups (8 ounces) hazelnuts,
   toasted and coarsely chopped

1 tablespoon butter, melted

1/4 cup light corn syrup

3 tablespoons honey

3/4 teaspoon curry powder

1/4 teaspoon salt

1/8 teaspoon cayenne pepper,
   ground

1 1/2 teaspoons butter

SALAD:

2 cups (4 ounces) spinach leaves,
   washed

1 1/2 cups (4 ounces) spring greens,
   washed and torn

1 1/3 cups (6 ounces) cranberries,
   sweetened and dried

1 Anjou pear, cored and cubed

1 yellow bell pepper, seeded and
   cut into thin strips

1/4 cup green onions,
   thinly sliced

DRESSING DIRECTIONS:
Process dressing ingredients in food processor or blender until smooth. Set aside.

HAZELNUT DIRECTIONS:
Preheat oven to 300 degrees. Place hazelnuts in large bowl. Pour melted butter in 9 × 9 × 2-inch pan; set aside. Stir corn syrup, honey, curry powder, salt, and cayenne pepper in small saucepan until boiling. Boil 2 minutes; do not stir. Stir in 1 1/2 teaspoons butter

Receipt - 6/22/2014

Three Rivers Public Library

Items Checked Out Today
Barcode: 292125
Title: 101 foods that could save your life!
Author: Grotto, David W
Due:7/13/2014

Barcode: 99995009
Title: Charlie [videorecording] : a toy story
Author: Waters, Drew
Due:6/29/2014

Barcode: 319289
Title: Ice age: Continental drift
[videorecording]
Author: Martino, Steve
Due:6/29/2014

Barcode: 310127
Title: The people's pharmacy quick & handy
home remedies : Q&As for your common
ailments
Author: Graedon, Joe.
Due:7/13/2014

until melted. Immediately pour over nuts. Stir until coated. Spread into prepared pan. Bake at 300 degrees for 15 to 20 minutes, stirring occasionally, until golden brown. Pour onto buttered baking sheet; cool. Break into small pieces. Makes 2½ cups.

SALAD DIRECTIONS:
Place salad ingredients in large bowl. Toss with dressing. Sprinkle on 1 cup curried hazelnuts.

BREAK IT DOWN . . .
Calories: 210; Total fat: 8.5g; Saturated fat: 1g; Cholesterol: 5mg; Sodium: 155mg; Total carbs: 34g; Fiber: 4g; Sugar: 26g; Protein: 4g.

Honey (Mellis)

BUSY AS A BEE
Did you know . . . that bees travel an average of 55,000 miles and need to tap over two million flowers just to bring you one pound of honey?

What's the Story?

Bees have been producing honey for at least 100 million years. Honey is produced as food stores for the long winter months ahead. European honey bees, genus *Apis Mellifera,* produce more than enough honey for their hive so that humans can harvest the excess. The color and flavor of honey differ depending on the bees' nectar source (the blossoms). In fact, there are more than three hundred unique kinds of honey in the United States alone, originating from clover, eucalyptus, orange blossom, and buckwheat. Lighter-colored honeys are milder in flavor, while darker honeys are usually stronger in flavor.

A Serving of Food Lore . . .

The benefits of honey can be traced as far back as the ancient writings of Sumerians, Babylonians, and the sacred Indian Vedas writings. Honey was used to bless buildings and homes—it was poured over thresholds and over bolts that were to be used in sacred buildings. Cleopatra of Egypt regularly took honey-and-milk baths to maintain her youthful appearance. Honey was so highly valued in ancient times that it was common to use it as a form of tribute or payment. In ancient Greece, honey was offered to the gods and to spirits of the dead. One of the first alcoholic beverages known was made with honey and was called mead, considered the "drink of the gods." European settlers introduced European honey bees to the United States around 1638.

Where Is Honey Produced?

The main producers of honey are Australia, Canada, Argentina, and the United States.

Why Should I Include Honey?

Honey is primarily composed of fructose, glucose, and water. It also contains trace enzymes, minerals, vitamins, and amino acids including niacin, riboflavin, pantothenic acid, calcium, copper, iron, magnesium, manganese, phosphorus, potassium, and zinc. Honey contains flavonoids and phenolic acids, and the darker the honey, the higher the level of antioxidants. Honey acts as a prebiotic and aids in the growth of friendly bifidobacteria, thus improving gut health.

Home Remedies

Greek and Roman athletes used honey to increase strength and stamina. Honey has been used as an effective antimicrobial agent, for treating minor burns and scrapes, and for aiding the treatment of sore throats and other bacterial infections.

Throw Me a Lifesaver!

CHOLESTEROL: A human study found that people with hyperlipidemia (elevated fats in the blood) who ate honey had a decrease in their triglycerides as opposed to those fed a sugar solution, which increased triglycerides.

COLITIS: A rat study found that honey conferred the greatest protection against colitis compared with other sugars. It was noted that enzymes that protect cells from being damaged were at their highest level in the honey-fed group.

CANCER: An article in the *Journal of the Science of Food and Agriculture* reported on a group of Croatian researchers who found significantly decreased tumor growth and spreading of cancer (metastasis) in mice when honey was ingested orally or given by injection. Honey was found to be an effective agent for inhibiting the growth of bladder cancer cell lines.

WOUND-HEALING: Honey has long been revered for its antibacterial and wound-healing properties. A special preparation of honey called Medihoney, known for its high antibacterial properties, was used in treating wound care in Children's Hospital in Bonn, Germany, for three years. Researchers observed significant reductions in even the most resistant wound infections as a result of using the honey preparation. Cancer treatment can often lead to side effects such as sores in the inside of the mouth; one study found that honey applied to the sores reduced discomfort.

Don't Throw Baby an Anvil!

Honey should not be fed to infants less than one year of age because they lack the ability to kill botulism spores that lie within.

Tips on Using Honey

SELECTION AND STORAGE:
- Honey comes in basically five different forms: comb honey, cut comb (liquid honey that has chunks of comb in it), liquid honey, crystallized honey, and whipped or "creamed" honey (the honey is the consistency of butter).
- To keep antioxidant content high, don't keep honey any longer than six months.
- Honey is best stored at room temperature. Do not refrigerate.
- If your honey crystallizes, simply place the honey jar in warm water and stir until the crystals dissolve.

PREPARATION AND SERVING SUGGESTIONS:

- When substituting honey for granulated sugar, replace sugar with half the amount of honey. If the recipe calls for one tablespoon of sugar, use just one half tablespoon of liquid honey.
- When baking with honey, remember to:
  - Reduce liquids by ¼ cup for each cup of honey used.
  - Add ½ teaspoon baking soda for every cup of honey.
  - Reduce oven temperature by 25 degrees to prevent over-browning.
- Coat the measuring cup with nonstick cooking spray or vegetable oil before adding the honey. The honey will slide right out.
- Tired of peanut butter and grape jelly? Have a peanut butter and honey sandwich. Or substitute another nut butter, like almond or cashew.
- Replace sugar in tea and coffee with clover honey. Or better yet, use orange blossom or buckwheat for a real taste treat.
- Use honey, soy sauce, pressed garlic, and olive oil as a glaze for barbecued anything!

Firefighter's Honey Muesli
by Dave Grotto
Servings: 1 • Prep time: 5 minutes

This recipe was created as part of a cholesterol-lowering program for Chicago firefighters. It's quick, simple, and tasty—perfect fuel for putting out whatever kind of "fire" you're fighting! This recipe contains four powerhouse foods.

INGREDIENTS:

1 teaspoon honey
½ cup rolled oats
½ cup skim milk or low-fat vanilla soy milk

1 ounce mixture of almonds, walnuts, and pistachios
⅛ cup dried cherries and cranberries

DIRECTIONS:

Mix all ingredients and eat immediately, or cover, refrigerate overnight, and eat the next day.

BREAK IT DOWN . . .

Calories: 330; Total fat: 8g; Saturated fat: 1g; Cholesterol: 0mg; Sodium: 90mg; Total carbs: 56g; Fiber: 6g; Sugar: 10g; Protein: 11g.

Horseradish (*Armoracia rusticana*) or Wasabi (*Wasabia japonica*)

THE OL' SWITCHEROO

Did you know . . . that most "wasabi" outside of Japan is really horseradish with green food coloring added to it? Real wasabi is one of the rarest, most difficult and expensive vegetables to grow in the world and is in limited supply. But the good news is, though entirely different plants, horseradish is much easier to find and shares many of wasabi's healthy characteristics.

What's the Story?

HORSERADISH: The English name "horseradish" was first thought to be a bungled twist on the German word *meerrettich,* interpreted as *mare* (female horse) *radish* (meaning root). However, several English plant names use the word "horse" to indicate that it is big or strong. Horseradish is a member of the cabbage family.

WASABI: There are several species of wasabi but the most commonly found is *Wasabia japonica.* Like horseradish, all are members of the cabbage family. Wasabi, also known as "Japanese horseradish," is not a root but rather a knotty stem or "rhizome." It is used predominantly as a spice and has a strong flavor, so much so that it is nicknamed "namida," which means "tears" in Japanese. Though it has "heat," it's more akin to a hot mustard than a chili pepper, irritating the sinus cavity rather than the tongue. Wasabi is a condiment traditionally served with raw fish (sushi and sashimi) and noodle (soba) dishes in Japan.

A Serving of Food Lore . . .

Horseradish was thought to have originated in the Mediterranian in 1500 B.C. and was one of the "five bitter herbs" Jews were told to eat at Passover. Popularity spread throughout Europe from 1300 to 1600 A.D. "Horseradish ale" was the rage in England and Germany from 1600 to 1700. European chefs found that horseradish went well with meat or seafood. German settlers brought horseradish with them to America in the 1700s. Today, the horseradish industry produces nearly six million gallons of prepared (containing vinegar and possibly other ingredients) horseradish annually.

WASABI: According to Japanese legend, wasabi was discovered hundreds of years ago in a remote mountain village by a farmer who decided to grow it. He reportedly showed it to Tokugawa Ieyasu, a Japanese warlord of the era. Ieyasu, who later became Shogun, liked it so much he declared it a treasure only to be grown in the Shizouka area. The use of wasabi dates back to the origins of sushi.

Where Are Horseradish and Wasabi Grown?

HORSERADISH: Collinsville, Illinois, and the surrounding area grows nearly sixty percent of the world's supply though it can be found growing throughout the world.

WASABI: Wasabi is an indigenous herb of Japan that grows along stream beds in mountain river valleys. Few geographical areas are suited for growing wasabi.

Why Should I Eat Horseradish and Wasabi?

HORSERADISH: Contains vitamin C and the minerals potassium, calcium, magnesium, and phosphorus. It is rich in glucosinolates, which are known cancer- and bacteria-fighters.

WASABI: Wasabi is high in fiber and vitamin C. It is a good source of potassium, calcium, and magnesium. It contains the phytochemicals isothiocyanates, which have antibacterial and anticancer properties.

Home Remedies

HORSERADISH: Used by early Greeks as a lower-back rub and aphrodisiac. Also used as a cough expectorant, and as treatment for food poisoning, scurvy, tuberculosis, and colic. In the southern United States, horseradish rubbed on the forehead was a popular method of getting rid of headaches.

WASABI: Wasabi's antibacterial properties were first documented in a tenth-century Japanese medical encyclopedia. It was believed to be an antidote to food poisoning, making it a natural accompaniment to raw fish.

Throw Me a Lifesaver!

HEART HEALTH: A rat study found that the isothiocyanates in Wasabi inhibit platelet aggregation and deaggregation. It was found that in the case of a heart attack, where aspirin is commonly prescribed, the isothiocyanates in wasabi had an immediate effect as opposed to thirty minutes for aspirin.

MELANOMA: Eighty-two percent of lung tumors resulting from metastatic melanoma were reduced in mice who were administered a component of wasabi.

BREAST CANCER: A human cell line study showed that a relatively small concentration of wasabi inhibited up to 50 percent of breast cancer cells.

CANCER: Both wasabi and horseradish inhibited the growth of colon, lung, and stomach cancer cells in a human cell study.

ORAL HEALTH: Wasabi has even been known to prevent tooth decay.

BACTERIA KILLER: Horseradish and wasabi root have components including isothiocyanates that are effective in killing *H. pylori* and other bacteria.

Tips on Using Horseradish and Wasabi

SELECTION AND STORAGE:

Horseradish:

- The vast majority of horseradish sold today is prepared horseradish that comes in jars, which will keep for a year unopened and for four months opened.

Wasabi:

PASTE:

- Wasabi will last up to two years if frozen.
- Refrigerated opened shelf life is approximately 30 days.

RHIZOMES:

- Keep refrigerated when not being used.
- Wrap in damp paper towels.
- Rinse in cold water once a week.
- Refrigerated shelf life is approximately 30 days.

PREPARATION AND SERVING SUGGESTIONS:

- Wasabi is prepared by grating the fresh rhizome against a rough surface. Some Japanese sushi chefs will only use a sharkskin grater. Grate in a circular motion.
- After grating, chop fresh wasabi with the backside of a knife. This will release more of the flavor.
- Compress the fresh wasabi into a ball and let stand for five to ten minutes at room temperature so that the sweetness and heat have time to develop.
- Spread a little on the fish and then dip the fish side of the sushi into soy sauce so that the sauce does not touch the wasabi.
- Mix wasabi paste with soy sauce, called "wasabi-joyu," and use this as a dipping sauce for the raw fish, or mix the wasabi directly into a bowl of noodles.
- Add a dash of horseradish to tomato juice.
- Perk up tuna and potato salad and coleslaw with a dab of horseradish.

Wasabi Asian Noodles
by Chef J. Hugh McEvoy

Servings: 8 (3 ounces each) • Prep and cooking time: 30 minutes

This recipe contains four powerhouse foods.

INGREDIENTS:

*½ teaspoon fresh wasabi, or
  horseradish paste*
1 cup enriched semolina flour
1 cup whole wheat flour
*½ cup enriched all-purpose
  unbleached white flour*

4 tablespoons egg yolks
½ cup water
3 tablespoons extra-virgin olive oil
1 teaspoon kosher salt

DIRECTIONS:

Assemble and prepare pasta machine for use. Mix together all ingredients in a stand mixer or food processor until dough begins to form a ball. Remove dough from mixer and knead gently on a floured marble or wooden surface. Use as little flour as possible to prevent dough from sticking. Knead until smooth, about 10 minutes. Wrap dough in plastic wrap and place in refrigerator 1 hour. Roll out pasta dough to ⅛-inch thickness. Cut into linguini or other flat noodle using a pasta machine. Cook noodles as soon as possible. Garnish (sprinkle) with sesame oil and toasted sesame seeds before serving. Serve as a bed for any favorite stir-fry entrée or as a separate side dish with any Asian meal.

BREAK IT DOWN . . .

Calories: 275; Total fat: 9g; Saturated fat: 2g; Cholesterol: 103mg; Sodium: 59mg; Total carbs: 40g; Fiber: 2g; Sugar: 3g; Protein: 8g.

Kale *(Brassica oleracea L. var. acephala)*

What's the Story?

Kale is a member of the "headless" cabbage family, which also includes broccoli, cauliflower, and brussels sprouts. Its specialty group includes a variety of other greens such as collards. There are many varieties to choose from: Curly or Scots kale; Plain Leaved; Rape kale; Leaf and Spear; Cavolo Nero, also known as dinosaur; Tuscan and Lacinato kale ("black cabbage"). "Salad Savoy" or ornamental kale is popular for landscaping use but it can make a tasty side dish too.

A Serving of Food Lore . . .

Kale is thought to have originated in Asia Minor (the Asian part of Turkey) and was brought to Europe over 2,500 years ago. Kale made its way to the United States with English settlers in the seventeenth century. Dinosaur kale was discovered in Italy in the late nineteenth century. Ornamental kale, called so because it was originally a garden plant, was first produced commercially in the 1980s in California. Today, kale is a traditional favorite in the southern United States and is growing in popularity in other regions.

Where Is Kale Grown?

Kale production is mainly found in the southeastern United States.

Why Should I Eat Kale?

Kale's nutrient density makes it one of the healthiest foods that you could add to your diet. It is an excellent source of vitamin A, vitamin C, and potassium. Kale is also a good source of calcium, iron, and folate. It contains a variety of phytochemicals including eyesight-promoting, cancer-fighting lutein.

Throw Me a Lifesaver!

CANCERS OF THE LUNG, ESOPHAGUS, MOUTH AND PHARYNX: Fruits and vegetables that are high in carotenoids, including leafy greens like kale, lower the risk of lung cancer, esophageal cancer, and mouth and pharynx cancers, according to the American Cancer Society.

BLADDER CANCER: In a study of 130 bladder cancer patients and an equal number of control subjects, those who had consumed kale regularly had a lower risk for bladder cancer.

Tips on Using Kale

SELECTION AND STORAGE:
- Smaller leaves are milder-flavored. Choose deeply colored leaves for tenderness and optimum flavor.
- Avoid dry, wilted, and limp leaves. Tiny holes in the leaves may be an indication of insect damage.
- Keep unwashed kale in a plastic bag and store in the refrigerator crisper. Place a damp paper towel in the bag to keep moist. Cook it within a few days of purchase.

PREPARATION AND SERVING SUGGESTIONS:
- Wash well to make sure all dirt is removed.
- Remove the center vein in the leaves and stems, as these tend to be tough to chew.
- Serve kale immediately after preparing to prevent it from becoming soggy.
- If using kale in a raw salad, do not chop or tear until you are ready to use. This preserves the vitamin C content.
- Kale can be steamed, simmered, blanched, braised, sautéed, and baked. Cooking kale takes about 8 to 15 minutes depending on the method.
- Serve kale with vitamin C–rich food such as citrus fruits, vinegar, peppers, and dried fruit to increase the absorption of iron.
- Use sautéed kale in casseroles, salads, pasta, and potato dishes.

• Simply sautéing kale with fresh garlic, olive oil, and lemon juice or balsamic vinegar makes a wonderful dish. Try sprinkling a little grated cheese on top.

Comforting Kale and Lentil Soup
by Rosalie Gaziano
Servings: 16 (1 cup) • Prep and cooking time: 75 minutes

This soup is easy to prepare and it's even better the next day. This recipe contains six powerhouse foods.

INGREDIENTS:

1 small onion, chopped
2 cloves garlic, minced
3 tablespoons olive oil
1 24-ounce can diced tomatoes
½ cup dried lentils
⅓ pound whole grain macaroni of
    your choice

1 pound fresh kale,
    chopped fine
3 quarts water
1 cup Parmesan cheese,
    freshly grated, to sprinkle
    on top
Salt and pepper to taste

DIRECTIONS:
Boil macaroni, rinse, and set to the side. Rinse lentils and add to a separate small saucepan with enough water to cover and cook until tender, about 20 minutes. Meanwhile, peel and chop onion, and mince garlic cloves. Add olive oil to soup pot and heat. Add garlic and onions to pot and sauté until translucent, being careful not to burn. Remove center vein from kale leaves and chop coarse. Add kale to onion and garlic mixture and sauté for 10 minutes. Add 1 can chopped tomatoes, salt, and pepper, and let simmer 10 minutes. Add water to kale mixture, bring to a boil, and let simmer 30 minutes. Add cooked lentils and macaroni to soup and let simmer together another five minutes. Serve hot with Parmesan cheese grated on top. Serve with crusty Italian or French bread.

BREAK IT DOWN . . .
Calories: 130; Total fat: 4.5g; Saturated fat: 1.5g; Cholesterol: 5mg; Sodium: 247mg; Total carbs: 16g; Fiber: 3g; Sugar: 3g; Protein: 6g.

Kiwi *(Actinidia)*

A LITTLE FUZZY

The Chinese gooseberry was renamed "kiwifruit" because it resembled the New Zealand kiwi bird, which also happens to be fuzzy, round, and brown.

What's the Story?

The Chinese gooseberry, or kiwifruit, is native to Southeast Asia. Of the more than fifty species of kiwi, the most common commercially grown variety is *Actinidia deliciosa* (cultivar "Hayward"). Kiwi has grown in popularity but still accounts for but a little over one percent of world fruit consumption. The biggest kiwifruit-consuming markets are in Europe, North and South America, Japan, and Asia.

A Serving of Food Lore . . .

The kiwi originated in the Yangtze River Valley of northern China and the Zhejiang province on the coast of eastern China. It has been considered a delicacy since its beginnings. During the nineteenth and twentieth centuries, the gooseberry made its way throughout the world. Missionaries exported the first plants into New Zealand and the United States in the early 1900s. Norman Sondag, an American importer, was instrumental in renaming the Chinese gooseberry when he observed that the fruit closely resembled the New Zealand kiwi bird. In 1974, "kiwifruit" was accepted internationally as the official name of the exotic fruit.

Where Is Kiwi Grown?

Italy and China are the world's leading producers of kiwifruit. It is also grown commercially in New Zealand, California, South Africa, and Chile, and, in much smaller quantities, throughout other countries in Europe and the United States.

Why Should I Eat Kiwi?

The kiwi is the most nutrient-dense of the twenty-seven most commonly eaten fruits. It has more vitamin C than any other fruit. Kiwis are high in fiber, potassium, and vitamin E. It also contains lutein, which is a phytochemical that may reduce the risk of cancer, heart disease, and cataracts. There is also limited production of a red-fleshed variety of kiwi that is rich in anthocyanin, a plant chemical often found in other red-, purple-, and blue-hued foods such as cherries, plums, currants, and blueberries. Anthocyanin offers potent antioxidant properties that are thought to provide protection against heart disease and cancer.

Throw Me a Lifesaver!

HEART DISEASE: A study out of the University of Oslo found that kiwifruit, added to a normal diet, helps a component of red blood cells called platelets become "less sticky." Kiwi also lowered triglycerides (fat in the blood).

FIGHTING CANCER: A leading nutrition scientist at the Rowett Research Institute has shown that eating kiwifruit daily can protect DNA against damage that may lead to cancer. More significantly, kiwifruit seems to help repair the damage caused to DNA. A variety of naturally occurring substances have also been discovered in kiwifruit that are effective in killing oral tumor cells.

MACULAR DEGENERATION: Kiwi is an excellent source of lutein and zeaxanthin, phytochemicals found in the human eye. Recent studies indicate that diets rich in lutein are protective against cataracts and other forms of macular degeneration.

Tips on Using Kiwi

SELECTION AND STORAGE:
- Select firm, unblemished fruit.
- To test for ripeness, press the outside of the fruit. If it gives in to pressure, the fruit is ripe and ready to eat. If the kiwi is not ripe when it is

first bought, place in a brown paper bag at room temperature and check daily for ripeness.

- Kiwi can be stored for days at room temperature. For longer storage, keep in the refrigerator for up to four weeks.

PREPARATION AND SERVING SUGGESTIONS:

- Did you know that kiwi can be eaten with or without the skin? The skin is an excellent source of nutrients and fiber.
- Besides peeling and slicing, "slooping" is another technique that is used. Simply cut the kiwi in half, scoop out fruit with a spoon, and dig in.
- Top waffles, French toast, or a bagel with sliced kiwi.
- Eat with cereal or cut up into oatmeal.
- Makes a great addition to salads and pastas!
- Use as a tenderizer. Since it is an acidic fruit, it makes an excellent marinade.
- Substitute kiwi for tomatoes on a sandwich.

Fun Fruit Kabobs

Adapted from *Lean Moms, Fit Family* by Michael Sena and Kirsten Straughan

Servings: 4 • Prep time: 15 minutes

This recipe is so simple to make, even for little kids. You might want to assist them in cutting up the fruit but they love being part of the assembly line, skewering the fruit. This recipe has seven powerhouse foods in it.

INGREDIENTS:

2 kiwis, sliced into fourths   *²/₃ cup pineapple chunks*
1 apple or pear, cut into chunks   *1 cup nonfat yogurt*
1 banana, cut into chunks   *¼ cup dried coconut, shredded*
¹/₃ cup red seedless grapes   *4 skewers*
½ cup sliced strawberries

DIRECTIONS:

Slide pieces of fruit onto each skewer and design your own kabob by putting as much or as little of whatever fruit you want. Do this until the stick is almost covered from end to end. Spread coconut onto a large plate and yogurt onto another large plate. Hold your kabob at the ends and roll it in the yogurt, so the fruit gets covered. Then roll it in the coconut. Try raisins, chopped nuts, low-fat granola, or a favorite breakfast cereal in place of coconut.

BREAK IT DOWN . . .
Calories: 150; Total fat: 3g; Saturated fat: 2g; Cholesterol: 0mg; Sodium: 50mg; Total carbs: 33g; Fiber: 4g; Sugar: 25g; Protein: 4g.

Lemons (*Citrus limon*)

LEMONADE'S FIRST STAND
Did you know . . . the earliest written evidence of lemonade comes from Egypt?

What's the Story?

The lemon is actually a hybrid citrus tree developed as a cross between a lime and a citron, an ancient fruit that is best known for its candied peel. The lemon is an oval-shaped fruit used primarily for its juice, though the pulp and rind zest are also used in cooking or mixing. There are several varieties, but the most popular are the Eureka, Lisbon, and Meyer.

A Serving of Food Lore . . .

Lemons are thought to have originated in either China or India some 2,500 years ago. Though their migration is uncertain, many believe that Arab traders introduced the lemon throughout the Mediterranean. Spain served as the lemon's gateway from Palestine in the eleventh century. From the Iberian Peninsula the fruit traveled throughout Europe. Lemons were introduced to North Africa at around this same time. Christopher Columbus brought lemons to the Americas on his second voyage to the New World in 1493. Lemons were highly prized by miners from the era of the California gold rush for their protection against scurvy. People were willing to pay up to one dollar per lemon, a high price today and a very high price back in 1849.

Where Are Lemons Grown?

The major producers of lemons today are the United States, Italy, Spain, India, Argentina, Greece, Israel, and Turkey. In the United States, Southern California, Arizona, and Florida are the main growers of lemons.

Why Should I Eat Lemons?

Lemons are an excellent source of vitamin C. They also contain vitamin A, folate, calcium, and potassium. Limonene, a compound shown to have anticancer properties in laboratory animals, is present in lemons. All citrus fruits are high in flavonoids, the most common antioxidant found in fruits and vegetables and thought to block substances that cause cancer and heart disease.

Home Remedies

Lemon juice in hot water has been widely advocated as a daily natural treatment for constipation. People drink lemon juice and honey (½ squeezed lemon and 1 teaspoon of honey), or lemon juice with salt or ginger, as a cold remedy. Any of the lemon-plus preparations are good substitutes for caffeinated hot beverages. Lemon has been revered as a key ingredient in various household cleaners for its fresh scent and stain-removal properties. Lemon also does a great job in removing odor from hands. Many claim that applying a little lemon juice mixed with water several times a day to blemishes will help them disappear.

Throw Me a Lifesaver!

RHEUMATOID ARTHRITIS: Vitamin C–rich foods provide protection against inflammatory polyarthritis, a form of rheumatoid arthritis involving two or more joints. A research study involving more than 20,000 subjects found that subjects who consumed the lowest amounts of vitamin

C–rich foods were more than three times more likely to develop arthritis than those who consumed the highest amounts.

CANCER: In laboratory tests, citrus limonoids have been shown to fight cancers of the mouth, skin, lung, breast, stomach, and colon, and human neuroblastoma tumors, which occur most often in children. Next to cranberries, lemons exerted the highest antiproliferation activities on in vitro human liver cancer cells. Because of limonoids' ability to stay in the bloodstream for an extended period of time, researchers believe that they may be better suited for supressing cancer cell growth than other nutrients. (In comparison, phenols in green tea typically stay in one's system for only four to six hours.)

Tips on Using Lemons

SELECTION AND STORAGE:
- Choose lemons that are bright yellow with smooth and glossy skin.
- Lemons will last for a week or two at room temperature. For extended storage, keep lemons Ziplocked in the fridge crisper for up to six weeks.

PREPARATION AND SERVING SUGGESTIONS:
- To yield the most juice, a lemon should be room temperature or warmer.
- Roll the lemon under your palm on a hard surface to soften it before juicing. A large lemon will yield about 3 to 4 tablespoons of juice.
- Just need a bit of juice? Make a toothpick hole in the skin through which to extract juice, and then leave the toothpick in the hole to "seal" it and maintain freshness.
- Add lemon juice, pulp, and rind into salads, soups, and anywhere that you want a fresh citrus taste.
- Lemon juice can be used to change milk into buttermilk.
- Lemon juice "cooks" fish without heat in traditional ceviche dishes.

Steamed Artichokes with Lemon Wasabi Sauce
by Chef Dave Hamlin
Servings: 2 • Prep time: 30 minutes

You can also substitute steamed asparagus for the artichokes. This recipe has seven powerhouse foods in it.

INGREDIENTS:

ARTICHOKES:

2 artichokes

1 lemon

1 tablespoon fresh garlic

½ teaspoon fresh cracked black pepper

LEMON WASABI SAUCE:

1 cup lite mayonnaise

¼ cup lite sour cream

1 teaspoon wasabi or horseradish

Juice of 1 lemon

Juice of ½ lime

1 tablespoon fresh basil, chopped

Fresh cracked black pepper to taste

Salt to taste

DIRECTIONS:

ARTICHOKE PREPARATION:

Cut stem off at base of artichoke and cut off bottom; peel skin off stem. Rub cut surfaces with fresh lemon to prevent browning. Peel outer leaves from artichoke. Cut top one-third off of artichokes. Rub all cut surfaces with fresh lemons. Squeeze the remaining juice and pulp of lemon down the center of the artichoke. Place artichokes in simmering water with the leftover whole lemon. Sprinkle 1 tablespoon of fresh garlic over the artichokes, and push down into leaves. Sprinkle the black pepper on top. Simmer for 25 to 30 minutes or until center is fork-tender. Remove and let rest for 5 minutes.

SAUCE PREPARATION:

Mix to sauce consistency and refrigerate until needed. Serve with steamed artichokes.

BREAK IT DOWN . . .

Calories: 100; Total fat: 3g; Saturated fat: 1.5g; Cholesterol: 10mg; Sodium: 710mg; Total carbs: 17g; Fiber: 4g; Sugar: 7g; Protein: 3g.

Limes *(C. aurantifolia and C. latifolia)*

WON'T SELL YOU A "LEMON"
Did you know . . . limes are not green lemons?

What's the Story?

Limes can be sour or sweet but usually possess a greater sugar and citric acid content than lemons and are more acidic and tart in taste. The two most common varieties of sour limes available are the Tahitian or Persian lime and the key lime.

A Serving of Food Lore . . .

Limes are thought to have originated in the southeastern region of Asia. Middle Eastern traders introduced lime trees from Asia into Egypt and Northern Africa around the tenth century. The Arabian Moors brought them to Spain in the thirteenth century, from whence limes spread throughout southern Europe. Limes were on board when Columbus traveled on his second voyage to the Americas in 1493. In the United States, limes were established in Florida by the sixteenth century when Spanish explorers brought the West Indies lime to the Florida Keys, where that species was renamed "key lime."

Where Are Limes Grown?

Today, Brazil, Mexico, and the United States are among the leading commercial producers of limes. In the United States, limes are grown in Florida, the Southwest, and California.

Why Should I Eat Limes?

Limes contain powerful phytochemicals known as flavonol glycosides. These include limonin glucoside and kaempferol, strong antioxidants that help to prevent oxidative damage of cells, lipids, and DNA. Kaempferol may help prevent arteriosclerosis and additionally may act as a chemopreventive agent to fight cancer.

Home Remedies

SCURVY: For hundreds of years, British sailors have eaten limes and their juice to prevent scurvy on long sea voyages. The British were nicknamed "limeys" because of this—now considered a derogatory term.

Throw Me a Lifesaver!

IMMUNITY: Research shows that consumption of vegetables and fruits high in vitamin C is associated with a reduced risk of death from numerous causes including heart disease, stroke, and cancer.

CANCER: Flavonol glycosides may prevent the division of cancer cells for many types of cancers. Lime's powerful antioxidant limonin was shown to stop cancer cell proliferation in one study.

ANTIBIOTIC EFFECTS: In West African villages where cholera epidemics occurred, using lime juice during the main meal of the day was determined to have been protective against the contraction of the disease.

Tips on Using Limes

SELECTION AND STORAGE:
- Choose firm and heavy limes for the most juice.
- Select limes that are glossy and light to deep green in color.
- Small brown areas on the skin should not affect flavor, but large blemishes or soft spots indicate a damaged lime. Hard, shriveled skin is a sign of dryness.
- Limes may be stored at room temperature or in the refrigerator (in a plastic bag) for up to 3 weeks. Limes store better in the refrigerator but those left at room temperature will yield more juice.

PREPARATION AND SERVING SUGGESTIONS:
- Depending on the type and size of the lime, it will take between six and nine to make one cup of fresh lime juice. To juice by hand, roll the lime on a firm surface before squeezing out the juice.
- Limes or lime juice are a great salt substitute and add a tangy flavor.

Black Bean Soup with Lime and Cumin
Courtesy of www.fruitsandveggiesmatter.gov
Servings: 6 • Prep and cooking time: 20 minutes

This soup recipe is simple to make, especially when using canned black beans. This recipe contains ten powerhouse foods.

INGREDIENTS:

4 cups black beans, cooked and
   rinsed
1 tablespoon extra-virgin olive oil
1 tablespoon cumin
1 cup white onions, chopped
1 cup carrots, chopped
2 cloves garlic, chopped
½ cup red bell pepper, chopped
3 cups vegetable stock, low-sodium

¼ cup chipotle chiles (or green
   chiles), chopped
¼ cup plus 2 tablespoons fresh-
   squeezed lime juice
6 slices lime
1 tablespoon sour cream,
   low-fat
Chopped cilantro garnish
Salt to taste

DIRECTIONS:
Heat olive oil in a nonstick frying pan over medium heat. Add cumin and brown it, taking care not to burn it. Add chopped onions, carrots, garlic, and bell pepper, and cook slowly until browned. Puree the beans with 3 cups stock in a blender or food processor. Add in vegetable mixture along with the chiles, add lime juice, and process until creamy. Return mixture to pot and reheat until thickened. Salt to taste, and top with sour cream. Garnish with a slice of lime and chopped cilantro.

BREAK IT DOWN . . .
Calories: 221; Total fat: 5g; Saturated fat: .5g; Cholesterol: 1mg; Sodium: 360mg; Total carbs: 39g; Fiber: 12g; Sugar: 5g; Protein: 12g.

Mango *(Mangifera indica L.)*

IT TAKES TWO TO MANGO

Did you know . . . the mango is considered sacred in India and symbolizes love, friendship, and fertility?

What's the Story?

Mango is a fruit that varies in shape ranging anywhere from oval to round to kidney-shaped. It is one of a family of seventy-two flowering plants that includes its cousins the cashew and the pistachio. There are six major varieties of mangoes available in the United States, of which the top four are Tommy Atkins, Haden, Keitt, and Kent.

A Serving of Food Lore . . .

The mango is native to southern and southeastern Asia, particularly eastern India, Burma, and the Andaman Islands. References to mango can be found in Hindu writings dating as far back as 4000 B.C. Buddhist monks considered the mango a sacred fruit because they believed (and do to this day) that Buddha often meditated under a mango tree. The Persians are said to have carried it to East Africa in around the tenth century A.D. In 1862 the first seeds were brought into Miami from the West Indies. Nearly twenty years later the mango was introduced to Santa Barbara, California.

Where Are Mangoes Grown?

India accounts for seventy-five percent of all mangoes grown today. Few of them reach North America or Europe because of import restrictions as a result of concern about bringing in "pests" along with the fruit. (This may soon change under new United States regulations that will permit irradiated fruit in.) Mexico and China compete for second place in production, followed by Pakistan, Indonesia, Thailand, Nigeria, Brazil, the Philippines, and Haiti. In the United States, Florida has been the main producer, but California is now beginning production in the Coachella Valley.

Why Should I Eat Mangoes?

Mangoes are an excellent source of vitamins A and C, potassium, and carotenes, including beta-carotene. The vitamin content varies depending on the maturity and variety of the fruit. Green mangoes contain more vitamin C (as it ripens, the amount of beta-carotene increases). The mango is also a good source of vitamin K and has a variety of antioxidant components.

Home Remedies

There are many health claims attributed to mangoes, ranging from improved digestion and immunity, to heart health, to lowered blood pressure, to curing asthma. Many believe that mangoes are both an aphrodisiac and an effective means of birth control.

Throw Me a Lifesaver!

HEART HEALTH: Fruits and vegetables high in potassium and antioxidants such as vitamin A, carotenoids, vitamin C, and flavonoids may help prevent or control hypertension and reduce the subsequent risk of stroke and heart disease. In addition, foods high in soluble fiber and pectin appear to lower the amount of cholesterol circulating in the blood.

DIGESTION: Mangoes are a good source of fiber and contain enzymes that aid in digestion.

CANCER: Deep yellow-orange vegetables and fruits are rich in beta-carotene, which may protect cell membranes and DNA from oxidative damage. A cell line study examined the anticancer activity of mango and found that it interrupted phases of growth throughout the life cycle of the tumor cell.

Don't Throw Me an Anvil!

Mangoes, when combined with blood-thinning medication, may make your blood too thin! Talk to your doctor, pharmacist, or a registered dietitian about including mangoes in your diet.

Tips on Using Mango

SELECTION AND STORAGE:

CAN YOU SMELL WHAT THE MANGO'S GOT COOKIN'?

When it's ripe, you will be able to smell the sweetness of the mango from the stem end of the fruit.

- Red and yellow are typically the color of ripeness but color is not always the determining factor. The skin should give a little when pressed.
- Avoid mangoes that are gray, pitted, or have black spots on the skin; those are sure signs of rotting.
- Mangoes can be eaten fresh, frozen, or dried. They also come in nectars and jams or jellies.
- Mangoes should be stored at room temperature but when ripe they can be stored in the refrigerator for up to five days. Frozen mango may be stored in an airtight container for up to six months.

PREPARATION AND SERVING SUGGESTIONS:

- Avoid eating the skin—it may make you ill!
- To peel off the skin and cut the fruit off the pit, you must first slice off both sides or "cheeks" of the mango, being careful to avoid the large fibrous pit in the middle of the fruit. Take one side, hold it skin-side down in the palm of your hand and cut four or five vertical slices into the fruit. Be very careful not to cut through the mango skin. With both hands, grasp each end of the cut mango and turn it inside out. Carefully cut the fruit away from the skin and keep in large juicy slices or cut into cubes.
- Want a lot? Waste not! In Mexico, a common practice is to make a "lollipop" out of the mango by piercing the pit with a fork and eating the remaining flesh like a lollipop.
- Mangoes make excellent desserts and a tasteful addition to any fruit salad.
- Use for making a marinade for fish and meats.
- Try grilling mangoes for a tropical barbecue twist.

Mango Slaw
Courtesy of Chef Allen Susser, author of *The Great Mango Book*
Servings: 8 (½ cup) • Prep time: 15 minutes (but chill for at least 1 hour)

This recipe contains ten powerhouse foods.

INGREDIENTS:

2 large mature green mangoes,
   peeled, cut from the pit, and
   shredded
1 large carrot, peeled and shredded
1 small red onion, thinly sliced
2 tablespoons chopped fresh mint
2 tablespoons chopped fresh basil
3 tablespoons chopped fresh
   cilantro

1 teaspoon minced garlic
¼ cup freshly squeezed lime juice
2 tablespoons sugar or agave
   syrup
1 teaspoon seeded and minced
   serrano chile
2 tablespoons Thai fish sauce

DIRECTIONS:

In a large bowl, combine the mangoes, carrot, and onion. Add the mint, basil, and cilantro and toss together. In a small bowl, combine the garlic, lime juice, sugar, chile, and fish sauce. Stir until the sugar is dissolved. Pour the lime mixture into the slaw and toss together, coating all the ingredients well. Cover and refrigerate for at least 1 hour, or up to 24 hours before serving.

BREAK IT DOWN . . .
Calories: 63; Total fat: 0g; Saturated fat: 0g; Cholesterol: 0mg; Sodium: 355mg; Total carbs: 16g; Fiber: 1.5g; Sugar: 13g; Protein: 0g.

Millet *(Panicum miliaceum L.)*

FOR THE BIRDS?

Did you know . . . more birds than people in the United States eat millet?

What's the Story?

Millet is a small yellow grain with a mild, sweet flavor and actually describes a group of grasses that are thought to be some of the oldest cultivated crops in the world. The five most popular millet varieties are proso, foxtail, barnyard, browntop, and pearl. Most people are familiar with millet because of its prominence in birdseed.

A Serving of Food Lore . . .

Millet is native to Africa and Asia and there is evidence of its being grown since the fifth century B.C. Millet slowly spread westward toward Europe, leading to proso's introduction into the United States in the eighteenth century. It was first grown along the Eastern Seaboard and was later introduced farther west into the Dakotas.

Where Is Millet Grown?

Foxtail millet is grown extensively in Africa, Asia, India, and the Near East. Proso millet is grown in the former Soviet Union, mainland China, India, and Western Europe. In the United States, both millets are grown, principally in the Dakotas, Colorado, and Nebraska.

Why Should I Include Millet?

Millet is a good source of fiber and protein, the vitamins thiamine and niacin, and the minerals magnesium, phosphorus, zinc, copper, and manganese. It is also a good source of the carotenoids lutein and zeaxanthin.

Home Remedies

Finger millet, otherwise known as African millet, is an age-old remedy for obesity. It is thought to be effective because it takes longer to digest.

Throw Me a Lifesaver!

HEART HEALTH: Scientists fed millet to rats for twenty-one days. By the end of the study, good cholesterol had increased without an increase in bad cholesterol.

DIABETES: Diabetic rats on a high-millet diet had decreased levels of insulin sensitivity and better glucose management compared to their control group.

Tips on Using Millet

SELECTION AND STORAGE:
- Millet comes in both packages and bulk. Beware of "webbing" in bulk bins, a sure sign of bug infestation!
- Store in a cool, dry place. Millet can also be kept in a sealed container in the refrigerator.

PREPARATION AND SERVING SUGGESTIONS:
- One cup of millet requires three cups of liquid; it should cook for 40 minutes. One cup dry will yield three cups cooked.
- Millet can be dry roasted to increase the nutty flavor of the grain.
- Millet is great when dry roasted, cooked, and then marinated.
- Use in place of rice.

Creamy Millet Pudding with Cinnamon Sugar

Adapted from *Gluten-Free 101* by Carol Fenster

Servings: 6 • Prep and cooking time: 35 minutes

This recipe contains four powerhouse foods.

INGREDIENTS:

2 cups 1% milk

2 tablespoons cornstarch

2 large eggs

¼ cup honey

¼ teaspoon salt

1 teaspoon vanilla extract

1 cup cooked whole grain millet

½ teaspoon granulated sugar
  (optional)

½ teaspoon ground cinnamon
  (optional)

DIRECTIONS:

In a medium-size heavy saucepan, stir together 1¾ cups of the milk, eggs, honey, and salt, and whisk until egg is thoroughly blended. To the remaining ¼ cup of milk, stir in cornstarch until smooth. Add to saucepan. Place saucepan over medium-high heat and cook, stirring constantly, until mixture thickens, about 5 to 7 minutes. Remove from heat and stir in vanilla extract and cooked millet. Divide mixture into six dessert bowls or wineglasses. Sprinkle sugar and cinnamon, if desired, on pudding. You can eat this immediately as a creamy, warm dessert or chill it for at least an hour for a cool treat.

How to Cook Whole Grain Millet

Rinse 1 cup whole grain millet. Combine with 3 cups water and ½ teaspoon salt in heavy medium-size pot. Bring to boil over high heat, reduce to low and simmer, covered, 30 minutes or until all liquid is absorbed. Remove from heat. This makes 3 cups of cooked millet—1 cup for this pudding and 2 cups left over to eat as a side dish with meals or as a hot breakfast cereal.

BREAK IT DOWN . . .

Calories: 150; Total fat: 2.5g; Saturated fat: 1g; Cholesterol: 65mg; Sodium: 165mg; Total carbs: 25g; Fiber: 1g; Sugar: 15g; Protein: 6g.

Mint *(Mentha)*

NOT IN MINT CONDITION!

Did you know . . . that the "Mint Julep," a popular drink from the southern United States, is mainly bourbon and sugar with only a few mint leaves added?

What's the Story?

There are at least 25 to 30 known mint species. Spearmint, peppermint, orange or bergamot mint, pineapple mint, and pennyroyal are the most widely grown and used species. Besides its varied culinary uses, the herb mint is used in gums, candies, toothpaste, pest repellents, medicines, and cosmetics.

A Serving of Food Lore . . .

Mint is thought to have originated in the Mediterranean Basin, where it was valued as a foundation in perfumes, food flavorings, and medicinal products. The Romans brought mint throughout Europe. In the 1790s, mint was being grown in Massachusetts, and by 1812 peppermint was cultivated commercially for oil in Ashfield, Massachusetts.

Where Is Mint Grown?

Mint is mainly grown in China, India, the Mediterranean, the Philippines, and Egypt. In the United States, peppermint is primarily grown for essential oil production. Mint is also commercially produced in Michigan, Indiana, Wisconsin, Oregon, Washington, and Idaho.

Why Should I Eat Mint?

Mint contains phenolic compounds that have strong antioxidant activity. Its many vitamins and minerals include vitamin A, calcium, folate, potassium, and phosphorus.

Home Remedies

Peppermint has been used to aid digestion for thousands of years. It is also a folk remedy for many intestinal ailments, including gas, indigestion, cramps, diarrhea, vomiting, irritable bowel syndrome, and food poisoning. It has also been used for respiratory infections and menstrual problems. There are many sprays and inhalants on the market that contain mint and are promoted to relieve sore throats, toothaches, colds, coughs, laryngitis, bronchitis, nasal congestion, and inflammation of the mouth and throat.

Throw Me a Lifesaver!

HEART HEALTH: In a study where herbs and spices were examined for their potential to inhibit LDL cholesterol's conversion into the more harmful form, mint was one of the most effective.

CANCER: Mint's phenolic phytochemicals may help prevent cancer. Fresh mint was found to have very strong scavenging activity. Mint is high in salicylic acid and it is thought to play a role in the prevention of colorectal cancer and atherosclerosis.

LUNG CANCER: Mint given to mice with lung cancer reduced tumors significantly. The effects were attributed to the antioxidative and radical scavenging properties of mint.

BACTERIA: Research indicates that some essential oils may reduce food-borne pathogens. In one study, the natural essential oils found in mint prevented E. coli bacteria from growing. Mint might provide an alternative to conventional antimicrobial additives in foods.

PINWORM: Mint was found to have significant killing effect on pinworms.

DIGESTIVE HEALTH: A clinical trial in England found that patients who had received peppermint oil before surgery had less nausea after their surgeries than those who did not receive it. Other studies have shown that peppermint oil relieved spasms during colonoscopies and has a soothing effect in patients who suffer from irritable bowel syndrome.

RESPIRATORY RELIEF: Researchers discovered a nerve ending that responded to cold and to menthol. This may explain the cooling sensation from menthol, as well as its common use as an inhalant to reduce congestion in the nose.

Tips on Using Mint

SELECTION AND STORAGE:
- Leaves should be tender and not wilted. Older leaves tend to be bitter and "woody" tasting.
- Keep fresh mint leaves refrigerated in a plastic bag for no more than two to three days.

PREPARATION AND SERVING SUGGESTIONS:
- Use young leaves pinched from stem tips for the best flavor.
- In fruit salads, mint is a great addition to apples, pears, or strawberries and in salad dressings.
- Add to flavor tea and marinades.
- Mint is a great addition to soups, salads, sauces, meats, fish, poultry, stews, chocolate dishes, and lemon desserts.
- Peppermint is usually used for teas and sweets. Spearmint is the mint that is commonly used for meat sauces and jellies.
- Fresh mint is ubiquitous in Middle Eastern dishes, including tabbouleh.

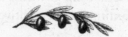

Spicy Japanese Mint Noodles
by Chef J. Hugh McEvoy

Servings: 13 (½ cup) • *Prep and cooking time: 1 hour, 20 minutes*
(includes 1 hour chill time)

This recipe contains five powerhouse foods.

INGREDIENTS:

2 tablespoons fresh mint leaves

16 ounces Japanese buckwheat soba noodles—dry

1 tablespoon soy sauce

2 teaspoons fish sauce

2 tablespoons organic sesame oil

2 tablespoons blackstrap molasses

¼ cup brown rice vinegar

¼ cup toasted sesame seeds

1 cup fresh green onion bulbs and tops, chopped

¼ cup fresh sweet red bell peppers, chopped

1 teaspoon crushed red pepper flakes

DIRECTIONS:

Whisk together molasses, soy sauce, fish sauce, rice vinegar, oils, and pepper flakes. Ensure all molasses has dissolved. Cook Japanese noodles in boiling water until al dente—just tender. Rinse cooked noodles under very cold water (to chill). Drain and blend noodles evenly with sauce. Chill for 1 hour. Just before serving, fold in mint, seeds, sweet peppers, and green onions. Garnish with whole mint leaves and chopped green onion. Serve with Japanese plum wine or saki.

BREAK IT DOWN . . .

Calories: 180; Total fat: 4g; Saturated fat: .5g; Cholesterol: 0mg; Sodium: 460mg; Total carbs: 32g; Fiber: 2g; Sugar: 2g; Protein: 6g.

Mushrooms *(Basidiomycota)*

RISKY BUSINESS!

Did you know . . . to the untrained eye, there are no easily recogniz-able differences between poisonous and edible mushrooms? My grandmother's "surefire" method was to have my grandfather try the wild mushrooms she picked first and if he suffered no ill effect, she then fed them to the family!

What's the Story?

Mushrooms are actually the "fruits" of fungus called *mycelium,* growing in soil, wood, or decaying matter. There are thousands of varieties of mush-rooms, ranging in size, shape, texture, and color. Some more popular types include black trumpet, chanterelles, cloud ears, lobster, morels, oys-ter, porcini, portobella, shiitake, truffles, white button, and wood ear mushroom. Mushrooms impart a fifth taste sense called *unami* in Japanese, translated to mean "savory" or "meaty." Not all edible mush-rooms are used in cooking; some are used for medicinal benefits and are sold in supplement form.

A Serving of Food Lore . . .

Mushrooms, in one variety or another, have been around since the very beginnings of vegetation. Eastern cultures have used mushrooms for both food and medicine for thousands of years. Ancient Egyptians believed that eating mushrooms would make you immortal. France became one of the first countries renowned for cultivation of mushrooms. After King Louis XIV's reign, mushroom cultivation gained popularity in England, and in the late nineteenth century, cultivated mushrooms came to the United States.

Where Are Mushrooms Grown?

China accounts for thirty-two percent of worldwide production. The United States cultivates sixteen percent of world output.

Why Should I Eat Mushrooms?

Though not generally thought of as "nutrition-packed" vegetables, many culinary mushrooms contain large amounts of selenium (in fact, more so than any other produce). Mushrooms are also a good source of B vitamins such as riboflavin and pantothenic acid. White, crimini, and portobella mushrooms are excellent sources of potassium. White button mushrooms start out as a good source of vitamin D, but if exposed to ultraviolet light for just five minutes after harvesting, a single serving will contain a powerhouse punch of 869 percent of the daily value of vitamin D! The benefit of this level of vitamin D is currently being investigated. Polyphenols are the main contributor to the antioxidant activity of mushrooms. Another antioxidant called ergothioneine, known for its anticancer properties, reaches its greatest value in fungi.

Home Remedies

Many species of mushrooms and fungi that have been utilized for thousands of years as folk medicines, for anything from warding off cancer to fighting heart disease, have come under intense study by ethnobotanists and medical researchers in recent years.

Throw Me a Lifesaver!

BREAST CANCER: A research study revealed that of seven vegetable extracts tested, white mushroom extract was the most effective in inhibiting aromatase, an enzyme associated with breast cancer growth.

PROSTATE CANCER: White button mushroom extract suppressed the growth of androgen-independent prostate cancer cells and decreased tumor size in a dose-dependent manner in in vivo and in vitro studies.

IMMUNE SYSTEM ENHANCEMENT: Mushrooms contain beta-glucans and other substances that may help the immune system recognize and devour abnormal cells that cause disease.

MIGRAINES: Psilocybin, originally an extract of certain psychedelic mushrooms, is being intensely studied for migraine headaches (as well as for illnesses like obsessive-compulsive disorder).

Tips on Using Mushrooms

SELECTION AND STORAGE:

- Wild mushrooms are available seasonally. You may find morels in the spring, chanterelles in midsummer, and porcini in the fall.
- For common mushrooms, choose those with a firm texture and even color with tightly closed caps.
- Store mushrooms partially covered in your refrigerator crisper. Use them within three days.
- Store dried mushrooms in an airtight container.

PREPARATION AND SERVING SUGGESTIONS:

- Dried mushrooms should be soaked in hot water or part of the recipe cooking liquid for about an hour before using. The liquid may be used for added flavor.
- Gently wipe mushrooms with a damp cloth or soft brush to remove occasional peat moss particles. Or, rinse with cold water and pat dry with paper towels.
- Mushrooms can be fried, sautéed, or stir-fried on their own and eaten as a side dish, or used to top an entrée.
- Mushrooms can be used in salads, soups, sauces, stir-fries, meat dishes, and other main courses.

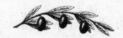

Portobella Mushrooms with Tiger Shrimp
by Chef J. Hugh McEvoy
Servings: 6 • Prep and cooking time: 35 minutes

To make this dish vegetarian, use "no-chicken" chicken stock by Natural Foods instead of regular chicken stock and omit the shrimp. This recipe features six powerhouse ingredients.

INGREDIENTS:

6 large portobella mushrooms
6 large (21/25 count) tiger shrimp
¾ cup whole wheat breadcrumbs
2 ounces shredded Parmesan
    cheese
⅓ cup sweet red bell pepper,
    chopped
⅓ cup fresh shallots, chopped

3 tablespoons fresh basil,
    chopped fine
3 tablespoons fresh cilantro,
    chopped fine
¾ cup chicken stock (low-salt)
3 tablespoons extra-virgin
    olive oil
Salt and pepper to taste

DIRECTIONS:

Remove stems from mushrooms. Using a heavy sauté pan, sauté mushroom caps in olive oil until lightly browned. Remove and set aside. Sauté peppers, shallots, and chopped mushroom stems in olive oil until lightly browned. Add breadcrumbs and heat through. Add chicken stock. Mix until evenly blended. Remove from heat. Add fresh chopped herbs and cheese to mixture. Fold together until evenly blended. Set aside. Steam tiger shrimp in shells. Peel and devein shrimp. Set aside. Stuff each mushroom cap three-quarters full with filling mixture. Do not overfill. Top each filled mushroom with steamed tiger shrimp. Curl shrimp inside mushroom cap. Brush each filled, topped mushroom with melted butter. Using a shallow baking pan, brown the stuffed mushrooms under a broiler until brown. Season with salt and pepper to taste. Garnish each cap with a fresh basil leaf. Serve immediately.

BREAK IT DOWN . . .

Calories: 200; Total fat: 12g; Saturated fat: 3g; Cholesterol: 20mg; Sodium: 35mg; Total carbs: 14g; Fiber: 3g; Sugar: 3g; Protein: 9g.

Oats *(Avena sativa)*

ANY WAY YOU SLICE IT . . .

Did you know . . . all forms of oats, whether old-fashioned, quick-cooking, steel-cut, or instant oatmeal, fall under the definition of whole grain? Because all three parts of the grain are preserved during the milling—no matter which variety—all provide the same nutrients in the same amounts. Bottom line . . . it's a matter of taste and texture! Eat the form that suits your taste and lifestyle!

What's the Story?

The seed portion of the oat plant is what we commonly refer to as "oats." After the inedible hull is removed, a "groat" remains. A variety of oat products are made from the groat, such as steel-cut oats (commonly known as "Irish oats"), old-fashioned oatmeal, quick oatmeal, instant oatmeal, oat flour, and oat bran. Oats in general have a mild, creamy, and somewhat floury texture.

A Serving of Food Lore . . .

Oats were one of the earliest cereals cultivated by humans. Many believe oats originated in Eurasia and were consumed in ancient China as long ago as 7000 B.C. The ancient Greeks were the first people known to have made porridge (cereal) from oats. In England, oats were considered an inferior grain, while in Ireland and Scotland they were used in a variety of porridges and baked goods. Cultivated oats came to America with the first British immigrants in the early 1600s. In fact, the British Quaker influence inspired the name "Quaker Oats" and the company remains the main supplier of oats to the United States today.

Where Are Oats Grown?

The top ten producers of grain include Russia, Canada, the United States, Poland, Finland, Australia, Germany, Belarus, People's Republic of China, and the Ukraine. Minnesota, Wisconsin, South Dakota, Iowa, and central Canada lead in oat production in North America.

Why Should I Eat Oats?

Oats contain healthy amounts of vitamin E, several B vitamins, the minerals calcium, magnesium, and potassium, and the trace minerals selenium, copper, zinc, iron, and manganese. They are rich in the phytochemicals 1,3-beta-glucan and avenanthramides. Oats contribute both soluble and insoluble fiber. Insoluble fiber benefits the digestive system. The soluble fiber found in oats works like a sponge by going after cholesterol and removing it before it has a chance to clog arteries and lead to heart disease.

Home Remedies

When oats first arrived on the scene in the American colonies, they were used to cure stomach discomfort and digestive ailments. Oats have also been reported to have antispasmodic, anti-inflammatory, diuretic, and stimulant properties and have also been used as a folk remedy for tumors. Externally, for centuries people have taken oat baths to help soothe itchiness, eczema, and other disorders of the skin.

Throw Me a Lifesaver!

HEART HEALTH: There are over forty clinical studies spanning forty years that confirm oats' ability to lower not only total cholesterol but also harmful LDL cholesterol, both significant risk factors for heart disease. The U.S. Food and Drug Administration approved the first food-specific health claim for use on oatmeal packaging and in advertising in 1997. Eating three grams of soluble fiber from oats as part of a low-fat and low-cholesterol diet has been shown to lower blood cholesterol and low-density lipoproteins (LDLs), the particles that carry cholesterol into your arteries. In a study in the *Australian Journal of Nutrition and Dietetics,* researchers found that a substance in oats called beta-glucans significantly reduced LDL ("bad") cholesterol.

HIGH BLOOD PRESSURE: In a study in the *Journal of Family Practice,* groups of men and women who had high blood pressure experienced significant reduction in blood pressure, the need for antihypertensive medication, and improved lipids and blood glucose, when oats were added to their diet.

WEIGHT MANAGEMENT: Research shows that beginning the day with a nutritious, fiber-rich diet can help you maintain a healthy weight. Oatmeal was found to have the highest satiety value out of all breakfast foods, providing a greater feeling of fullness.

DIABETES: Several long-term studies show that people with high whole grain intake had from twenty-eight to sixty-one percent lower risk for developing type 2 diabetes compared with those with the lowest intakes.

Tips on Using Oats

SELECTION AND STORAGE:
- Look for tightly sealed boxes or canisters. Avoid bulk cereals; grains in open bins may be exposed to moisture, mold, and insect contamination.
- Keep oats in an airtight and moisture-proof container to prevent bugs from getting in and mold/fungi growth from forming.
- Properly stored and dry, rolled oats may keep for as long as a year.

PREPARATION AND SERVING SUGGESTIONS:
- Oats can be prepared in a variety of different ways. They can be processed into cereals and snacks, made into beer, and baked into cookies, muffins, and breads.
- For creamier-style oatmeal, bring the oats, milk or soy beverage, or water to a boil, then simmer.
- The most popular oatmeal toppings are: milk, sugar, and fruit such as raisins and bananas.
- Try them in meatloaf and meatballs, or as a coating for chicken and fish.
- Quick or old-fashioned oats can be substituted for up to one-third of the flour called for in recipes for muffins, biscuits, pancakes, loaf-type quick breads, coffee cakes, yeast breads, cookies, and bars.
- Oatmeal cookies are the number one non-cereal usage for oats.

Ina's Whole Wheat Oatmeal Pancakes
by Ina Pinkney

Servings: 12 pancakes • Prep time: 8+ hours—oats have to refrigerate overnight
Cooking time: 5 minutes

I made these pancakes for my wife on Mother's Day. She exclaimed that hands down, these were the best pancakes she had ever had! Their creator, Ina Pinkney, is the chef and owner of the renowned Ina's Kitchen in Chicago. Ina says the test of a good pancake is how it tastes unadorned, on its own. I couldn't agree more! These whole wheat oatmeal pancakes are great straight up but they also taste great with slices of bananas or a few blueberries placed on the pancake before flipping it over. Just a little pure maple syrup drizzled over the top is needed to bring out the rich flavors contained within! This recipe contains three powerhouse foods.

INGREDIENTS:

¾ cup old-fashioned rolled oats
2 cups buttermilk, low-fat
¼ cup whipping cream, light
1 egg
2 tablespoons brown sugar

2 tablespoons canola oil
½ cup whole wheat flour
½ cup all-purpose flour
½ teaspoon salt
1 teaspoon baking soda

DIRECTIONS:
Combine rolled oats, buttermilk, and cream in a mixing bowl, cover, and refrigerate overnight. The next day, beat egg with brown sugar and oil in a mixing bowl. In another bowl, combine flours, salt, and baking soda. Stir into egg mixture along with the oats soaked in buttermilk and cream. Batter will be thick. Coat a large, nonstick pan with cooking spray. Add batter, measuring ¼ cup for each pancake. Pancakes should be about 4" across. Cook for 3 to 4 minutes on the first side, until tiny bubbles appear and the surface loses its sheen. Flip. Cook second side, 2 to 3 minutes, until cooked through. Repeat until all batter is used.

BREAK IT DOWN . . .
Calories: 120; Total fat: 5g; Saturated fat: 1.5g; Cholesterol: 30mg; Sodium: 250mg; Total carbs: 15g; Fiber: 2g; Sugar: 5g; Protein: 4g.

Olives *(Olea Europaea)*

WHEN FRESH IS NOT BEST!
Did you know ... fresh olives off the tree taste horrible!
Commercially available olives are brine-, salt-, or olive oil–cured
first before they ever meet human lips.

What's the Story?

Olives are fruits that grow on trees, contain a single pit, and have flesh
filled with oil. The ripe fruits are either pressed to extract oil or sold
whole. There are dozen of cultivars of olives but some of the most popular are Ascolano, Barouni, Gordal (one of the most popular table olives
from Spain), Manzanillo, Mission (most widely used for cold-pressed
olive oil in California), Picholine, Rubra, and Sevillano (the largest
California commercial variety).

> Did you know ... that green and black olives are really the same
> olive and only vary in the degree of ripeness—black being the most
> ripe?

A Serving of Food Lore . . .

The olive has a very long history dating back to biblical times. The olive
branch, a symbol of peace known worldwide, was brought back to Noah
by a dove signifying the end of God's wrath. In fact, carbon-dating of an
olive seed found in Spain suggests an age of eight thousand years old!
Besides the Mediterranean region, olives are thought to also have originated in tropical and central Asia and various parts of Africa. Olives were
grown in Crete as long ago as 2500 B.C. Olives spread to Greece and other
parts of the Mediterranean area. Olive trees first appeared in California in
the late 1700s.

Where Are Olives Grown?

According to the International Olive Oil Council, Spain is the largest producer of olive oil, followed by Italy and then Greece. Tunisia, Turkey,

Syria, Morroco, and Portugal round out the next highest group for production. These eight countries combined account for over ninety percent of world olive oil production.

Why Should I Eat Olives?

Olive oil contains seventy-five percent heart-healthy monounsaturated fat and only thirteen percent from saturated fat. Many of olive oil's health benefits come from active compounds such as oleocanthal, which has a strong anti-inflammatory action to fight heart disease and cancer. The flavonoid polyphenols in olive oil are natural antioxidants that boast a host of beneficial effects, from healing sunburn to lowering cholesterol, blood pressure, and risk of coronary disease. Many other nut and seed oils have no polyphenols whatsoever.

Home Remedies

A few drops of warmed olive oil, also known as sweet oil, placed in the ear canal has been known to help alleviate earaches.

Throw Me a Lifesaver!

CANCER PREVENTION: Epidemiological evidence suggests that olive and olive oil consumption as part of a Mediterranean diet has cancer-protective properties.

COLON CANCER: Spanish researchers found that the active ingredients maslinic and oleanolic acids in olive oil prevented human colon cancer cells from multiplying and restored apoptosis (programmed cell death).

HEART DISEASE: The United States Food and Drug Administration (FDA) in clear, albeit careful, terms has stated: "Limited and not conclusive scientific evidence suggests that eating about two tablespoons (23 grams) of olive oil daily may reduce the risk of coronary heart disease due to the monounsaturated fat in olive oil. To achieve this possible benefit, olive oil is to replace a similar amount of saturated fat and not increase the total number of calories you eat in a day."

HIGH BLOOD PRESSURE: In 2007, the *Journal of Nutrition* reported the findings of researcher Isabel Bondia-Pons from the University of Barcelona. She and her colleagues evaluated the effects of moderate consumption of olive oil (about two tablespoons a day) by non-Mediterranean men who typically consumed very low levels of olive oil. They experienced a modest reduction in their systolic blood pressure which was attributed to the increase of heart-healthy oleic fatty acids in their diet.

Tips on Using Olives

SELECTION AND STORAGE:
- For the highest antioxidant content, choose "extra-virgin" or "virgin" oil, the least-processed forms.
  - Extra-virgin olive oil: comes from the first pressing of the olives and is favored for its superior taste.
  - Virgin olive oil: has a greenish tint, is obtained by pressing crushed fruit in coarse bags and removing the oil. It has a stronger taste than extra-virgin.
  - Except in a pinch, you should avoid bottles and containers labeled "refined oil," "pomace olive oil," or "light oil."
- Transfer olive oil to a sealable container and refrigerate. It will become solid but rapidly reliquefies if left at room temperature for a few minutes.
- Store oil away from light and heat to maintain phytochemical content.

PREPARATION AND SERVING SUGGESTIONS:
- Use olive oil for lower-temperature cooking. The particles found in extra-virgin olive oil cause it to burn and smoke at higher temperatures. Once the oil burns, many of the health benefits go POOF—up in smoke!
- Use to flavor sauces and gravies or as a dressing on salads and vegetables. Olive oil infused with fresh herbs also makes a delicious dip for hot, crusty Italian bread! *Mangia, Mangia!*
- Place a medium black olive on each fingertip and you will have exactly one fat serving (give or take a finger). They are fun to eat that way too.

Honey-Balsamic Dressing
by Dave Grotto
Servings: 12 • Prep time: 10 minutes

This recipe contains three powerhouse foods.

INGREDIENTS:

½ cup extra-virgin olive oil

½ cup balsamic vinegar

2 tablespoons honey

1 teaspoon lemon juice

1 teaspoon black pepper

½ teaspoon salt

DIRECTIONS:

Whisk together vinegar, honey, lemon juice, salt, and pepper until well blended. Slowly add olive oil while whisking. Serve over salad or hot vegetables, or use as a dip for bread.

BREAK IT DOWN . . .

Calories: 100; Total fat: 9g; Saturated fat: 1.5g; Cholesterol: 0mg; Sodium: 100mg; Total carbs: 5g; Fiber: 0g; Sugar: 4g; Protein: 0g.

Onions (Allium cepa)

DON'T BE THICK-SKINNED!

Did you know . . . the thickness of an onion's skin has been used to predict how bad the next winter may be? Thin skins mean a mild winter is coming, while thick skins indicate a rough winter ahead.

What's the Story?

Onions are a member of the lily family and there are two basic types:
- Bulb-forming:
  - Storage, fall/winter onions: Examples include white, yellow, and Spanish.
  - Fresh, spring/summer onions: Examples include Maui, Vidalia, Walla Walla, Grand Canyon, and Texas SuperSweet.

- Perennial—produce clusters of onions that can be replanted for another crop. Varieties include Egyptian onions, shallots, and potato
onions.

A Serving of Food Lore . . .

The origin of the onion is thought to be in Asia, where onion gardens have
been excavated dating as far back as 5,000 years ago. Pharaohs were buried
with onions as a sign of eternity. The Romans believed the onion could
cure whatever ailed them. Well into the twentieth century, the three main
vegetables of European cuisine were beans, cabbage, and onions. During
the Middle Ages, onions were an acceptable form of currency used to pay
rent, and they were always a welcome wedding gift!

Onions were growing wild in the United States long before the first
Pilgrims arrived. The Native Americans used wild onions for cooking and
seasonings, in syrups, and in dyes. Onion cultivation in the United States
began in 1629 and it is now one of the top ten vegetables grown in this
country.

Where Are Onions Grown?

The world's leading producers are China, India, United States, Turkey, and
Pakistan. In the United States, Idaho, Oregon, Washington, California,
and Texas are the largest producing states.

Why Should I Eat Onions?

Onions contain quercetin, a powerful flavonoid antioxidant. Onions are
an excellent source of fiber, vitamin C, and folate. Green onions (scallions)
have moderate amounts of vitamin A. Phytochemicals found in onions,
particularly allyl sulfides, appear to reduce the risk of some cancers.

Home Remedies

In many parts of the world, onions have been used to heal blisters, boils,
and damaged skin. In the United States, products that contain onion extract are used in the treatment of topical scars; however, in a side-by-side
test, onion extract did not perform any better than a petrolatum salve.

Throw Me a Lifesaver!

CANCER: In a study that evaluated the top ten vegetables consumed in the United States, yellow onions were the third highest in phenolic (a type of antioxidant) content and were fourth highest in anticancer-growth activity. The National Cancer Institute has found that onions have a modest level of cancer-protective activity.

LUNG CANCER: Onions are rich in the phytochemical quercetin, which has been shown to have beneficial effects against lung cancer. A case-controlled study of 582 subjects found that people who increased their onion consumption decreased their risk of developing cancer. In a Finnish study, men who ate foods high in quercetin had a sixty-percent-reduced incidence of lung cancer.

COLON AND LIVER CANCER: Researchers at Cornell University found that strong-tasting onions—particularly New York bold, western yellow, and shallots—do a better job of inhibiting the growth of liver and colon cancer cells than do milder-tasting onions.

PROSTATE CANCER: A U.S. researcher found that the strongest risk reduction factors for prostate cancer were onions, cereals and grains, beans, fruits, and vegetables.

HEART HEALTH: Allyl sulfides, found in onions, decrease the tendency of blood clots to form, significantly lowering total LDL cholesterol levels. A study of Japanese women found that those with the highest onion intake had the lowest LDL cholesterol. University of Wisconsin–Madison researchers found that the stronger-tasting and -smelling onions made blood platelets less sticky, thus reducing risk for atherosclerosis, cardiovascular disease, heart attack, and stroke.

BONE HEALTH: A study published in the *Journal of Agriculture and Food Chemistry* reported that onion consumption increased bone density in rats, possibly decreasing the risk for osteoporosis.

Tips on Using Onions

SELECTION AND STORAGE:
- Onions are available in fresh, frozen, canned, and dehydrated forms.
- An onion shouldn't smell like an onion until you cut it.
- Avoid onions that are sprouting, are soft, or whose skin is wet.
- If stored at 55 degrees, they may retain all their vitamin C content for as long as 6 months.

PREPARATION AND SERVING SUGGESTIONS:
- Slicing an onion causes its cell walls to tear, which releases a sulfur compound called propanethial-S-oxide, which in turn causes eye irritation. Place the onion in the refrigerator about 1 hour before cutting to reduce this effect. Cutting an onion under running water also helps reduce irritation to the eyes.
- Cooking onions gives them more of a sweet taste. "Caramelizing" onions occurs when prolonged heat causes the sugars to brown the onion.
- Popular onion uses include being employed as an ingredient in casseroles, pizzas, soups, stew, salads, onion rings, and as a garnish.

Simple Southern Italian Onion, Tomato, and Basil Salad
by Rosalie Gaziano
Servings: 4 • Prep time: 10 minutes

This salad is especially good when kept in the refrigerator for a few hours or even overnight. This recipe includes five powerhouse foods.

INGREDIENTS:

4 red tomatoes, ripe

1 medium Vidalia or sweet onion

2 tablespoons extra-virgin olive oil

1 pinch crushed red pepper
   to taste

1 large bunch fresh basil (½ cup
   when chopped)

Salt to taste

A few whole leaves of basil to
   garnish

DIRECTIONS:

Cut wedges of fresh tomatoes into clear glass or favorite colorful salad bowl. Peel and wedge onion into same bowl. Pour olive oil, salt, pepper, and basil, and toss well. Chop fresh basil and garnish with one or more sprigs for color.

BREAK IT DOWN . . .
Calories: 110; Total fat: 8g; Saturated fat: 1g; Cholesterol: 0mg; Sodium: 15mg; Total carbs: 9g; Fiber: 2g; Sugar: 6g; Protein: 2g.

Oranges *(Citrus sinensis)*

CITRUS KING
Did you know . . . oranges are the largest citrus crop in the world?

What's the Story?

Oranges fall into two categories: sour oranges and sweet oranges. There are many different varieties and subvarieties of sweet orange. The navel is the most popular eating orange in the world; the Florida and California Valencia is mostly juiced. Other popular varieties include the blood or pigmented orange such as the Ruby, and the acidless orange, more native to the Mediterranean region. Mandarins or tangerines, *Citrus reticulata,* are considered distinct from the sweet orange but there are hybrids, such as the Temple orange, that combine the best of sweet and tangerines.

A Serving of Food Lore . . .

Sour varieties of oranges were cultivated well before the Middle Ages. The sweet varieties have only been around since the fifteenth century. The origins of the orange are thought to be in Southern Asia and from there, it spread to Syria, Persia, Italy, Spain, and Portugal. Columbus brought them to the West Indies, and Spanish explorers brought them into Florida, where they were first planted around 1875. Spanish missionaries were responsible for introducing them to California.

Where Are Oranges Grown?

Brazil is the leading orange-producing country in the world, followed by the United States, Mexico, Spain, Italy, China, Egypt, Turkey, Morocco, and Greece. Florida and California are the leading orange-producing states in the U.S.

Why Should I Eat Oranges?

Oranges are a great source of potassium, a mineral that's important for heart health, and an excellent source of vitamin C, providing one hundred thirty percent of the recommended daily value (RDA) per orange. Oranges are also a good source of the B vitamin folate, which helps protect against heart disease and birth disorders. Phytochemically speaking, oranges are a rich source of flavanones, a specialty group of the flavonoid family of antioxidants which offer cell protection against a host of diseases. A four-ounce glass of orange juice is equivalent to one fruit serving.

Home Remedies

Oranges, orange juice, and orange rind have been used as home remedies for a variety of conditions including coughs and the common cold, constipation, toothaches, cataracts, and anorexia. Orange is applied topically for acne.

Throw Me a Lifesaver!

HEART HEALTH: The Food and Drug Administration advises that "Diets containing foods that are good sources of potassium and low in sodium may reduce the risk of high blood pressure and stroke."

WEIGHT CONTROL: Fibers found in the white layer of an orange curb appetite and suppress hunger levels for up to four hours after eating. Studies show that people who eat fruit such as oranges tend to eat less at subsequent meals compared to people who eat snacks such as chips, snack crackers, desserts, or candy.

ANXIETY: Patients awaiting dental procedures who were exposed to the odor of orange had reduced anxiety and improved mood compared to the control group.

KIDNEY STONES: In a randomized study, researchers found that orange juice, more than any other citrus juice, boosted levels of citrate in the urine, necessary to stop kidney stones from forming.

Tips on Using Oranges

SELECTION AND STORAGE:
- Fruit: Look for fruits that are firm and heavy for their size, with bright, colorful skins. Avoid fruit with bruised, wrinkled, or discolored skins; this indicates the fruit is old or has been stored incorrectly.
- Juice: Drink orange juice by the sell-by date on the carton and within one week after opening the carton.
- Oranges will keep at room temperature for several days. But for best results, store in a plastic bag or the crisper drawer of your refrigerator.
- Oranges can be frozen, too.

PREPARATION AND SERVING SUGGESTIONS:
There are several ways to peel oranges:
- The "basketball" peeling method: Slice off the stem end of the fruit. Without cutting into the "meat" of the fruit, score the peel with a knife or a citrus peeler into quarters like a basketball. Pull away the peel.
- The "round and round" peeling method: Using a slight sawing motion, cut only the outer, colored peel away in a continuous spiral, leaving the white membrane. Cutting lengthwise with the curve of the fruit, remove the white membrane.
- Add orange segments to a parfait or to a salad with red onions and romaine lettuce.
- Use orange juice as a meat tenderizer, as a component of marinade, or in dressings.

Orange and Dried Pear Compote
by Ina Pinkney
Servings: 6 (⅓ cup servings) • Prep and cooking time: 30 minutes

This recipe contains six powerhouse foods.

INGREDIENTS:

½ cup water
½ cup orange juice
¼ cup honey
1 large orange, peeled and
    sectioned with seeds removed
¼ cup lemon juice

6 ounces dried pears, sliced into
    thin strips
2 tablespoons mint, fresh, finely
    chopped
1 teaspoon coriander seeds,
    toasted and ground

DIRECTIONS:

In a heavy saucepan, combine water, orange juice, and honey and bring to a boil. Add the orange segments, lemon juice, and pears. Reduce the heat to a simmer and stir occasionally until the fruit is plump and tender, 15 to 20 minutes. Remove from the heat and stir in the herbs. Let cool to room temperature, cover, and refrigerate for at least one hour. Can be served cold or at room temperature.

BREAK IT DOWN . . .
Calories: 140; Total fat: 0g; Saturated fat: 0g; Cholesterol: 0mg; Sodium: 0mg; Total carbs: 37g; Fiber: 3g; Sugar: 30g; Protein: 1g.

Oregano (Origanum)

HAPPILY EVER AFTER . . .

Did you know . . . ancient Romans and Greeks would crown a bride and groom with oregano during a wedding ceremony because the herb was believed to banish sadness?

What's the Story?

Oregano, also called Greek oregano, wild marjoram, mountain mint, and known by some as "Joy of the Mountains," is a member of the mint family. There are over twenty different species of oregano.

A Serving of Food Lore . . .

Oregano originated in the Mediterranean and was traded as a spice. It came with European colonists to North America, where it was grown in gardens and grew in the wild as well. Originally, oregano was used in the United States for medicinal purposes, until after World War II, when soldiers returning from the Mediterranean brought back a taste for the herb as a seasoning.

Where Is Oregano Grown?

Oregano is mostly grown in Asia, Europe, North Africa, and North America.

Why Should I Eat Oregano?

Did you know that a tablespoon of oregano packs the same antioxidant strength as an apple?

One tablespoon of oregano also has about the same antioxidant capacity as one banana or a cup of string beans or one half cup of steamed carrots. It contains many vitamins, minerals, and phytochemicals that act as strong antioxidants. It is also a good source of the carotenoids lutein, zeaxanthin, and beta-carotene.

Home Remedies

Ancient Greeks applied oregano leaves to soothe aching muscles. The Romans would use oregano for scorpion and spider bites. In the United States, oregano was used for chronic coughs, asthma, and to help relieve toothaches. Men turned to a mixture of olive oil and oregano as a scalp treatment in hopes of revitalizing hair growth. The same olive oil and oregano combination has been applied to rheumatic limbs and sprains with success. (At least, with greater success than as a cure for baldness.)

Throw Me a Lifesaver!

CANCER: Oregano contains important phenolic acids that have strong free radical–scavenging activity, which can help prevent certain types of cancers from forming. Indian oregano was shown to have protective properties against radiation-induced DNA damage in an animal cell study.

ANTIBACTERIAL, ANTIFUNGAL, ANTIPARASITIC ACTIVITY: In a cell study, oregano oil caused damage to *E. coli* bacteria within one minute. Oregano was found in another study to cause irreparable damage to *Giardia lamblia,* a nasty little parasite that causes diarrhea and abdominal pain.

ULCERS: Combining cranberry extract and oregano extract was more effective in killing *h. pylori* than either cranberry or oregano extract alone. Researchers believe that therein lies a synergistic effect of oregano and cranberry phenolics, nicely illustrating the benefit of combining many of the 101 foods!

Tips on Using Oregano

SELECTION AND STORAGE:
- Choose fresh oregano that is bright green and not wilted; avoid oregano leaves and stems that are blackened or yellowed.
- The smell should be sweet, with an aromatic flavor.
- Fresh oregano can be kept in the refrigerator up to three days.

PREPARATION AND SERVING SUGGESTIONS:
- Oregano can be chopped fresh or dried and used in a variety of recipes.
- Oregano can be used to add flavor to yeast breads, marinated vegetables, black beans, zucchini, eggplant, roasted meats, and fish; it also enhances cheese and egg dishes.
- Try it in stews and soups too!
- Garlic, thyme, parsley, and olive oil complement the flavor of oregano.

Broiled Bufala Mozzarella, Tomato, and Oregano on Garlic Whole Wheat Crostini
by Dave Grotto
Servings: 4 • Prep and cooking time: 15 minutes

This recipe contains six powerhouse foods.

INGREDIENTS:

1 clove garlic
2 tablespoons olive oil
1 large tomato, sliced
4 slices whole wheat crostini

4 ounces bufala mozzarella, sliced in four pieces
2 tablespoons fresh oregano
1 tablespoon fresh basil
Salt and pepper to taste

DIRECTIONS:
Preheat broiler. In a bowl, combine oregano, basil, salt, and pepper; mix and set aside. Rub crostini with garlic clove and brush on olive oil. Toast crostini until slightly browned. Place tomato slice and then cheese slice on top of crostini. Sprinkle on herb mixture. Place crostini on a cookie sheet and broil for approximately 3 to 4 minutes or until cheese is bubbly and browned.

BREAK IT DOWN . . .
Calories: 220; Total fat: 14g; Saturated fat: 5g; Cholesterol: 22mg; Sodium: 190mg; Total carbs: 16g; Fiber: 2g; Sugar: 2g; Protein: 8g.

Papaya *(Carica papaya linn.)*

LIKE BUTTA'

Did you know . . . papain, a naturally occurring digestive enzyme in papaya, is often used as a meat tenderizer?

What's the Story?

The papaya fruit "tree" is, in reality, a large herb that can reach up to 20 to 30 feet. The papaya is also known as "Papaw" or "Paw Paw" in Australia and *Mamao* in Brazil. Individual fruits can weigh up to 20 pounds!

There are two types of papayas, Hawaiian and Mexican. Most papaya found in grocery stores is the sweeter, pear-shaped, yellow-orange skinned (when ripe) Hawaiian type, and the flesh of the Hawaiian papaya is usually orange or pinkish with small black seeds in the center. Mexican papayas are much larger than the Hawaiian variety and can weigh up to 10 pounds.

A Serving of Food Lore . . .

The origins of papaya are unknown but it is thought to have come from southern Mexico and neighboring Central America. Spaniards carried papaya seeds throughout Central and South America and later to the Philippines in the mid-1500s to 1600s. Today, the papaya is grown in most tropical regions throughout the world.

Where Is Papaya Grown?

Commercial production of the papaya is primarily in Hawaii, tropical Africa, the Philippines, India, Ceylon, Malaya, and Australia. Small-scale production also occurs in parts of Latin America, such as Mexico. Forty percent of Mexico's papaya crop is produced in the state of Veracruz.

Why Should I Eat Papaya?

One half of a small papaya provides 150 percent of the daily value of vitamin C. Papayas are also a good source of vitamin A, potassium, folate, and fiber. They contain carotenoids, mainly cryptoxanthin, which may reduce the risk of lung and colon cancer and possibly benefit rheumatoid arthritis. Papaya is known for its protein digestive enzyme, papain. Besides being an aid to digestion, it is also commonly used in commercial food processing, as a meat tenderizer, and as a beer stabilizing agent.

Home Remedies

In many tropical regions, the latex found in the papaya plant is used as a vermifuge to rid the body of parasites. Parts of the root are used to expel roundworms. The latex is also used as a way to heal boils and warts, and remove freckles.

Throw Me a Lifesaver!

HUMAN PAPILLOMAVIRUS (HPV): Women who had an increased consumption of beta-cryptoxanthin and lutein/zeaxanthin, and increased intake of vitamin C, had lower rates of infection by HPV, the cervical cancer virus, according to one research study. The researchers concluded that women who consumed at least one papaya (rich in all of the aforementioned nutrients) or more per week had lower risk of contracting the HPV infection than those who didn't.

BURN/WOUND-HEALING: Russian scientists have found that the antioxidants and natural enzymes in papaya can accelerate the healing of burns and wounds. Rats treated with papaya-based medicine had wounds that were half the size of those not given the treatment.

DECREASED RISK OF AGE-RELATED MACULAR DEGENERATION: Phytochemicals such as lutein, cryptoxanthin, and zeaxanthin, present in papaya, may help maintain better eyesight longer in older people.

Tips on Using Papaya

SELECTION AND STORAGE:
- Papayas that are hard and green are immature and will never properly ripen. Look for papayas that are mostly or completely yellow.
- The papaya should give slightly to pressure, but should not be soft at the stem end.
- Avoid buying fruit that is bruised, shriveled, or has soft spots.
- Store unripe papayas at room temperature until they are fully golden all over.
- To ripen quickly, place papayas at room temperature in a brown paper bag. Then transfer to the refrigerator for up to 5 days.

PREPARATION AND SERVING SUGGESTIONS:
- Wash papaya under cool running water, cut in half, and spoon out seeds.
- Blend with milk, yogurt, or orange juice for a smoothie.
- Puree papaya to make salad dressing or a base for ice cream.
- Add papaya slices to make any type of fruit salad.
- Papayas can be used to make hot and spicy salsa.
- Papaya seeds taste like peppercorns and can be dried and ground and used in salads or other dishes.
- Immerse tough meat in papaya juice overnight to tenderize.

Ginger Papaya Cocktail
by Lisa Dorfman

Servings: 2 • Prep time: 10 minutes

All five ingredients (including the garnish but not the vodka in the alcohol option) are powerhouse foods.

INGREDIENTS:

*1 large ripe papaya, deseeded and
    peeled*
Juice of 2 key limes
3 tablespoons ginger, grated
**For an evening cocktail add
    2 ounces of vodka.*

2 tablespoons agave syrup
2 mint leaves

DIRECTIONS:
Puree papaya flesh in a food processor or blender. Add lime juice and grated ginger. Continue to blend. Garnish with mint leaf.

BREAK IT DOWN . . . (NONALCOHOLIC VERSION)
Calories: 170; Total fat: 0g; Saturated fat: 0g; Cholesterol: 0mg; Sodium: 10mg; Total carbs: 46g; Fiber: 6g; Sugar: 28g; Protein: 2g.

Parsley *(Petroselinum crispum)*

ODOR EATERS

Did you know . . . parsley is traditionally added on the plate as a garnish of both beauty and function? The function is to eliminate strong odors on the breath after a meal.

What's the Story?

Parsley belongs to the *Umbelliferae* family that includes celery and carrots. *Petroselinum* is derived from the Greek word *petros* which means "stone," referring to the plant's preference for growing in rocky places. Among several varieties in cultivation, the most popular two are the curled-leaved, also known as "curly" leaf (crispum) and the broad-leaved Italian, also known as "flat" leaf (*P. neapolitanum*). Curled-leaved parsley is most often used as a garnish.

A Serving of Food Lore . . .

Parsley's origins appear to be from the Mediterranean region where it has been cultivated for more than 2,000 years. The variety crispum was mentioned by the Roman philosopher Pliny. Greeks valued parsley for its culinary and medicinal uses and symbolic value. They often adorned their victors in battle and sport and their heroes in death with ornamental parsley.

Where Is Parsley Grown?

Parsley is grown all over the world. In the United States, it is mostly grown commercially in California and Florida but is readily available from other states depending on the season.

Why Should I Eat Parsley?

Parsley is a source of vitamin C, iodine, iron, and many other minerals. Parsley has potent phytoestrogenic activity, equal to that found in soybeans, suggesting possible cancer-preventative properties. There are many volatile oils and flavonoid phytochemicals in parsley, all having cancer-protective attributes.

Home Remedies

Parsley is one of the medicinal herbs used by diabetics in Turkey. It is valued as a breath-freshener, due to its high concentration of chlorophyll, and in tea form, parsley is often used as a diuretic.

Throw Me a Lifesaver!

DIABETES: The Turks were on to something! In a study testing parsley's benefits with diabetic rats, researchers found that the rat subjects who were given parsley experienced lowered blood glucose while their GSH (a cell protector) levels increased. Parsley extract was also found to have a protective effect comparable to the diabetic medication, glibornuride, against liver toxicity caused by diabetes.

CANCER: Myristicin, a phytochemical that has been isolated in parsley, is an effective inhibitor of tumors in mice.

Tips on Using Parsley

SELECTION AND STORAGE:
- Parsley comes in both dried and fresh forms.
- Choose fresh parsley that does not have wilted or yellow leaves—a sure sign that it is not fresh!

- Trim off any wilted parts before storing fresh parsley refrigerated in a plastic bag.
- Curled-leaved parsley can be frozen.

PREPARATION AND SERVING SUGGESTIONS:
- Wash fresh parsley by swishing it around in a bowl of water. Drain and repeat.
- When trimming, keep some of the stem with the head of parsley.
- Recipes commonly call for parsley to be sautéed at the beginning of the dish. Save half of the parsley and add it at the end of the cooking process for best taste and nutritional value.
- Italian flat-leaf parsley is best for hot dishes.
- Parsley is the cornerstone ingredient in the Middle Eastern dish made from bulgur wheat called tabbouleh.
- Add parsley to soups and sauces, vegetable and grain dishes, meat and fish, or use to garnish salads.

Green Eggs and Ham
by Chef J. Hugh McEvoy
Servings: 4 • Prep and cooking time: 20 minutes

The original recipe called for ham, eight whole eggs, and three tablespoons of butter. By swapping out four of the whole eggs with egg whites, replacing the ham with "wham," and replacing butter with far less canola oil, you save 100 calories, 268 milligrams of cholesterol, ten grams of fat, and seven grams of saturated fat! And best yet, no sacrificing TASTE! This recipe contains seven powerhouse foods.

INGREDIENTS:

2 tablespoons fresh parsley, chopped

1 tablespoon fresh basil, chopped

1 tablespoon fresh cilantro, chopped

2 ounces (2 slices) Worthington Wham (veggie ham) or honey ham, chopped

1 tablespoon sweet red bell peppers, chopped

1 tablespoon fresh shallots, chopped

2 ounces Brie cheese—$\frac{1}{4}$" cubes

1 tablespoon canola oil

$\frac{1}{8}$ teaspoon sea salt

$\frac{1}{8}$ teaspoon black pepper

1 pound white asparagus

4 eggs

4 egg whites

4 tomato slices (optional)

DIRECTIONS:

Trim asparagus. Steam just until tender and set aside. Using heavy sauté pan, lightly brown wham/ham, shallots, and sweet peppers in canola oil. Beat eggs into a froth in a small bowl. Add eggs to sauté pan mixture. Blend while cooking only until set. Add cheese. Fold until just evenly mixed. Remove from heat. Add coarse chopped herbs. Fold gently into eggs. Do not overmix. Keep colors separate! Season with salt and pepper to taste. This dish can be served by itself or over toast points, beside the white asparagus over fresh red tomato slices.

BREAK IT DOWN . . .
Calories: 220; Total fat: 13g; Saturated fat: 4g; Cholesterol: 195mg; Sodium: 380mg; Total carbs: 6g; Fiber: 3g; Sugar: 3g; Protein: 17g.

Passion Fruit *(Passiflora edulis)*

LOVE AT FIRST BITE
Did you know . . . in some cultures, a popular belief is that after eating passion fruit, you will fall in love with the next person you meet?

What's the Story?

Passion fruit comes from the passionflower plant and is part of the genus *Passiflora.* There are two main types of passion fruit commonly used for commercial purposes: the New Zealand purple passion fruit and the Hawaiian yellow passion fruit. The taste of the yellow and purple passion fruit is similar; both are sweet and tart, but the purple passion tends to be less acidic and is juicier than the yellow variety.

A Serving of Food Lore . . .

The purple passion fruit is thought to be native to Brazil, possibly from the Amazon, but no one knows for sure. The purple passion fruit was mainly grown in Australia before the 1900s. Seeds were brought to Hawaii in 1801.

Where Is Passion Fruit Grown?

Passion fruits can be found in most tropical regions but the main commercial growers are located in South America, the Caribbean, Brazil, Florida, Hawaii, Australia, East Africa, and South Africa.

Why Should I Eat Passion Fruit?

Passion fruit is a good source of vitamin A and an excellent source of vitamin C (supplying nearly seventy percent of the daily allowance) as well as potassium, calcium, and iron. One passion fruit also contains about fifteen percent of the recommended daily allowance of iron. When eaten with the seeds, a serving is an excellent source of fiber (about fifteen grams). It is also rich in a number of phytochemicals including passi-florine, lycopene, and carotenoids.

Home Remedies

Puerto Ricans eat passion fruit to lower blood pressure. Brazilians eat the seeds to induce sleep. The Spanish discovered that passion fruit was used as a sedative in many folk medicine practices throughout South America. In Madeira, the juice is taken to aid in digestion and also used as a treatment for gastric cancers. Passionflower has been used to treat nervous and easily excited children, bronchial asthma, insomnia, nervous gastrointestinal disorders, and menopausal problems.

Throw Me a Lifesaver!

CANCER: Phytochemicals found in passion fruit were able to increase apoptosis (programmed cell death) in a line of cancer cells. The common phytochemicals thought responsible were carotenoids and polyphenols.

HYPERTENSION: An extract of passionflower significantly lowered systolic blood pressure in hypertensive rats.

HEART HEALTH: Passion fruit seeds were shown to reduce total lipids, triglycerides, and cholesterol in hamsters.

Tips on Using Passion Fruit

SELECTION AND STORAGE:
- Choose large, heavy, and firm fruit.
- When passion fruit are ripe, the outside will turn from green to a deep purple, red, or yellow color.
- If purchased unripe, leave at room temperature until ripe; the skin will wrinkle but the fruit will not soften too much. Once at desired ripeness, place in the refrigerator for up to one week.

PREPARATION AND SERVING SUGGESTIONS:
- Cut the passion fruit in half lengthwise and scoop out the seedy pulp with a spoon.

- To remove seeds, strain in a nonaluminum sieve or use cheesecloth, squeezing to extract the juice.
- The seeded pulp can be made into jelly or combined with pineapple or tomato in making jam.
- Spoon the pulp over other soft fruits or ice cream.
- The pulp makes a delicious jam or jelly and the seeds add a nice crunch!
- Add passion fruit to mixed green salads or fruit salads for a new taste.
- Top chicken, fish, or pork with a spoonful of passion fruit for a fruitful change.
- Add passion fruit and fruit juices to any fruit salad or smoothie for a refreshing new taste.
- In Australia they eat the pulp with cream and sugar on it.
- In Venezuela, passion fruit is used to make ice cream and added to rum cocktails.

Passion Fruit Sorbet
by Chef J. Hugh McEvoy
Servings: 14 • Prep time: 15 minutes
"Cooking" time: 6½ hours

This recipe contains four powerhouse foods.

INGREDIENTS:

2 cups fresh purple passion fruit juice

20 ounces fresh purple passion fruit

½ cup white granulated sugar

½ cup water

1 tablespoon fresh lime juice

2 tablespoons fresh grated orange peel

2 tablespoons mint leaves for garnish

DIRECTIONS:

Using a heavy saucepan, bring water and sugar to a boil. Dissolve sugar completely. Add lime juice and passion fruit juice—bring back to boil. Remove from heat. Add passion fruit pulp including seeds. Transfer mix to a freezer-safe container. Chill in refrigerator for at least six hours—do not freeze yet. Using a home ice-cream maker, churn the chilled mix into sorbet until almost solid. Add grated orange zest and blend evenly. Put in freezer and freeze until solid. Serve garnished with mint leaves.

BREAK IT DOWN . . .
Calories: 78; Total fat: 0g; Saturated fat: 0g; Cholesterol: 0mg; Sodium: 12mg; Total carbs: 20g; Fiber: 4g; Sugar: 17g; Protein: 1g.

Peanuts *(Arachis hypogaea)*

GET YOUR PEANUTS!
Did you know . . . that 2.4 billion pounds of peanuts are consumed in the United States each year—about half of it in the form of peanut butter?

What's the Story?

The peanut is not really a nut at all. It is technically a legume along with its cousins beans and peas, all belonging to the *Leguminosae* family. Legumes are edible seeds enclosed in pods. Peanuts grow underground, unlike "tree nuts" such as walnuts, almonds, and pistachios. Virginias, Runners, and Spanish peanuts are the three main types grown in the United States. Virginias (cocktail nuts) are large-kerneled. Medium-size kernels are called Runners and small-size kernels are called Spanish peanuts. A fourth type, Valencia peanuts, characterized by three or four small kernels in a long shell, are grown less frequently in the U.S.

A Serving of Food Lore . . .

The peanut is grown mainly in tropical and subtropical regions throughout the world but is thought to be native to the Western Hemisphere, most likely originating in Brazil or Peru. Spaniards brought the peanut to Europe; Portuguese explorers transplanted it to Africa, and from there it was brought back to the Americas. Peanuts were consumed by soldiers during the Civil War as a cheap source of protein. George Washington Carver, considered by many to be the father of the peanut industry, was the one who suggested to farmers that they rotate their cotton plants and cultivate peanuts. He also developed more than 300 uses for peanuts ranging from food uses to industry applications.

Where Are Peanuts Grown?

China and India are the largest producers of peanuts. In both countries, most nuts are processed for oil and sold locally. The United States, Argentina, Sudan, Senegal, and Brazil are the major producer–exporters. In the United States, peanuts are grown mainly in Georgia, Texas, Alabama, North Carolina, Florida, Virginia, and Oklahoma.

Why Should I Eat Peanuts?

Scientists at the University of Florida found that peanuts rival fruits in their levels of antioxidants. The Florida researchers identified high concentrations of polyphenols, particularly p-coumaric acid. Roasting can increase the level of the polyphenols, boosting overall antioxidant content by as much as twenty-two percent. Peanuts are an excellent source of beta-sitosterol, known to have anticancer properties. They are also a good source of resveratrol, an antioxidant also found in red wine that may help fight heart disease.

Home Remedies

GUM IN HAIR: Smearing peanut butter on hair that has gum stuck in it helps with the gum's removal.

STICKER AND INK REMOVER: Same deal—just smear peanut butter on surfaces containing unwanted ink and stickers and they should come off!

Throw Me a Lifesaver!

HEART HEALTH: The U.S. Food and Drug Administration approved a qualified health claim for peanuts in 2003: "Scientific evidence suggests but does not prove that eating 1.5 ounces of most nuts, such as peanuts, as part of a diet low in saturated fat and cholesterol may reduce the risk of heart disease." A study in the *Journal of the American College of Nutrition* showed that regular consumption of peanuts lowered triglycerides and improved diet quality by increasing nutrients associated with the prevention of cardiovascular disease.

TYPE 2 DIABETES: Study subjects who ate half a serving of peanut butter or a full serving of peanuts five or more times a week had up to a twenty-seven percent reduced risk of developing type 2 diabetes.

WEIGHT MANAGEMENT: A USDA survey found that peanut eaters were better able to meet their needs for vitamin A and E, folate, calcium, magnesium, zinc, iron, and fiber. The participants in this survey had lower BMIs (Body Mass Index—a measurement used to determine obesity) than non–peanut eaters.

COLON CANCER: A study found that female subjects who frequently consumed peanuts and peanut products had reduced risk for colorectal cancer.

Tips for Using Peanuts

SELECTION AND STORAGE:
- Look for peanuts either shelled or unshelled, as oil, as peanut butter (with or without additives like sugar and salt, smooth, creamy, chunky, super-chunky, and more), and as an ingredient in confections or sauces—you name it!
- Peanuts can turn rancid quickly so try to taste one before you buy them.
- Shelled peanuts can be stored up to three months in the refrigerator and up to six months in the freezer.

PREPARATION AND SERVING SUGGESTIONS:
- Make your own peanut butter in a food processor.
- Toss chopped peanuts on a salad.
- Use peanut oil in a vegetable stir-fry.
- Try a peanut butter and banana sandwich for a change of taste.

Aztec Cocoa Fire Peanuts

by Chef J. Hugh McEvoy

Servings: 18 • Prep and cooking time: 18 minutes

This recipe definitely has a grown-up taste, with a slight cocoa flavor and not overtly sweet. This is a great snack to serve by itself but it also makes a great topping on salads for added crunch. *Tasty tip:* Omit the cayenne pepper and substitute hot cocoa mix for dark cocoa powder for more kid appeal. This recipe contains four powerhouse foods.

INGREDIENTS:

1 pound dry-roasted peanuts
2 tablespoons granulated sugar
2 tablespoons egg whites
½ teaspoon sea salt

¼ teaspoon cayenne pepper (optional)
3 tablespoons of dark cocoa powder

DIRECTIONS:

Beat egg whites, cayenne pepper, salt, and sugar in a small mixing bowl. Blend in peanuts and coat evenly. Spread evenly on a greased or papered baking sheet. Roast nut mixture at 350 degrees for 4 minutes. Take out of oven and stir and coat evenly again. Return to oven for another 4 minutes (do not overbake). Cool nuts at least 15 minutes. Mix well to separate nuts. Dust peanuts with unsweetened cocoa mix. Dust again. Serve with plenty of refreshing beverages.

BREAK IT DOWN . . .

Calories: 160; Total fat: 13g; Saturated fat: 2g; Cholesterol: 0mg; Sodium: 70mg; Total carbs: 7g; Fiber: 2g; Sugar: 3g; Protein: 6g.

Pears *(Pyrus L.)*

What's the Story?

Pears are part of the rose family. There are over 3,000 known varieties but
only three species of pear trees bear the fruit we typically consume today.
The Anjou, Bartlett, Bosc, Comice, Seckel, and Forelle pear varieties are
the most popular in the United States.

A Serving of Food Lore . . .

It is thought that the pear was used as a source of food during the Stone
Age. The pear's likely place of origin was Asia and southeastern Europe.
Records of cultivation can be traced as far back as 5000 B.C. in China.
Around the seventeenth century, pears became popular in Europe. The
pear tree was immortalized alongside a partridge in the eighteenth-
century Christmas carol "The Twelve Days of Christmas." An attempt at
planting the first pear tree in the northeastern American colonies failed
due to a poor growing climate in 1620. Pear trees did much better farther
west in Oregon and Washington and have flourished there since the 1800s.

Where Are Pears Grown?

The leading pear-producing countries are China, the United States, Italy,
Spain, Germany, Belgium, and France. More than ninety-five percent of
the pears sold in the United States are grown in Washington, Oregon, and
Northern California.

Why Should I Eat Pears?

One medium-size pear contains as much vitamin C and potassium as one
half cup of orange juice. An average pear contains about four grams of

fiber, much of which is made up of soluble pectins and lignans. It is also packed with powerful phytochemical antioxidants.

Home Remedies

Pears have been used throughout history for a variety of health challenges such as digestive disorders and spasms, and for reducing fevers. Topically, pear fruit has been used as an astringent.

Throw Me a Lifesaver!

REDUCED COUGH WITH PHLEGM: A study conducted in Singapore found an association between increased dietary fiber from fruit and reduced risk of certain types of lung disease. There was an inverse relationship between cough with phlegm and fruits particularly high in flavonoids, such as quercetin and catechins found in pears.

WEIGHT LOSS: A study found that diets high in fruits, such as pears and apples, helped women between the ages of 30 and 50 to lose weight. After 12 weeks, those women who ate pears and apples lost on average over three pounds. This study also found a significant decrease in overall blood glucose and cholesterol in the women who consumed the two fruits.

Tips on Using Pears

SELECTION AND STORAGE:
- Pears are one of the only fruits that will ripen best off the tree.
- Choose firm and unblemished pears.
- To ripen pears quickly, place in a brown paper bag and store at room temperature.
- Bartlett pears will turn from green to yellow when they are ripe.
- To check for ripeness, press your thumb against the stem end of the pear (when slightly soft to the touch the pear is ready to eat).
- Pears should be stored at room temperature until ripe.
- Ripe pears can be stored in the refrigerator for about 3 to 5 days.

PREPARATION AND SERVING SUGGESTIONS:
- Wash and eat. . . . Eating the skin will provide your body with more fiber!
- Dried pears have higher fiber and potassium, lower vitamin C.
- Slice a ripe juicy pear into oatmeal or place in yogurt or a fruit smoothie.
- Add pears to your favorite green salad or fruit salad.
- Bake pears in the oven and sprinkle with cinnamon for a sweet-tasting treat.

Simple Baked Pear
by Cynthia Sass
Servings: 2 • Prep and cooking time: 40 minutes

This recipe contains three powerhouse foods.

INGREDIENTS:

1 ripe medium pear
1 tablespoon maple syrup
1 ½ tablespoons water
1 tablespoon raisins
Pinch freshly grated cloves and nutmeg

DIRECTIONS:
Preheat oven to 375 degrees. Combine maple syrup, water, and spices in a small bowl so raisins are fully covered. Soak raisins in maple solution for 20 minutes. Wash and core pear. Remove raisins and stuff into center of pear. Drizzle maple solution over top and sides of pear. Bake in glass baking dish covered loosely with foil at 375 degrees for about 20 minutes or until tender.

BREAK IT DOWN . . .
Calories: 90; Total fat: 0g; Saturated fat: 0g; Cholesterol: 0mg; Sodium: 0mg; Total carbs: 23g; Fiber: 2g; Sugar: 18g; Protein: 0g.

Pecans *(Carya illinoinensis)*

YOU CRACK ME UP

Did you know . . . that the name "pecan" is a Native American word that was used to describe nuts requiring a stone to crack?

What's the Story?

The pecan tree belongs to the hickory family and is one of the largest fruit-bearing trees known. There have been over 1,000 varieties created, of which only 500 now exist; and only a handful of varieties are commonly used today. The most popular pecan varieties include the Cape Fear, Desirable, Elliott, Schley, and the Sumner. The pecan is the only tree nut that is truly native to the United States.

A Serving of Food Lore . . .

Pecans were first "discovered" growing in North America and parts of Mexico by European colonists in the 1600s. America's President, Thomas Jefferson, loved pecans and had trees imported from Louisiana planted in his Monticello orchards. One of the origin tales of the pecan pie recounts that pecan pie was created by a French person who settled in New Orleans, and was introduced to the nut by Native Americans.

Where Are Pecans Grown?

Eighty percent of the world's pecans comes from the United States, with Georgia leading the nation in production. Other states that grow pecans include Louisiana, Mississippi, Alabama, Texas, New Mexico, Arizona, Oklahoma, Florida, North Carolina, South Carolina, Arkansas, California, and Kansas. Pecans are also grown in Mexico, Australia, Israel, Peru, and South Africa.

Why Should I Eat Pecans?

Pecans are a source of thiamine, gamma-tocopherol (a type of vitamin E), magnesium, protein, and fiber. They ranked fourteenth in total antioxidant capacity according to a 2004 report in the *Journal of Agricultural and Food Chemistry* and eighth out of fifty foods according to a report from the Institute of Basic Medical Sciences at the University of Oslo in Norway. They are also rich in the heart-healthy phytochemical beta-sitosterol. Pecans are also a rich source of heart-healthy oleic acid, the same type of fat found in olive oil.

Throw Me a Lifesaver!

HEART HEALTH: Researchers from Loma Linda University and New Mexico State University discovered that adding 1½ ounces of pecans a day (27 to 30 pecan halves) as part of a heart-healthy diet reduced LDL ("bad") cholesterol twice as much as those who did not add pecans to their American Heart Association Step I diet. Triglycerides were also reduced and HDL ("good") cholesterol rose for those who consumed the pecans. Another study from Loma Linda showed that adding just a handful of pecans into one's diet each day dramatically increased levels of gamma-tocopherol, a type of vitamin E thought responsible for reducing lipid oxidation. Study subjects who had normal lipid levels ate a little over two ounces of pecans per day for eight weeks and showed significant decreases in LDL and total cholesterol.

Tips on Using Pecans

SELECTION AND STORAGE:
- When selecting pecans, look for plump nutmeats that are fairly uniform in color and size.
- Unshelled pecans can be stored in a cool, dry place for three to six months.
- Shelled pecans need to be refrigerated in airtight containers and can be kept up to nine months. Pecans stored in freezer bags can be frozen for up to two years.

PREPARATION AND SERVING SUGGESTIONS:
- Basic toasted pecans: Preheat oven to 300 degrees. Place ½ cup of shelled pecans on a baking sheet in a single layer. Roast for approximately seven minutes but be careful not to burn them.
- Sprinkle chopped pecans on salads and fruit salads.
- Throw some on cold or hot cereal, whole wheat pancakes or waffles.
- Add chopped pecans to just about any side dish—they really add flavor to pilafs.
- Use crushed pecans as an alternative to breading meat or fish.

Black Cherry, Gingersnap, and Pecan Parfait
Courtesy of the Georgia Pecan Commission
Servings: 4 • Prep time: 10 minutes

This wonderful dessert is best made at least thirty minutes ahead of serving, allowing time for the gingersnap crumble to soften slightly. My kids, who are not exactly *nuts* about nuts, enjoyed this dessert. This recipe contains four powerhouse foods. The "ginger" snaps don't count but they sure make the dish yummy!

INGREDIENTS:

8 gingersnaps
½ cup pecan halves, toasted if desired
2 (6 ounces each) containers nonfat black cherry yogurt
⅔ cup fat-free whipped topping
2 kiwis, peeled and chopped
1 black cherry for garnish (optional)

DIRECTIONS:
In a medium-size resealable plastic bag, combine gingersnaps and ¼ cup pecans; seal bag. With a rolling pin or large heavy spoon, gently pound mixture to crumble cookies and pecans. (The mixture should be somewhat coarse, not finely ground.) Set aside. In a small bowl, mix all yogurt together. Add whipped topping and gently fold in to blend. Do not overmix. To assemble in individual 6- to 8-ounce glass serving pieces, spoon 2 tablespoons gingersnap-pecan mixture into bottom of each glass. Top each with ¼ cup yogurt mixture. Portion the chopped kiwi into each glass and top with remaining yogurt mixture. Top each serving with remaining gingersnap-pecan

mixture. Coarsely chop remaining ¼ cup pecan halves and sprinkle on top for garnish. Refrigerate parfaits at least 30 minutes or up to two hours. Serve chilled.

BREAK IT DOWN . . .
Calories: 254; Total fat: 9g; Saturated fat: .5g; Cholesterol: 1mg; Sodium: 150mg; Total carbs: 30g; Fiber: 2.5g; Sugar: 16g; Protein: 6g.

Peppers *(Capsicum)*

WOULDN'T YOU RATHER EAT A PEPPER TOO?
Did you know . . . red and green bell peppers are one and the same? A red bell is a riper version of the green but has twice as much vitamin C and eleven times more beta-carotene!

What's the Story?

The *Capsicum* umbrella of peppers includes varieties from the sweet bell (red, yellow, green, and purple) to hot chili peppers. There are several varieties of chili peppers and each differs in flavor and heat intensity. The pain caused by the heat of the pepper is actually a group of phytochemicals called capsaicinoids, which act on pain receptors in the mouth and throat. Capsaicin is the primary capsaicinoid and can be found in varying degrees throughout the pepper. William Scoville, a chemist, developed a heat-ranking scale based on the amount of capsaicin a pepper has. Bell peppers rank a zero (no capsaicin) while the habanero varieties may go well beyond 350,000! In general, larger chilies are milder because they contain fewer seeds and white membrane (the hottest part of the chili) in proportion to their size. Most pepper varieties can be found dried, canned, or fresh.

A Serving of Food Lore . . .

Peppers have been traced back 6,000 years ago in Central and South America. Columbus brought pepper seeds back to Spain in 1493.

Where Are Peppers Grown?

China, Turkey, Spain, Romania, Nigeria, and Mexico are the main producers of bell peppers. India, Mexico, Indonesia, China, and Korea are the leading hot pepper producers.

Why Should I Eat Peppers?

Peppers are rich in vitamin C and a good source of beta-carotene and B vitamins. They also contain flavonoids and capsaicinoids, inflammation-reducing phytochemicals.

Home Remedies

Heat up cold feet with a pinch of cayenne pepper in each sock. (Can you smell what the sock's got cookin'?) You'd think the last thing you might want to swallow is hot peppers when you have a sore throat, but because of its anti-inflammatory effects, cayenne pepper may be soothing instead.

Throw Me a Lifesaver!

SKIN CANCER: There appear to be other capsaicinoids beyond hot capsaicin that have health benefits. A mouse study showed that capsiates in sweet pepper induced cell death (apoptosis) in skin cancer cells.

PROSTATE CANCER: Capsaicin, found in red peppers, had an antiproliferative effect on both androgen-positive and -negative prostate cancer cells when fed to mice with prostate cancer.

ARTHRITIS: A task force found that out of seventeen evaluated treatment types for hand arthritis, only six of them were supported by research evidence. The use of topical capsaicin (a phytochemical in hot pepper) cream was one of them.

Tips on Using Peppers

SELECTION AND STORAGE:
- Bell peppers come in a variety of colors.
- Choose peppers with tight skin and that are firm to the touch.

- Store unwashed bell peppers in a plastic bag in the refrigerator. They will stay fresh for about a week. Sweet peppers can be frozen without being blanched.
- Green bell peppers will stay fresh a little longer than the yellow and red ones.

PREPARATION AND SERVING SUGGESTIONS:
- Cut top off of peppers and remove seeds.
- Grill peppers until skin becomes blackened. Place peppers in a Ziploc bag for 15 minutes to allow them to steam. Remove pepper from bag and scrape the skin off. Remove stem and core, and remove seed from pepper.
- Add a dash of cayenne pepper to your favorite sauce or side dish to spice it up!
- Grilled sweet bell peppers are delicious on sandwiches.
- Chop up a little jalapeño or serrano pepper and add it to chopped tomatoes, onions, garlic, and green pepper for a tasty salsa cruda.

Red Pepper Hummus on Zahtar Whole Wheat Pita
by Dave Grotto
Servings: 8 • Prep and cooking time: 15 minutes

Zahtar is a Middle Eastern seasoning consisting of sesame seeds, sumac, and thyme. It is easy to make but much easier to buy at a specialty store. This recipe contains five powerhouse foods.

HUMMUS INGREDIENTS:

1 can garbanzo beans, drained	2 cloves garlic
1/3 cup sesame tahini	3/4 cup (1 large) roasted
2 tablespoons extra-virgin olive oil	red pepper

ZAHTAR PITA INGREDIENTS:

2 tablespoons zahtar	2 whole wheat pitas
1 teaspoon extra-virgin olive oil	

DIRECTIONS:

Roast red pepper over open flame until charred. Remove black skin. Core and remove seeds. Slice into medium pieces. Combine red pepper and all other ingredients in a food processor and blend until creamy. Set aside. Brush olive oil on pita bread. Sprinkle zahtar seasoning liberally over pita. Toast until browned. Cut into triangles and serve with hummus.

BREAK IT DOWN . . .
Calories: 210; Total fat: 11g; Saturated fat: 1.5g; Cholesterol: 0mg; Sodium: 90mg; Total carbs: 22g; Fiber: 5g; Sugar: 1g; Protein: 7g.

Persimmon *(Diospyros kaki L.)*

HEAVENLY FRUITING BODY
Did you know . . . the Greek word *diospyros* means "food of the gods"?

What's the Story?

More than two thousand different varieties of persimmons exist today! Persimmon, also known as "Sharon fruit" or "Kaki," can be classified into two general categories: those that bear astringent fruit until they are soft-ripe and those that bear nonastringent fruits. The shape of the fruit varies from spherical to acorn to flattened or squarish, and the color can range anywhere from light yellow-orange to dark orange-red. The size can be as little as a few ounces to more than a pound. The entire fruit is edible except for the seed and calyx.

An astringent cultivar must be jelly-soft before it is fit to eat and includes varieties such as Eureka, Hachiya, Honan Red, Saijo, Tamopan, Tanenashi, and Triumph. A nonastringent persimmon can be eaten when it is crisp as an apple and includes varieties such as Fuyu (Fuyugaki), Gosho/Giant Fuyu/O'Gosho, Imoto, Izu, Jiro, Maekawajiro, Okugosho, and Suruga. Then, a third category is seedless astringent varieties, which include Chocolate, Gailey, Hyakume, Maru, and Nishimura Wase. The Hachiya type makes up approximately ninety percent of the available fruit and can be identified by its acornlike shape.

A Serving of Food Lore . . .

The Asian persimmon is native to China, where it has been cultivated for centuries. It then spread to Korea and Japan many years ago, where additional cultivars were developed. The plant was introduced to California in the 1880s when a United States naval commander brought back a native Japanese persimmon variety to Washington, D.C.

Where Are Persimmons Grown?

The largest producers are China, Brazil, Japan, Italy, and Korea. The majority of persimmons in the United States are grown in California and they are also grown to a lesser extent in Hawaii, Texas, and some other southern states.

Why Should I Eat Persimmons?

Persimmons are an excellent source of vitamin A, a good source of vitamin C, and rich in fiber. They contain a variety of phytochemical antioxidants such as proanthocyanidin, epicatechin, gallic, and p-coumaric acids. One study found persimmons to be higher in soluble and insoluble dietary fibers, total phenols, and many minerals than apples.

Home Remedies

The leaves of the persimmon have been used in Chinese medicine for a variety of conditions: as a poultice for snakebites and skin irritations, as a beverage made from boiled leaves for hypertension, for reducing blood clotting, and to fight cancer.

Throw Me a Lifesaver!

LEUKEMIA: Two human cell line studies showed that persimmon extract strongly inhibited the growth and induced apoptosis (programmed cell death) of leukemia cells.

CHOLESTEROL: Rats who had a persimmon-supplemented diet had significantly less total cholesterol, LDL cholesterol, triglycerides, and lipid peroxides compared to rats who didn't eat persimmons.

Tips on Using Persimmons

SELECTION AND STORAGE:

- Look for persimmons that are round and plump, and have smooth, glossy skin and deep red undertones. Avoid fruits that are missing the green leaves at the top.
- Unless you are planning to eat them right away, buy firmer fruits and allow them to ripen.
- Ripe Fuyu persimmons look like flattened tomatoes and are crisp, while the acorn-shaped Hachiya is very soft and juicy.
- Store them in the refrigerator when ripe.
- Eat the fruit as soon as possible. Overripe persimmons quickly turn mushy.

PREPARATION AND SERVING SUGGESTIONS:

- Wash Fuyu variety persimmons, remove core and leaves, and slice or eat whole.
- Rinse Hachiya persimmons and slice in half. Remove seeds and spoon fruit out of skin.
- Add firm Fuyu persimmon slices to salads, pancakes, waffles, and hot or cold cereal.
- Puree Hachiya persimmon flesh and add it to drinks, smoothies, or fresh fruit sauces. You can also use the puree to make cookies.
- Slice Fuyu and spread with lime juice, salt, and chili powder. Eat with a slice of low-fat cheese.
- Make salsa with a twist—add Fuyu, onion, tomatillo, cilantro, and chili serrano, and mix together.

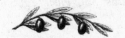

Persimmon Muffins
by Chef J. Hugh McEvoy
Serves: 12 • Prep and baking time: 20 minutes

This recipe contains eight powerhouse foods.

INGREDIENTS:

8 ounces fresh persimmon

1 cup enriched all-purpose
　　unbleached white flour

1 cup whole wheat flour

⅓ cup agave syrup

¼ cup canola oil

¼ cup yellow raisins

¼ cup seedless California
　　raisins

4 ounces dry-roasted pecans,
　　unsalted

2 large whole eggs

⅛ teaspoon ground allspice

⅛ teaspoon ground cloves

½ teaspoon ground cinnamon

¼ cup water

1 teaspoon baking powder

1 teaspoon baking soda

DIRECTIONS:

Presoak raisins in water. Preheat oven to 375 degrees. Using a food processor, blend persimmon pulp, agave, eggs, canola oil, spices, baking powder, and baking soda until smooth. Transfer to a hand mixing bowl. Add flour and hand-mix just until smooth. Drain water from raisins into muffin mixture. Add raisins and nuts, gently fold until evenly mixed. DO NOT overmix. Portion into medium-size muffin pan (¾ full). Bake until done; a toothpick should come away clean—about 12 to 14 minutes. Dust with powdered sugar when cool.

BREAK IT DOWN . . .

Calories: 270; Total fat: 13g; Saturated fat: 1g; Cholesterol: 32mg; Sodium: 159mg; Total carbs: 36g; Fiber: 3g; Sugar: 19g; Protein: 4g.

Pineapples *(Ananas comosus)*

MACHINE CORE

Did you know . . . though canned pineapple was sold in 1901, it wasn't widely available until engineer Henry Ginaca invented a machine in 1911 that could remove the outer shell, inner core, and both ends of 100 pineapples in under sixty seconds?

What's the Story?

Pineapple is related neither to the pine tree nor the pine nut nor the apple. Pineapple is the only edible member of the *Bromeliaceae* family. Also known as Ananas, Nanas, and Pina, pineapples take a full eighteen months to grow and must be grown from the crowns or tops of other pineapples and are only harvested when ripe. Popular varieties include the Smooth Cayenne, Red Spanish, Sugar Loaf, and the Golden Supreme, with a golden yellow flesh that has a sweeter taste than all of the other varieties.

A Serving of Food Lore . . .

The pineapple is native to southern Brazil and Paraguay. The name "pineapple" came from European explorers who thought the fruit resembled a cross between a pinecone and an apple. Christopher Columbus was the first person to introduce pineapples to Europe after discovering them on the Caribbean island of Guadeloupe in 1493.

Where Are Pineapples Grown?

Besides Hawaii, pineapple is also grown in Costa Rica, Honduras, Brazil, Mexico, the Dominican Republic, El Salvador, Ecuador, Nicaragua, the Philippines, Thailand, and China.

Why Should I Eat Pineapples?

Pineapples are a good source of vitamin C, vitamin B6, manganese, and copper. They also contain a group of digestive enzymes called bromelain that have anti-inflammatory properties.

Home Remedies

Pineapple peel may be effective in removing corns by softening and breaking down the dead skin. Possibly this may be due to the activity of bromelain, a protein-digesting enzyme. However, no research studies have been conducted.

Throw Me a Lifesaver!

Much of the research surrounding pineapple is really focused on the protein digestive enzyme bromelain, which naturally occurs in pineapple. Bromelain's properties include:

- Interference with growth of malignant cells and tumors
- Inhibition of platelet aggregation
- Fibrinolytic activity
- Anti-inflammatory action
- Skin debridement properties
- Enhanced absorption of drugs (amoxicillin)

Dr. Andrew Weil, considered the "father of alternative medicine," reports that bromelain is an effective treatment for severe bruises and hematomas and can promote healing of injuries by reducing pain and swelling. He also relays that bromelain:

- Reduces postoperative swelling
- Helps relieve symptoms associated with sinusitis
- When combined with antibiotics and trypsin (an enzyme), can also help control the symptoms of urinary tract infections
- May help relieve symptoms of rheumatoid arthritis

Results of several clinical trials indicate that bromelain acts as a blood-thinner and can help relieve the symptoms of angina and thrombophlebitis.

CANCER PREVENTION: Cornell University food scientists found that eating pineapples reduced the formation of nitrosamines (potential carcinogens) in humans.

Tips on Using Pineapples

SELECTION AND STORAGE:
- Look for one that is heavy for its size, free of soft spots and bruises, and has a sweet smell at the stem end.
- Most canned pineapple comes packed in its own juice so there is no need to purchase pineapple in heavy or even "light syrup" varieties.
- They can be left at room temperature for one to two days or in a plastic bag in the refrigerator for three to five days.
- If the pineapple is already cut, store it in an airtight container with some of its own juice to stay fresher.

PREPARATION AND SERVING SUGGESTIONS:
- To prepare a pineapple, first use a knife to remove the base and crown. Then cut it into quarters, remove the core, and make slices in the quarters by cutting from flesh to rind, and separate the fruit from the rind.
- Pineapple corers are also available.
- Pineapple juice makes a great base for most marinades. Because of the protein digestive qualities of bromelain, pineapple juice makes a great meat tenderizer.
- Fruit salads—pineapple is a great addition to salads, especially those with other tropical fruits.
- Pineapple juice and sparkling water combined make a refreshing beverage.

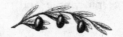

Grilled Pineapple and Chili Pork Tenderloin
with Mesclun Greens
by Chef Dave Hamlin
Servings: 4 • Prep and cooking time: 35 minutes

This recipe has an amazing twelve powerhouse foods!

INGREDIENTS FOR CHUTNEY:

¼ cup red pepper, diced small

¼ cup green pepper, diced small

¼ cup red onion, diced small

1 cup fresh pineapple, diced small
(reserve the remaining
pineapple)

½ teaspoon fresh ginger, minced

½ teaspoon fresh garlic, minced

2 scallions, diced

1 teaspoon cilantro, minced

½ teaspoon chili powder

¼ teaspoon cumin

3 tablespoons rice wine vinegar

INGREDIENTS FOR TENDERLOIN:

1 pound pork tenderloin

1 teaspoon extra-virgin olive oil

4 1" pineapple slices

3 cups mesclun greens

½ teaspoon chili powder

Salt and pepper to taste

DIRECTIONS:

Mix all ingredients for chutney together and reserve. Prepare chutney while grill is heating up. Rub tenderloin with small amount of olive oil. Season with salt and pepper. Sprinkle with chili powder. Slice reserved pineapple into ½"-thick slices. Grill pork tenderloin on all sides on medium-high heat to an internal temperature of 150 degrees (about 10 to 12 minutes). While pork is grilling, grill the pineapple slices. Remove pineapple and pork and let rest for approximately 5 minutes.

TO PLATE:

Lay down a bed of mesclun greens. Shingle the grilled pineapple slices over the greens. Slice pork on the bias in ¼"-thick slices and shingle in the center of the plate against the grilled pineapple. Spoon chutney over sliced pork.

BREAK IT DOWN . . .
Calories: 350; Total fat: 11g; Saturated fat: 3.5g; Cholesterol: 105mg; Sodium: 240mg; Total carbs: 27g; Fiber: 3g; Sugar: 21g; Protein: 36g.

Pistachios *(Pistacia vera)*

SEEING RED

Did you know . . . pistachios from outside the United States were originally dyed red to hide imperfections resulting from crude harvesting methods? But natural pistachios grown in the U.S. today are harvested with state-of-the-art equipment that preserves their natural beauty. "Red" pistachios are still available for those who prefer them.

What's the Story?

Pistachios are related to the cashew, peach, and mango family. They grow on trees in grapelike clusters and it takes about ten to fifteen years for a tree to mature enough to yield a good crop. Harvesting is still done by hand in Turkey, where workers shake the trunks of the pistachio trees by hand, whereas large machines are used to shake pistachio trees in California.

A Serving of Food Lore . . .

Evidence from excavations has shown that tribes in the Near East gathered pistachios as far back as 20,000 B.C. Archaeologists discovered remnants of pistachios in Turkey dating as far back as 7000 B.C. Pistachios are also mentioned in the Bible (Genesis 43:11). The Queen of Sheba was so enamored with pistachios that she was known to have claimed exclusive rights to all pistachio production. In ancient Persia (Iran), couples met underneath the pistachio tree on moonlit nights listening to ripe nuts crack open in hopes that good fortune would be released upon them.

Prior to 1976, all pistachios consumed in the U.S. were from the Middle East; the first commercial crop of California pistachios was produced that year.

Where Are Pistachios Grown?

Iran and California currently compete as the world's largest producer and exporter of pistachios in the world. Turkish and California pistachios are the predominant pistachios in the United States as the tariffs on Iranian pistachios make it cost-prohibitive to carry in the U.S. The variety most commonly grown in the United States is a descendent from the Kerman region in Iran.

Why Should I Eat Pistachios?

Pistachios are high in fiber and, in fact, a serving of pistachios contains more fiber than half a cup of broccoli. They are a good source of protein, supplying six grams per ounce (about 49 kernels). A one-ounce supply provides as much potassium as half of a large banana and contains good amounts of other minerals such as magnesium, copper, and phosphorus. They are a good source of thiamine, vitamin B6, and the gamma-tocopherol form of vitamin E.

Pistachios are the richest source of phytosterols—which may have anticancer and heart-health properties—amongst all of the tree nuts. They are also high in the amino acid arginine, which may help dilate blood vessels to enhance blood flow to all areas of the body, and are the richest source of the phytochemical lutein, excellent for eye health, compared to any other tree nut.

Throw Me a Lifesaver!

CANCER: The pistachio is second only to wine as a tremendous source of the plant chemical resveratrol. This substance may play a role in fighting cancer and heart disease.

HEART HEALTH: Because of pistachio's "quad-combo" of heart-healthy substances—high phytosterol (279mg/100g), gamma tocopherol, arginine, and high monounsaturated fat content—they are an excellent addition to the diet to help fight heart disease and improve circulation. Healthy subjects who ate twenty percent of their calories as pistachios for three weeks had decreased oxidative stress and total cholesterol with improved HDL levels.

MACULAR DEGENERATION: Pistachios are the highest tree-nut source of lutein.

Tips on Using Pistachios

SELECTION AND STORAGE:

- Look for shells that are already cracked open. Closed shells usually contain immature kernels and should be discarded.
- Pistachios draw moisture from the air, which causes them to eventually lose their crunch. To maintain freshness, store them in an airtight container in the refrigerator.
- Pistachios will maintain their freshness in the freezer for at least a year.

PREPARATION AND SERVING SUGGESTIONS:

- Slightly split shells can be opened by wedging one half of the shell from an already-opened pistachio into the split and turning it until you can retrieve the kernel.
- If a recipe calls for 1 cup of shelled pistachios, use two cups of unshelled.
- You can remove the skin from shelled nuts by blanching the nuts for one minute, then dry in the oven on low heat for fifteen minutes, or you can remove the skin by toasting them.
- Add pistachios to muffins; either in the batter or crumbled on top.
- Throw a handful into cold or hot cereal or make a trail mix of pistachios, dried fruit, and chocolate chips.
- Chopped pistachios make a great coating for fish, chicken, or meat.

Pistachio Dover Sole

by Chef J. Hugh McEvoy

Servings: 6 • Prep and cooking time: 30 minutes

This recipe contains six powerhouse foods.

INGREDIENTS:

36 ounces Dover Sole fish fillets
1 cup dry-roasted pistachios,
    shelled
½ cup olive oil
¼ cup fresh basil, chopped
¼ cup fresh parsley, chopped

2 tablespoons fresh shallots,
    chopped
1 fresh garlic clove,
    chopped
¼ teaspoon sea salt
¼ teaspoon black pepper

DIRECTIONS:

Preheat oven to 400 degrees. Using a food processor, chop nuts slightly, add fresh herbs, all but one tablespoon of the olive oil, shallots, salt, and pepper. Blend into a chunky/smooth emulsion. Set aside. Using remaining olive oil, lightly sauté fish fillets in a pan over medium heat. Do not fully cook fish. Place browned fillets into a buttered baking dish or pan. Spread a thick layer of pistachio coating over each fish fillet. Bake fish until crisp-crusted and cooked just until fish flakes.

BREAK IT DOWN . . .

Calories: 415; Total fat: 27g; Saturated fat: 11g; Cholesterol: 122mg; Sodium: 320mg; Total carbs: 7g; Fiber: 2g; Sugar: 0g; Protein: 37g.

Plums aka "Prunes" (Prunus domestica)

MONKEY BUSINESS

Did you know . . . in 1905, a plum grower from California decided to "hire" five hundred monkeys to pick his plums? Unfortunately, the cost savings in labor he thought would happen didn't really materialize. His new "hired hands" ate all of the plums they picked!

What's the Story?

Prunes are dried plums like raisins are dried grapes. Four of the most common varieties are French, Imperial, Italian, and Greengage. In recent years, the term "dried plums" has been used by industry on packaging in place of prunes, which carries some stigma among the last few generations of Americans. It takes 3 pounds of fresh plums to produce one pound of dried plums.

A Serving of Food Lore . . .

The idea to preserve the fresh fruit by drying in the sun probably began in the Caspian Sea region. In California in the mid-nineteenth century, Louis Pellier planted plum tree cuttings from France.

Where Are Plums Grown?

Nearly one hundred percent of plums grown in the United States and seventy percent of the world's supply are from California.

Why Should I Eat Plums?

Plums are a rich source of fiber and contain important nutrients such as potassium, vitamin K, and minerals such as iron. They also contain caffeoylquinic acid, a phenolic compound, which has high antioxidant activity. In fact, the antioxidant content of fresh plums doubles when they become prunes.

Home Remedies

Whether stewed or dried, plums have always been mom's first choice in relieving constipation. A large German study found that plums were most effective for relieving constipation in those patients suffering from chronic constipation and those diagnosed with irritable bowel syndrome (IBS). Plums also contain sorbitol, a naturally occurring sugar alcohol which tends to promote laxation.

Throw Me a Lifesaver!

BONE HEALTH: A study of rats that were fed plums showed reduced bone loss.

CHOLESTEROL: Men who ate twelve plums daily in addition to their diet had significant lowering of LDL cholesterol.

CANCER: Plums contain ursolic acid, which interferes with cell-signaling pathways and thus may protect against some forms of cancer.

COLON CANCER: A study using rats fed varying amounts of a plum diet found a significant decrease in colon cancer risk factors.

Tips on Using Plums

SELECTION AND STORAGE:
- Plums should be plump, shiny, free of mold, and somewhat soft.
- Extend their freshness by storing them in an airtight container in the refrigerator where they will last up to six months.

PREPARATION AND SERVING SUGGESTIONS:
- Soak plums that are very dry in hot water for a few minutes. If cooking plums, soaking them beforehand in water or juice will cut down on cooking time.
- Trail mix—dice up prunes and mix with a variety of other dried fruits and nuts.
- Baking—cut down on fat and increase moistness by substituting an equal amount of plum puree for fat in the recipe.
- Top pancakes or waffles with stewed or soaked plums.
- Stuffing—add plums to your favorite stuffing.

Breakfast Pudding
from *Stealth Health* by Evelyn Tribole
Servings: 6 • Prep and cooking time: 45 minutes (refrigerate for at least two hours)

If you have kids who are not too thrilled about eating plums, try this recipe. The taste is wonderful. Garnish the pudding with fresh berries and serve chilled. . . . Yum! This recipe contains four powerhouse foods.

INGREDIENTS:

1 (12-ounce package) pitted plums
   (about 2 cups)
1½ cups orange juice
1 teaspoon cinnamon

¼ teaspoon nutmeg
2 (8-ounce) containers nonfat
   vanilla yogurt

DIRECTIONS:

Combine the plums, orange juice, cinnamon, and nutmeg in a medium saucepan; bring to a boil over medium heat. Remove from heat, cover, and set aside for 30 minutes or longer. Puree the plums with all of the orange juice in two batches in a food processor or blender. Gently fold in the vanilla yogurt until blended. Stir in the cinnamon and nutmeg. Transfer to six 6-ounce custard cups. Cover and refrigerate at least 2 hours or overnight.

BREAK IT DOWN . . .
Calories: 230; Total fat: 1.5g; Saturated fat: .5g; Cholesterol: 5mg; Sodium: 60mg; Total carbs: 53g; Fiber: 4g; Sugar: 41g; Protein: 5g.

Pomegranate *(Punica granatum L.)*

FOR IT IS WRITTEN . . .
Did you know . . . pomegranates are traditionally eaten on the Jewish holidays of Rosh Hashanah and Sukkot? The number of seeds found in the fruit is the exact same number of commandments in the Torah—613!

What's the Story?

The name "pomegranate" is a combined form of the latin words *pomum,* meaning "apple," and *granatum,* meaning "grainy" or "seeded." There are about fourteen varieties of pomegranate that are consumed throughout the world. "Wonderful" is the best known variety in the United States. Other popular varieties include "Grenada," "Early Foothill," and "Early Wonderful."

A Serving of Food Lore . . .

Pomegranates are one of the oldest known fruits and are thought to have originated in Iran and northern India. The pomegranate appears in Egyptian mythology and art, and was carried by Egyptians in the desert because of its thirst-quenching juice. The ancient city of Granada in Spain was renamed after the fruit during the Moorish period. Spanish conquistadors brought the fruit to the Americas in the early 1500s.

Where Are Pomegranates Grown?

Pomegranates grow abundantly throughout Asia, the Middle East, the Mediterranean region, and the United States. California's San Joaquin Valley is home to most pomegranate orchards.

Why Should I Eat Pomegranates?

Pomegranates are rich in vitamin C and many different types of antioxidants. The major antioxidant activity of pomegranates comes from three anthocyanidins: delphinidin, cyanidin, and pelargonidin. The polyphenol content in pomegranate juice is three times that found in green tea and red wine. Polyphenol research is most promising in the areas of heart disease and cancer prevention.

Home Remedies

In India, pomegranates are used for preserving food, and as an antiseptic and disinfectant. The Greek physician Dioscorides often prescribed pomegranate for oral and gastric disorders. Pomegranate juice can help those who suffer from chronic diarrhea.

Throw Me a Lifesaver!

ANTIMICROBIAL: Pomegranates have been found to be effective in killing a variety of life-threatening bacteria in laboratory experiments.

CARDIOVASCULAR DISEASE: Different studies with humans and mice found that supplementation with pomegranate juice helped prevent the development of fatty streaks in arteries. In another heart-related study published in the *American Journal of Cardiology,* researchers noted that patients who drank pomegranate juice daily for three months had improved heart function.

CANCER: A cell study using human breast cancer cells found that treatment with pomegranate extract significantly inhibited cancer cell growth and increased cell apoptosis (cell death). Another cell study found that pomegranate juice reduced inflammatory cell signaling in colon cancer cells. Men with rising prostate-specific antigen (PSA) scores after receiving radiation therapy who consumed pomegranate juice daily had an increase in cell apoptosis (cell death) and a decrease in cell proliferation. And other research points to pomegranate's ability to inhibit protaste tumor growth.

HYPERTENSION: A human study involving hypertensive patients who consumed eight ounces of pomegranate juice for fourteen days showed a decrease in systolic blood pressure and a thirty-six percent decreased risk of stroke.

BONE LOSS: An animal study found that those mice given pomegranate extract for two weeks showed a significant decrease in bone loss.

Tips on Using Pomegranates

SELECTION AND STORAGE:
- Pick one that is heavy for its size, with taut, thin, shiny, smooth skin.
- Pomegranates should be stored in a cool, dark place, where they will last for about a month. If refrigerated, they can keep for about two months.
- Seeds can be stored in the refrigerator for about three days and can be frozen in an airtight container for about six months.
- Pomegranate juice can be kept in the freezer for about six months.

PREPARATION AND SERVING SUGGESTIONS:
- To remove the seeds, slice off the crown end and score the rind vertically from top to bottom.
- Place the pomegranate in a bowl of water and break the sections apart. The seeds will sink to the bottom and the membranes and rind will float.
- To make juice, put the seeds in a food processor until juice is formed and strain the seeds through a fine-mesh sieve.
- Topping: Sprinkle pomegranate seeds on desserts and salads.
- Pomegranate juice can be used to make marinades, sauces, vinaigrettes, jelly, and juice.

Pomegranate/Cranberry Sauce for Chicken or Turkey
by Chef Kyle Shadix
Servings: 12 (¼ cup) • Prep and cooking time: 22 minutes

This sauce is delicious over ANYTHING! Three-quarters of a cup of agave syrup can be substituted for the honey, if desired. This recipe is a grand slam, with all five ingredients being powerhouse foods.

INGREDIENTS:

2 cups 100% pomegranate juice   ½ cup pomegranate seeds
1 cup honey   Zest of 1 lemon or orange
One 12-ounce bag fresh or frozen
     cranberries (3 cups)

DIRECTIONS:

Pour pomegranate juice and honey in a saucepan and bring to a boil. Add cranberries and simmer, stirring occasionally, until berries just pop, 10 to 12 minutes. Stir in zest and pomegranate seeds, and chill.

BREAK IT DOWN . . .
Calories: 210; Total fat: 0g; Saturated fat: 0g; Cholesterol: 0mg; Sodium: 0mg; Total carbs: 57g; Fiber: 1g; Sugar: 52g; Protein: 0g.

Potatoes *(Solanum tuberosum L.)*

CHIP ON HIS SHOULDER

Did you know . . . in 1853, railroad tycoon Commodore Cornelius Vanderbilt was displeased with a chef who cut his potatoes too thick? Chef George Crum mockingly sliced the commodore's potatoes paper-thin, fried them, and sent them back to him. Vanderbilt loved his new potatoes and named them "Saratoga Crunch Chips," the forerunner of today's potato chip.

What's the Story?

There are over 500 varieties of potatoes grown worldwide and fifty different varieties typically consumed in the United States. Most U.S. supermarkets only carry five to seven different varieties. The starchy, brown-skin, white-flesh Russet is the most widely used potato variety in the United States. Waxy Round Whites have a smooth, light tan-colored skin with white flesh. Long Whites are medium starch, oval-shaped, and have thin, light tan skin. These potatoes have a firm, creamy texture. Red-skinned potatoes have rosy red skins and white flesh. These waxy tubers are often referred to as "new potatoes." Starchy Yellow Flesh are popular in Europe and becoming increasingly popular in the United States. They have a dense, creamy texture. They look buttered when cooked. Finally, Blue and Purple, originally from South America, have a nutty flavor and flesh that ranges from dark blue or lavender to white.

A Serving of Food Lore . . .

Inca Indians in Peru were the first to cultivate potatoes, around 200 B.C. In 1536, Spanish conquistadors brought them back to Europe and it was Sir Walter Raleigh who introduced them to Ireland in 1589. However, Europeans first considered potatoes "evil" due to their similarities to the potentially poisonous nightshade family (mandrake and belladonna are members). Potatoes were brought to colonial America in 1621 and the first potato patches in North America were established in New Hampshire in 1719. A terrible fungus destroyed the potato crops in Ireland in 1856, devastating the economy in what has now become known as "The Great Irish Potato Famine."

Where Are Potatoes Grown?

Potatoes are mainly grown in Poland, India, the Russian Federation, China, and the United States.

Why Should I Eat Potatoes?

A medium-sized potato contains nearly half of the daily recommended intake of vitamin C, and with the skin on, potatoes supply twenty-one percent of the daily value of potassium. By comparison, the potato has as much vitamin C as a medium tomato and twice as much potassium as a banana. Potatoes of color, particularly red- and purple-skin and -flesh potatoes, contain the highest levels of antioxidants, especially carotenoids and anthocyanins.

NOT JUST SKIN DEEP

A popular belief is that all of the nutrition is contained within the skin of the potato. More than fifty percent of the overall nutrition content can be found in the potato itself! But why sell yourself short? Eat the whole thing!

Home Remedies

The Incas placed potatoes on broken bones to promote healing. Whole potatoes were carried to prevent rheumatism, and eaten with other foods to prevent indigestion. Washing your face with cool potato juice clears up blemishes. Carrying a potato in your pocket was thought to make tooth pain go away. An old remedy for sore throat was placing a slice of baked potato in a stocking and tying it around the throat.

Throw Me a Lifesaver!

CANCER: Human case studies have shown that lectins, such as those found in potatoes, attach to receptors on cancer cell membranes, leading to apoptosis and cytotoxicity, and inhibiting tumor growth.

CARDIOVASCULAR HEALTH: A long-term study that followed 84,251 women found that eating potatoes may be heart-healthy.

DIABETES: Potato peel added to the diet of diabetic rats was found to significantly reduce plasma glucose and drastically reduce frequent urination complication attributed to diabetes. The total food intake was significantly reduced too.

HYPERTENSION AND STROKE: According to the Food and Drug Administration, "Foods, such as potatoes, that are good sources of potassium and low in sodium may reduce the risk of high blood pressure and stroke."

Tips on Using Potatoes

SELECTION AND STORAGE:
- Select firm, smooth potatoes. Avoid those with wrinkled or wilted skins, soft dark areas, cut surfaces, or those green in appearance.
- Potatoes will keep for several weeks when left in a cool, dark place with good ventilation. But don't store potatoes in the refrigerator because they will become dark when cooked.

PREPARATION AND SERVING SUGGESTIONS:
- Waxy type potatoes are ideal for salads, boiling, or roasting. Starchy types are great for baking and mashing.
- Trim off green areas and sprouts ("eyes") but leave the skins on for more nutrition!
- Wash potatoes thoroughly before eating, scrubbing with a vegetable brush.
- Pierce several times and microwave until tender, turning halfway through cooking time.
- Serve baked, mashed, roasted, or fried. Potatoes are even delicious raw!

Art's Vesuvio Potatoes
by Arthur Grotto aka "Noni"
Servings: 12 • Prep and cooking time: 90 minutes

This recipe contains three powerhouse foods.

INGREDIENTS:

3 pounds Russet potatoes	½ teaspoon salt
½ cup olive oil	½ teaspoon black pepper
1 tablespoon rosemary	½ cup dry white wine
1 tablespoon sage	

DIRECTIONS:
Preheat oven to 400 degrees. Lightly coat roasting pan with olive oil. Slice potatoes into quarters. Brush each slice with olive oil. Place in roasting pan. Sprinkle pepper, salt, sage, and rosemary over potato spears, covering well. Place roasting pan in oven, uncovered. Cook

for approximately one hour or until pierced easily with a fork. Sprinkle spears with wine and cook until golden brown.

BREAK IT DOWN . . .
Calories: 180; Total fat: 9g; Saturated fat: 1.5g; Cholesterol: 0mg; Sodium: 105mg; Total carbs: 21g; Fiber: 2g; Sugar: 1g; Protein: 2g.

Pumpkin *(Cucurbita maxima)*

THE GREAT PUMPKIN

Did you know . . . the heaviest pumpkin in the world weighed in at 1,469 pounds?

What's the Story?

Pumpkin comes from the Greek word "pepon" or "big melon." Cantaloupe melon, cucumber, and squash are also related to the pumpkin. Pumpkins best suited for carving on Halloween are not necessarily the best for making pumpkin pie. In fact, there are basically two different categories of pumpkin: canning pumpkins and carving pumpkins. And orange is not the only color choice, either. There's white, Australian Blue, and a red variety from Europe called Rouge D'Etant.

A Serving of Food Lore . . .

Pumpkin seeds found in Mexico were estimated to be at least 7,500 years old. Pumpkins were a mainstay in Native American culture and in fact, the entire pumpkin was used not only for food, but Native Americans would also make mats and other products from the shell. The first pumpkin pie was made by early settlers by filling a hollowed-out pumpkin shell with honey, milk, and spices and then baking it.

Where Are Pumpkins Grown?

The biggest producers of pumpkins include the United States, India, China, and Mexico. The "Pumpkin Capital of the World" is in Morton, Illinois, where Libby's pumpkin processing plant is located.

Why Should I Eat Pumpkins?

Pumpkin is a good source of fiber, potassium, selenium, vitamin A, beta-carotene, alpha-carotene, beta-cryptoxanthin, and lutein. Pumpkin seeds are a good source of omega-3 fats and an excellent source of phytosterols, which may benefit enlarged prostate glands. In fact, the use of pumpkin seeds for enlarged prostate dates back over 100 years. Plant phytosterols are helpful in lowering cholesterol, too.

Home Remedies

Folk medicine suggests consuming pumpkin seeds for reducing enlarged prostate glands. Pumpkin is one of the traditional Chinese medicines used to alleviate some of the complications and chronic diseases caused by diabetes. Eating unroasted pumpkin seeds with the onset of nausea helps alleviate motion sickness.

Throw Me a Lifesaver!

CANCER: A long-term Japanese study involving 1,988 gastric, 2,455 breast, 1,398 lung, and 1,352 colorectal cancer patients and 50,706 non-cancer outpatients showed that frequent consumption of pumpkin was associated with decreased risk for all four types of cancer.

PROSTATE CANCER: A correlation study found that those subjects who consumed pumpkin regularly had a decreased risk of developing prostate cancer.

DIABETES: A Japanese case-control study involving 133 participants with a history of diabetes mellitus found that those who ate a good amount of pumpkin had better blood glucose control.

HYPERTENSION: Hypertensive rats that were treated with pumpkin seed oil had reduced progression of hypertension.

ASTHMA: Diets high in omega-3 fatty acids, like those found in pumpkin seeds, may be beneficial to asthma sufferers.

Tips on Using Pumpkins

SELECTION AND STORAGE:
- For baking, look for "pie pumpkin" or "sweet pumpkin," which are sweeter and less watery than jack-o'-lantern pumpkins.
- Choose one that is heavy and has a good shape.
- Store in a cool, dry place. But once cut, pumpkin must be cooked that same day.

PREPARATION AND SERVING SUGGESTIONS:
- Remove the stem with a sharp knife and cut the pumpkin in half.
- Remove all of the seeds and stringy mess (save the seeds to roast later, if desired).
- Boil or steam: Cut the pumpkin into large chunks, rinse them, place them in a large pot with approximately one cup of water (the water doesn't need to cover the pieces), cover, and boil for 20 to 30 minutes until tender, or steam for 12 minutes.
- Oven: After you have cut the pumpkin in half, rinse with cold water, place the cut side down on a large cookie sheet, and bake at 350 degrees for one hour until tender.
- Microwave: Cut pumpkin in half, place cut side down on microwave-safe plate, microwave on high for 15 minutes until tender.
- Dice pumpkin, steam, and sprinkle nutmeg on it.
- Puree pumpkin and carrots, sliced onions, leeks, and chopped celery and parsley for a simple soup.
- Roast pumpkin seeds by first rinsing seeds well and then spreading them on a cookie sheet. Roast at 375 degrees for 20 to 30 minutes until dry; cool and serve. Sprinkle on salt, if desired.

Baby Roasted Pumpkins with Pink Potatoes
by Chef J. Hugh McEvoy
Serves: 9 • Prep and baking time: 90 minutes

This recipe contains four powerhouse foods.

INGREDIENTS FOR PUMPKINS:

9 (6 pounds) whole mini   3 tablespoons canola oil
   pumpkins   1 teaspoon sea salt

INGREDIENTS FOR SMASHED POTATOES:

2 pounds fresh red potatoes
  with skin

1 pound sweet potatoes baked
  in skin

¼ cup fresh green onions bulbs
  and tops, chopped

¼ cup unsalted butter

DIRECTIONS:

Remove tops from pumpkins and save. Remove seeds and threads. Cut level bottoms for stable baking. "Paint" the pumpkins with canola oil inside and out. Bake in a 350-degree oven for approximately 1 hour or until lightly brown and tender. Cut potatoes with skins on into even cubes. Steam until tender. Mash gently using a wire masher. Add butter and a bit of milk if needed. Add chopped green onion. Fill baked pumpkins with mashed potatoes. Brush potatoes and pumpkins with melted butter. Return to oven until golden brown, about 10 minutes. Serve covered with pumpkin tops as "hats."

BREAK IT DOWN . . .
Calories: 280; Total fat: 8g; Saturated fat: 2g; Cholesterol: 5mg; Sodium: 270mg; Total carbs: 52g; Fiber: 5g; Sugar: 26g; Protein: 6g.

Quinoa *(Chenopodium quinoa Willd)*

FOOD FIGHTER

Did you know . . . a mixture of quinoa and fat was used to sustain Incan armies, which frequently marched for many days? The mixture was known as "war balls."

What's the Story?

Quinoa (pronounced *keen-wa*) refers to the seed, about the size of millet, of the Chenopodium or "Goosefoot" plant. It is a relative of spinach and Swiss chard and comes from the Andes Mountains region of South America. There are over 1,800 known varieties of quinoa with color ranges from pale yellow to red to brown to black. The grain is soft and creamy but has a "tail" that is crunchy. Quinoa is available as a grain, flour, pasta, and cereal.

A Serving of Food Lore . . .

Quinoa was a staple food of both the Aztecs and the Incas that can be traced back some 5,000 years. It has been cultivated in the South American Andes since at least 3000 B.C. With the advent of the Spanish conquest in the 1500s, what was once a major crop headed toward a four-hundred-year decline in production. For quite some time, quinoa was only grown by peasants in remote areas for their own consumption. Now quinoa is making a resurgence as a valued crop for its nutrition value.

Where Is Quinoa Grown?

Most quinoa is imported from South American countries such as Peru, Bolivia, and Ecuador, although it is also being cultivated in the Colorado Rockies in the United States.

Why Should I Eat Quinoa?

Nutritionally, quinoa is an amazing grain! The nutritional quality has been compared to that of dried whole milk by the Food and Agriculture Organization (FAO) of the United Nations. Quinoa contains more protein than any other grain. Some varieties of quinoa have more than twenty percent protein! And what is unique about the protein in quinoa is that it is complete, containing all essential amino acids, being especially high in the amino acids lysine, methionine, and cystine. By adding it to other grains, those proteins become complete too. It also complements soy, which is lower in methionine and cystine. Quinoa is rich in iron, potassium, and riboflavin as well as B6, niacin, and thiamin. It is also a good source of magnesium, zinc, copper, and manganese, and has some folate (folic acid). Quinoa contains at least sixteen different triterpine saponins which may have anticancer and anti-inflammatory properties and inhibit cholesterol absorption.

Throw Me a Lifesaver!

WEIGHT MANAGEMENT: Compared to rice and wheat, quinoa was found to offer greater satiety, thus making it an ideal food for fighting obesity.

VACCINE HELPER: Quinoa enhanced antibody responses to antigens that were introduced into mice. The study showed the potential of quinoa saponins as "helpers" for vaccines.

Tips on Using Quinoa

SELECTION AND STORAGE:
- Quinoa products on the market include flour, pasta, flakes, brown, black, and red one hundred percent grain.
- Quinoa flour and grains should be stored in a sealed container in the refrigerator. Use the grains within a year and flour within 3 months.

PREPARATION AND SERVING SUGGESTIONS:
- Rinse quinoa before use to remove any of the powdery residue (saponin) that remains on the seeds. You may see "suds" when the seeds are swished in water—that is the saponins being removed. In South America the saponin which is removed from the quinoa is used as detergent for washing clothes and as an antiseptic to promote healing of skin injuries.
- Toast the grain in a dry skillet for five minutes before cooking to give it a delicious roasted flavor.
- Be careful not to add too much water or cook it too long, since quinoa can become mushy. Quinoa only takes about fifteen minutes to cook!
- It is excellent in hot casseroles, pilafs, soups, stews, and stir-fries, or cold in salads.
- Quinoa's light texture makes it an ideal choice as a base for salad. Mix cooled, cooked quinoa with chopped raw or cooked vegetables and fresh herbs, then toss it with a vinaigrette or soy sauce dressing.

Caribbean Quinoa
by Dawn Jackson Blatner

Servings: 6 • Prep and cooking time: 30 minutes

According to Dawn Jackson Blatner, spokesperson for the American Dietetic Association, quinoa is a "delicious, nutritious, and quick-cooking grain." When you try her recipe, I think you will agree! This recipe contains seven powerhouse foods.

INGREDIENTS:

1 cup quinoa
2 cups water
4 green onions, chopped
2 mangoes, diced
¼ cup sliced almonds
¼ cup dried cranberries

3 tablespoons fresh cilantro,
  chopped
1 lime, juiced
1 cup white balsamic vinegar
Salt and pepper to taste

DIRECTIONS:

Rinse and drain quinoa. Toast quinoa in a hot empty pan for about 5 minutes. Add 2 cups water. Bring to a boil, cover, and simmer over medium heat about 15 minutes until all water is absorbed. Let quinoa cool. Gently stir remaining ingredients into quinoa. Serve as a room temperature or cold salad.

BREAK IT DOWN . . .
Calories: 190; Total fat: 4g; Saturated fat: 0g; Cholesterol: 0mg; Sodium: 20mg; Total carbs: 36g; Fiber: 3g; Sugar: 14g; Protein: 5g.

Raspberries (Rubus)

HOW SWEET IT IS!
Did you know . . . xylitol, a popular sugar alternative, is made from raspberries?

What's the Story?

There are over two hundred known species of raspberries that range in color from red (*Rubus ideaus*) and black (*Rubus occidentalis*) to the less familiar orange, purple, and yellow varieties. Raspberries have similarities to both of their cousins: the blackberry and the strawberry. Raspberries and blackberries are collectively known as "bramble" fruits, which are fruits formed by the aggregation of several smaller fruits called drupelets.

A Serving of Food Lore . . .

Raspberries are native to Asia Minor and North America. Earliest recordings show that raspberries were popular around the time of Jesus Christ. Romans are thought to have begun the domestication of raspberries around the fourth century and spread raspberry cultivation throughout Europe. The British are credited with popularizing raspberries, especially in jam and jelly form, and for bringing the plants to New York in the mid-1700s. Cultivation of the native American black raspberry began in the 1800s.

Where Are Raspberries Grown?

The leading producers are Poland, Russia, Germany, Yugoslavia, Chile, and the United States.

Why Should I Eat Raspberries?

Raspberries are a good source of fiber, phosphorus, and selenium, and an excellent source of vitamin C. Raspberries are rich in a variety of antioxidants and phytochemicals associated with fighting disease. Flash freezing and processing raspberries into preserves destroys much of the vitamin C, but luckily most of the other antioxidants remain.

Home Remedies

Raspberry leaf tea is used to treat nausea and vomiting associated with morning sickness. Fresh raspberries, which are high in vitamin C, have been used to treat and prevent sinus infections.

Throw Me a Lifesaver!

CANCER: There are several recent studies that look at different cancers and the benefits of using raspberries or raspberry extract for potential treatments. A study using a rat model of human esophageal cancer cells found that a diet containing black raspberries significantly reduced tumor cell growth. A case-control studying using hamsters found that black raspberries will inhibit oral tumor formation. A cell study using the phytochemicals ferulic acid and beta-sitosterol, commonly found in black raspberries, stopped the growth of both premalignant and malignant oral cancer cell growth. A study observing the effects of raspberry extracts on human liver cancer cells found that the more extract that was used, the less replication of cells occurred.

DIABETES: Anthocyanins, powerful compounds found in raspberries, reduce blood glucose levels after starch-rich meals.

OBESITY AND FATTY LIVER: A study using mice fed high-fat diets and varying amounts of raspberries discovered that raspberries helped prevent and improve fatty liver and also reduced obesity.

Tips on Using Raspberries

SELECTION AND STORAGE:
- Avoid spoilage by making sure there are no signs of moisture and that they are not packed too tightly.
- Remove any berries that are spoiled or moldy, and place the un-washed berries back into their original container.
- Raspberries will keep fresh in the refrigerator for about two days.
- To freeze raspberries, rinse, pat dry, place them on a cookie sheet, and put them in the freezer. Transfer to a plastic bag. Frozen raspberries will keep for up to one year.

PREPARATION AND SERVING SUGGESTIONS:
- Gently wash them and pat dry.
- Top your cereal, salads, yogurt, ice cream, waffles, or pancakes.
- Raspberries are a great addition to fruit smoothies.

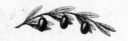

Raspberry-Peach Melba Tart

Adapted from *Healthy Homestyle Desserts* by Evelyn Tribole

Servings: 10 • Prep and cooking time: 20 minutes

This recipe contains three powerhouse foods.

INGREDIENTS:

1 whole wheat pie shell, prepared and cooled

FILLING:

8 ounces fat-free cream cheese
4 ounces light cream cheese

½ cup powdered sugar
1 teaspoon vanilla

PEACH GLAZE:

⅓ cup granulated sugar
1 tablespoon cornstarch

One 6-ounce can peach nectar

FRUITS:

2 kiwis, thinly sliced
1 peach, peeled and thinly sliced

One 6-ounce basket fresh
raspberries

DIRECTIONS:

In a small bowl, beat together the cream cheeses, powdered sugar, and vanilla. Spread the mixture on the cooled crust. Chill for 30 minutes. In small pan, stir together granulated sugar and cornstarch, and gradually add in peach nectar. Cook and stir over medium-high heat until the mixture begins to bubble. Cook and stir for 1 minute more. Remove from heat and cool at least 5 minutes. Using a pastry brush, apply a thin layer of glaze over the cream-cheese filling. Add kiwi slices. Add a thin layer of glaze. Add peaches and glaze. Top with raspberries and remaining glaze.

BREAK IT DOWN . . .

Calories: 220; Total fat: 9g; Saturated fat: 3g; Cholesterol: 0mg; Sodium: 180mg; Total carbs: 30g; Fiber: 3g; Sugar: 19g; Protein: 6g.

Rice, Brown

HERE COMES THE BRIDE!
Did you know ... the ancient ritual of throwing rice symbolized prosperity, abundance, and fertility—wishing the intended the blessing of many children?

What's the Story?

Rice is actually a grass and refers to two different species, *Oryza sativa* and *Oryza glaberrima*, with the first being most predominant. There are thousands of varieties of rice in existence with white being the most commonly consumed. However, white rice doesn't start off white—it becomes white from processing whole grain rice. Whole grain brown rice comes in Basmati, Texmati, short sweet, short, medium, and long grain versions. Whole grain rice also comes in black, red, and purple varieties.

A Serving of Food Lore ...

Rice is the most consumed grain in the world and is grown on every continent except for Antarctica. It has been part of the staple diet in Eastern countries for thousands of years. Recordings of rice consumption date back some 5,000 years ago in China. Rice arrived in Egypt in the fourth century B.C. and around that time India was exporting it to Greece and throughout Europe and eventually to the United States. Rice production has been part of U.S. agriculture since the late seventeenth century.

Where Is Brown Rice Grown?

China, India, Indonesia, and Bangladesh make up two-thirds of the world's rice production. The United States ranks eleventh in production but is a major exporter. In the U.S., the top rice producers include Arkansas, California, Louisiana, Mississippi, and Texas.

Why Should I Eat Brown Rice?

Rice is often the first solid food offered to an infant. It is the least allergenic grain and that is why it is often recommended as a first introductory food. Whole grain brown rice contains all three layers of the kernel—the bran, germ, and endosperm—which provides superior nutrition value over white rice. Brown rice is rich in lignans, phytoestrogens, and phenolic compounds that are high in antioxidant activity. Whole grain brown rice contains important nutrients such as thiamine, niacin, phosphorus, potassium, iron, riboflavin, and five times the fiber of white rice. The germ provides natural vitamin E. The bran of rice contains the phytochemicals that may reduce cholesterol.

Home Remedies

Japanese farmers ate mochi, a chewy cake made from brown rice, on cold winter days to increase their stamina.

Throw Me a Lifesaver!

HEART HEALTH: A small, randomized study examined the effects of adding rice bran oil to the diet. While the control diet did not lower cholesterol, the one containing rice bran oil lowered LDL cholesterol by seven percent. In studies of Finnish men, intake of brown rice is inversely related to not just cardiovascular-related death, but to all causes of death.

CANCER: Brown rice contains plant lignins, especially enterolactone, that help establish healthy flora in the human intestines credited with protecting against breast and other hormone-dependent cancers as well as heart disease. According to a Danish study of 857 postmenopausal women, those eating the most whole grains, including brown rice, were found to have significantly higher blood levels of enterolactone.

ALZHEIMER'S: Researchers discovered in animal experiments that eating brown rice reduced learning and memory deficits brought about by beta-amyloid protein, considered to be one of the leading contributors to Alzheimer's dementia.

Tips on Using Brown Rice

SELECTION AND STORAGE:

- Long grain rice produces light, dry grains that separate easily.
- Short grain rice produces almost-round grains that have higher starch content than either the long or medium grain varieties, and that stick together when cooked.
- Medium grain rice has size and texture characteristics between short and long.
- Brown rice has a shelf life of three to six months but can be extended by storing uncooked portions in the refrigerator.
- Refrigerate cooked brown rice for up to one week in a tightly covered container or in the freezer for approximately six months.

PREPARATION AND SERVING SUGGESTIONS:

- It takes approximately forty-five to fifty minutes to cook brown rice. There are instant and parcooked versions that take considerably less time but are equally nutritious.
- Rice cookers with timers are great to use to make perfect rice anytime.
- Use brown rice as a healthful filler in meat loaf, burgers, or other ground meat dishes.
- Use a half-and-half combination of brown rice and white rice. Mixing the two is also a good way to encourage kids to eat brown rice.
- Top a serving of brown rice with steamed vegetables and tofu, lean meat, poultry, or fish.

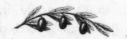

Bi Bim Bop
by Dave Grotto
Servings: 6 • Prep and cooking time: 30 minutes

Believe me: This dish is a meal in itself. The red bean paste added at the end really makes this recipe come to life. This recipe has eight powerhouse foods.

INGREDIENTS:

*1 pound beef, chicken, or seitan,
   cut in strips*
1 small yellow squash, julienned
1 large carrot, julienned
½ package bean sprouts
*2 dried shiitake mushrooms,
   rehydrated in hot water*
1 cup green onions, chopped
1 bag spinach

4 fried eggs (optional)
4 cups precooked brown rice
2 tablespoons sesame oil
¼ cup reduced-sodium soy sauce
¼ cup water
½ cup agave syrup
5 cloves minced garlic
Red bean paste to taste

DIRECTIONS:
Combine seitan (or meat), garlic, water, ¼ cup soy sauce, ¼ cup agave syrup, and 1 tablespoon of sesame oil in a medium bowl. Cover and refrigerate for at least 3 hours, preferably overnight. Julienne squash, carrots, and mushrooms. Start water boiling in a pot for spinach and bean sprouts. Add 1 tablespoon of sesame oil to a large frying pan and heat. Cook carrots, squash, green onions, and mushrooms separately. Add 1 tablespoon soy sauce and 2 tablespoons of agave syrup to each vegetable. Sauté until tender. Place in separate bowls. Cook meat/seitan with marinade in a large frying pan until well browned and meat starts to carmelize. Place in a separate bowl. Cook spinach for a minute, just enough to wilt. Cook sprouts for two minutes and set aside in bowl. Fry eggs, leaving yolk a little runny.

Add 1 cup of cooked brown rice to each individual serving bowl. Place a layer of spinach on top of the rice. Arrange portions each of mushrooms, carrots, sprouts, squash, onions, and meat on top of spinach. Top off with a fried egg. Add desired amount of red bean paste and serve. This dish tastes best when the egg is cut up and all ingredients are well mixed with the bean paste before eating.

BREAK IT DOWN . . .

Calories: 420; Total fat: 10g; Saturated fat: 2g; Cholesterol: 165mg; Sodium: 409mg; Total carbs: 57g; Fiber: 6g; Sugar: 25g; Protein: 29g.

Romaine Lettuce *(Lactuca sativa L.)*

"LETT-UCE C ABOUT THAT!"

Did you know . . . romaine is the most nutritious of all lettuces and is an excellent source of vitamin C (more than five times that of iceberg lettuce)?

What's the Story?

Romaine lettuce, known to the Romans as *Cappadocian* lettuce and to the Greeks as *Cos* lettuce, named after the Greek island that was the birthplace of Hippocrates, is a member of the sunflower family. Romaine lettuce has a stronger flavor than iceberg and is more tender and sweet and less bitter than other lettuce varieties. Lettuce is the second most popular vegetable consumed in the United States.

A Serving of Food Lore . . .

Lettuce is one of the oldest known vegetables and is believed to be native to the Mediterranean area. Romaine has been cultivated and eaten cooked or raw for almost 5,000 years and might be the oldest form of cultivated lettuce. Egyptian tombs reveal paintings of lettuce resembling romaine. Romaine lettuce was introduced to the United States from England in the 1600s.

Where Is Romaine Lettuce Grown?

Most lettuce in the United States is grown in California and Arizona but the main grower of romaine is Florida. About 18 million metric tons of lettuce are produced throughout the world.

Why Should I Eat Romaine Lettuce?

In addition to its high vitamin C content, romaine lettuce is also an excellent source of vitamin A. However, there is research that suggests that it's best to skip the no-fat dressing and opt for the full-fat version if you want to absorb any vitamin A from romaine! It is also a rich source of folic acid, supplying thirty-eight percent of the daily value in just one serving. Romaine also contains phosphorus, potassium, and fiber. Phytochemically, romaine lettuce is a good source of lutein and zeaxanthin—these phytochemicals are important antioxidants that battle many diseases. Romaine lettuce also contains a significant amount of lactucaxanthin, which is a rare dietary carotenoid that was found to suppress the Epstein-Barr virus, often associated with mononucleosis ("mono").

Home Remedies

Early Romans ate romaine at the end of the meal to aid in digestion and to promote sleep. Many Europeans still eat lettuce this way, but most Americans who eat romaine and other lettuces do so at the beginning of the meal. Caesar Augustus even built a statue praising lettuce because he believed it cured him of an illness.

Throw Me a Lifesaver!

MACULAR DEGENERATION: Romaine lettuce is rich in lutein and zeaxanthin, which are carotenoids found naturally in the eye that fight age-related macular degeneration, the leading cause of irreversible vision loss in the elderly.

WEIGHT MAINTENANCE: In a study conducted by Barbara Rolls, PhD, from Penn State, she found that starting off a meal with a low-calorie salad gave a sense of fullness and reduced subsequent calorie intake, which may be an effective way for managing weight.

REDUCED INFLAMMATION/HEART DISEASE/CANCER: Salicylic acid, a main compound found in aspirin, which is used to treat inflammation, has been found in romaine lettuce. Salicylic acid is a cyclooxygenase-2 (COX-2) inhibitor, a key enzyme involved in inflammation, certain cancers, and the promotion of heart disease.

Tips on Using Romaine Lettuce

SELECTION AND STORAGE:
- Look for large, unwilted, and darker-green outer leaves.
- Store lettuce in a plastic bag and place in the refrigerator crisper. Romaine lettuce will last for up to ten days.

PREPARATION AND SERVING SUGGESTIONS:
- Rinse lettuce under cold running water; you may also soak the leaves in the sink or in a large bowl. Dry leaves in a lettuce spinner or with a towel.
- When tearing leaves for salad, avoid bruising (which causes the leaves to discolor).
- Use as a base for a salad in addition to or as a replacement for other lettuces.
- Mix in with apple slices, raisins, dried cranberries (or your other favorite dried fruit), oranges, grapes, and pineapple.
- Serving a salad the next day, otherwise known as a "wilted" salad, may increase the absorption of nutrients.
- It's okay to cook lettuce (see below)! Try marinating romaine lettuce with a little soy sauce, dry white wine, brown sugar, and olive oil, and grill for a few minutes.

Romaine Sesame Stir-Fry
by Chef J. Hugh McEvoy
Serves: 6 • Prep and cooking time: 10 minutes.

This recipe contains five powerhouse foods.

INGREDIENTS:

1 pound romaine lettuce, chopped	½ tablespoon agave syrup
1 tablespoon garlic cloves, chopped	½ teaspoon toasted sesame oil
1½ tablespoons canola oil	½ teaspoon toasted whole sesame seeds
1 tablespoon light soy sauce	Kosher salt to taste
1 tablespoon Japanese rice wine	

DIRECTIONS:

Mix soy sauce, rice wine, agave, and salt in a small bowl and set aside. Preheat a large sauté pan [12 to 14 inch] or wok over high heat. Add canola oil. Immediately add garlic and stir-fry for a few seconds. Add chopped romaine. Stir-fry for about 1 minute, just until hot. Stir in the premixed sauce. Fold/stir-fry ingredients for 30 to 45 seconds. Lettuce should still be bright green and a bit crisp. Do not overcook. Remove/transfer into a large serving bowl. Drizzle with sesame oil and sprinkle with sesame seeds. Serve on a "bed" of raw, room-temperature romaine leaves and tomato slices. Serve with warm saki or chilled plum wine.

BREAK IT DOWN . . .

Calories: 56; Total fat: 4g; Saturated fat: 0g; Cholesterol: 0mg; Sodium: 180mg; Total carbs: 4g; Fiber: 2g; Sugar: 1g; Protein: 1g.

Rosemary *(Rosmariunus officinalis)*

ROSEMARY'S NO BABY

Did you know . . . rosemary is associated with longevity? Not so surprising, as some plants have been known to survive in the same location for as long as thirty years!

What's the Story?

Rosemary is an herb that has leaves resembling evergreen needles and belongs to the mint family. There are many varieties of rosemary that are available for both culinary and ornamental use but the popular cultivars for cooking are "Tuscan Blue," "Miss Jessup," and "Spice Island." The name "rosemary" is derived from the Latin name *rosmarinus* which means "dew of the sea"—rosemary commonly grows near the sea. Besides being used as an herb in flavorful dishes, rosemary is also used in cosmetics, disinfectants, shampoos, herbal medicine, and as a potpourri. The oil of rosemary is formed either from distilled flowering tops or from the stems and leaves. About 100 pounds of flowering tops yields about eight ounces of oil.

A Serving of Food Lore . . .

Rosemary is native to the Mediterranean area. Many cultures view rosemary as a symbol of love and fidelity. Brides have often worn a wreath of rosemary during their wedding ceremony. Guests attending the service would also receive a branch of rosemary as a symbol of love and loyalty. Rosemary is also used in funerals and other religious ceremonies as incense.

Where Is Rosemary Grown?

France, Spain, and the United States, specifically California, are the main growers of rosemary.

Why Should I Eat Rosemary?

A large number of polyphenolic compounds with antioxidant activity have been identified in rosemary that inhibit oxidation and bacterial growth.

Home Remedies

Rosemary tea is often used to ease headaches. In olden days, sprigs of rosemary were used to ward off "evil spirits" and nightmares. It was said that a sprig placed beneath the pillow would produce restful sleep. In Spain and Italy, many believed that the Virgin Mary had hidden in a rosemary bush for shelter. The scent of rosemary is supposed to be a memory-stimulant. In some countries, it is a custom to burn rosemary alongside the bed of sick patients and in some French hospitals, rosemary was burned with juniper berries to purify the air and prevent infection. Rosemary is often used to deter moths from invading clothing.

Throw Me a Lifesaver!

CANCER: Rosemary extract had a protective effect on human blood exposed to gamma rays (radiation). Rosemary also showed strong antimutagenic effects which may help prevent certain types of cancer.

Albino mice were fed an extract of rosemary for fifteen weeks. The number and size of papillomas were reduced in the treated animals. Carnosic acid, the main polyphenol antioxidant in rosemary, combined with vitamin D, enhanced cell differentiation and reduced human leukemia cancer cell spread in a cell line study. Similar results were achieved in mice.

PREVENTION OF BACTERIAL GROWTH: Rosemary oil was found to be highly effective against *E. coli* bacteria and may prevent the formation of certain types of bacterial growth in foods.

LUNG PROTECTION: Mice who were pretreated with an extract of rosemary prior to being exposed to diesel exhaust fumes had significantly less lung inflammation than those mice who were not pretreated.

Tips on Using Rosemary

SELECTION AND STORAGE:
- Rosemary is available in dried, oil, or fresh forms. Fresh is preferable because it loses most of its flavor when it is dried.

SERVING SUGGESTIONS:
- Fresh and dried leaves are commonly used in traditional Mediterranean cuisine as a flavor-enhancing herb.
- Rosemary is used to season poultry, lamb, fish, rice dishes, soups, and vegetables.
- The herb is often used to flavor wine and ales.

Rosemary-Garlic and Artichoke-Bean Spread
by Dave Grotto
Servings: 8 • Prep time: 20 minutes

This recipe contains nine powerhouse foods.

INGREDIENTS:

1 cup artichoke hearts
1 cup navy or any white bean
½ cup onions, chopped
⅛ cup extra-virgin olive oil
2 cloves garlic, minced
1 teaspoon fresh rosemary sprigs,
*   chopped*

1 tablespoon sweet chili sauce
¼ cup sun-dried tomatoes in oil,
*   drained and chopped*
1 teaspoon lemon zest
2 tablespoons fresh-squeezed
*   lemon juice*
Salt and cayenne pepper to taste

DIRECTIONS:
Combine all ingredients in a food processor and blend for approximately 30 seconds or until well-blended. Add cayenne pepper for a spicy version. Serve on celery sticks, with whole grain crackers, or as a sandwich spread.

BREAK IT DOWN . . .
Calories: 90; Total fat: 4g; Saturated fat: .5g; Cholesterol: 0mg; Sodium: 290mg; Total carbs: 11g; Fiber: 2g; Sugar: 2g; Protein: 4g.

Rye *(Secale cereale)*

FINNISH YOUR RYE!
Did you know . . . Finns eat approximately 110 pounds of bread per person every year, and one-third of that is made from rye?

What's the Story?

Rye is a cereal grain that is closely related to wheat and barley and varies in color from yellowish brown to grayish green. Rye is the main ingredient in making pumpernickel bread. Its gluten is less elastic than wheat, which makes breads made with rye more dense and compact. Rye can be found whole, cracked, as flour, or as flakes.

A Serving of Food Lore . . .

Rye probably first grew wild among barley and wheat fields in southwest Asia. It eventually made its way to eastern and northern Europe where it was first cultivated in Germany in 400 B.C. Rye continues to remain a staple food in Eastern European and Scandinavian countries.

Where Is Rye Grown?

Nearly 95 percent of the world's rye is grown in the area between the Ural Mountains and the Nordic Sea. The top rye growers are the Russian Federation, Belarus, Poland, and Germany.

Why Should I Eat Rye?

Whole grain rye contains many important vitamins and minerals, such as B vitamins, vitamin E, calcium, magnesium, phosphorus, potassium, iron, zinc, and folate. The insoluble fiber found in whole grain rye has a high concentration of lignans—more than any other cereal crop—which may offer cancer and heart-protective benefits.

Home Remedies

Rye cereal grain in its natural state has long been used to promote energy.

Throw Me a Lifesaver!

DIGESTIVE HEALTH: According to one study, the fiber from rye appears more effective than that from wheat in overall improvement of bowel health.

BREAST CANCER: A Finnish study involving 194 breast cancer patients and 208 control subjects found that high serum levels of enterolactone were associated with high intake of rye products and were inversely related to the risk of breast cancer.

CARDIOVASCULAR DISEASE: From 1989 to 2000, 3,588 elderly men and women took part in a long-term health study. Among the wealth of data were indications that consumption of rye bread, along with other dark breads, was associated with a lower risk of incident cardiovascular disease.

TUMORS: A cell line study showed that phytoestrogen and lignan extracts from rye significantly inhibited cancer cell proliferation.

PROSTATE CANCER: A rye bran diet was fed to mice that had developed prostate cancer. Apoptosis (cell death) increased over thirty percent and tumor cell reduction increased over twenty percent in the mice fed rye bran.

COLON CANCER: Another mouse study found that feeding mice with colon cancer a balanced high-fat diet with rye bran supplementation for 12 to 31 weeks was associated with a significant decrease in the number of tumors.

GALLSTONES: A hamster study found that when their diet was supplemented with rye bran, a lower frequency of gallstones occurred.

Tips on Using Rye

SELECTION AND STORAGE:
- Avoid rye that has evidence of moisture or webbing.
- If buying bread, read the label carefully on the ingredient list to see that rye is a predominant ingredient.
- Keep in an airtight container in a dark, dry, and cool place, preferably refrigerated, where it will keep for several months.

PREPARATION AND SERVING SUGGESTIONS:
- Before cooking rye, rinse it under running water to remove any dirt.
- Add one part whole rye to four parts boiling water with a pinch of salt. When the water boils, turn it down, cover, and simmer for about one hour.
- Soak the rye grains overnight and cook them for two to three hours for a softer texture.

- Use rye flour to make muffins and pancakes.
- Try rolled rye flakes for a tasty, hot breakfast cereal.
- Use rye bread to breathe new life into your favorite sandwich.

Rye Pizza Dough or Rolls
by Chef J. Hugh McEvoy
Servings: 8 • Prep and cooking time: 1 hour

This recipe contains two powerhouse foods.

INGREDIENTS:

I cup light rye flour
2 cups white bread flour
I cup water
2 teaspoons active dry baker's
* yeast*

I teaspoon kosher salt
¼ teaspoon maple sugar
* or syrup*
I tablespoon extra-virgin
* olive oil*

DIRECTIONS:
Place warm water, maple sugar, and yeast in a medium-large bowl. Let it stand until the yeast begins to grow. Stir in ⅓ of flour, and the oil and salt. Mix for a minute until evenly blended. Blend in remaining flour ¼ cup at a time. Dough will be very soft but should not be too sticky. Turn out onto a well-floured wooden cutting board. Knead dough for 5 minutes. Place in a buttered bowl, cover, and let the dough rise until doubled in bulk. Punch down the dough in bowl. Return dough to the floured cutting board. Knead again for one minute. Place back in bowl, cover, and allow to rise again. Dough is ready for pizza when it has doubled in size again.

BREAK IT DOWN . . .
Calories: 202; Total fat: 3g; Saturated fat: .5g; Cholesterol: 0mg; Sodium: 55mg; Total carbs: 38g; Fiber: 3g; Sugar: 5g; Protein: 6g.

Salmon *(Salmonidae)*

NOT WILD ABOUT IT?

Did you know . . . fat composition and contaminants of both farmed and wild salmon can vary widely, depending on species and the area they come from? Simply removing the skin after cooking may reduce many of these contaminants by up to fifty percent!

What's the Story?

Salmon is the common name for many different types of fish belonging to the family *Salmonidae.* Some of the fish within this family are salmon, while others are called trout. Some common Atlantic Ocean species include Atlantic salmon, landlocked salmon, and trout. Some common Pacific Ocean species include sockeye, chinook, pink, humpback, coho, cherry, and chum. Salmon are typically born in freshwater and migrate to the ocean; they return to the freshwater to reproduce. Pacific salmon typically die within a few days or weeks of spawning.

A Serving of Food Lore . . .

Research shows that at least ninety percent of salmon spawning in the same stream were born there. Salmon aquaculture is the major economic contributor to the world production of farmed finfish, representing over $1 billion in the United States annually.

Where Do Salmon Come From?

Salmon live in the Atlantic and Pacific Oceans, the Great Lakes, and other lakes throughout the world. The Kamchatka Peninsula in eastern Russia contains the world's greatest salmon sanctuary. The majority of Atlantic salmon in today's market is typically farmed (ninety-nine percent), while the majority of Pacific salmon is caught in the wild (eighty percent). Salmon farming is popular in Norway, Sweden, Scotland, Canada, and Chile; this type of salmon is most commonly consumed in the United

States and Europe. Most canned salmon in the United States is wild Pacific salmon; Alaskan salmon is always wild.

Why Should I Eat Salmon?

Salmon is a rich source of omega-3 fatty acids, which are necessary for proper brain functioning as well as a healthy cardiovascular system. Salmon is rich in protein and vitamin A. The flesh is usually orange or red due to the carotenoids found there. The main carotenoids found in salmon skin include astaxanthin and canthaxanthin. Salmon gain these carotenoids through their diets; wild salmon eat krill and tiny shellfish and farmed salmon get them from their feed. Astaxanthin is a natural antioxidant that is used as a coloring agent to give farm-raised salmon their namesake color, otherwise they would look somewhat gray. Salmon also contains important minerals including calcium, phosphorus, potassium, iron, magnesium, selenium, and zinc.

ANOTHER FISHY STORY?

Wild or farmed? Will the most nutritious version please raise their fin? Farm-raised get less exercise than wild salmon so they tend to be more fatty. And by being more fatty, they contain more omega-3 fats than their wild counterparts . . . but not by much. Either choice fits well in your diet!

Throw Me a Lifesaver!

OVERALL HEALTH: A review of observational studies suggests that the inclusion of fatty fish, such as salmon, along with fruit, vegetables, whole grains, nuts, and seeds, reduces the risk of cancer, heart attack, stroke, and diabetes. The omega-3 fats found in salmon have also shown benefit in improving heart health and fighting depression, asthma, and cancer.

Tips on Using Salmon

SELECTION AND STORAGE:
- Salmon comes fresh, frozen, canned, and smoked.
- Fresh wild-caught are only available for a few months out of the year. Farm-raised are available year-round.

- Fresh salmon should either be eaten or frozen within two days after purchase.

PREPARATION AND SERVING SUGGESTIONS:
- The skin should be removed, along with the bones.
- Be careful not to overcook salmon!
- Omega-3 fats can be destroyed by exposure to air, light, and heat, but freezing salmon will cause minimal loss.
- Salmon may be baked, broiled, fried, grilled, smoked, and even served raw as sushi.
- Common herbs that complement salmon include dill and rosemary.

Grilled Salmon with Cranberry-Cherry Salsa
Adapted from *The Golden Door Cooks Light and Easy* by Chef Michel Stroot
Servings: 4 • Prep and cooking time: 20 minutes

This is a family favorite. When I first prepared this dish at home, two of my daughters asked for seconds—that's a first! Though they love salmon, the cranberry salsa topping really made it extra special for them. Michel Stroot has married cranberries and cherries for great flavor and excellent health properties. This is a great anti-inflammatory dish with the featured ingredients of salmon, cranberries, cherries, and ginger! This recipe contains seven powerhouse foods.

INGREDIENTS FOR GINGERED CRANBERRY-CHERRY SALSA:

½ cup sweetened dried cranberries
½ cup cherries, pits removed
2 tablespoons sugar
2 tablespoons apple juice
2 tablespoons candied ginger, minced
1 teaspoon orange peel

INGREDIENTS FOR SALMON:

4 (4 ounces each) salmon fillets
1 teaspoon thyme or lemon thyme, dried
1 teaspoon salt, if desired
½ teaspoon black pepper, ground, if desired
12 whole chives, if desired

DIRECTIONS:
Preheat grill, stovetop grill, or broiler on high. Simmer cranberries, cherries, sugar, apple juice, candied ginger, and orange peel in medium saucepan over medium heat for 5 minutes or until cranberries are plump and soft. Remove salsa from heat and cool. Season salmon fillets with thyme, salt, and black pepper, if desired. Grill or broil for 3 to 5 minutes on each side until medium done. (Cooking time will vary with thickness of fillets.) Spoon ⅓ cup salsa on plate. Place salmon fillet in the center of plate; garnish with chives, if desired. Keep extra salsa in airtight container for up to 3 days.

BREAK IT DOWN . . .
Calories: 260; Total fat: 12g; Saturated fat: 3.5g; Cholesterol: 55mg; Sodium: 640mg; Total carbs: 16g; Fiber: 1g; Sugar: 14g; Protein: 23g.

Sardines *(Sardinops sagax caerulea)*

SNACK ATTACK!
Did you know . . . Saint Anthony's Day in Lisbon, Portugal, is one of the most popular festival days of the year? People take to the streets, where grilled sardines are the snack of choice.

What's the Story?

There are more than twenty species of sardines sold worldwide. The definition of sardines is somewhat vague and can refer to any number of small fish, but typically the ones sold in the United States are either sprats or herring. Much of the world supply of sardines is used as bait to catch larger fish.

A Serving of Food Lore . . .

In the nineteenth century, Napoleon realized the need to preserve food, and thus the first sardine was preserved in oil or tomato sauce. They used to be abundant off the coast of Sardinia, a Mediterranean island, and that's how they got their name. Sardines are also known as Atlantic or sea herring or pilchards.

Where Do Sardines Come From?

Sardines are found throughout the oceans of the world. Many of the fresh and canned sardines come from Portugal.

Why Should I Eat Sardines?

Sardines are coldwater fish that are good sources of omega-3 fatty acids, protein, and calcium (due to the small bones in the fish). A three-ounce serving supplies just as much calcium as a cup of milk—300 milligrams!

Home Remedies

Sardines are a good source of omega-3 fatty acids, which have been linked to alleviating depression.

Throw Me a Lifesaver!

HEART HEALTH: An animal study found that feeding sardines that were canned in olive oil to rats with high cholesterol was more effective at normalizing cholesterol than giving rats pure fish oil alone.

BREAST MILK ENHANCEMENT OF OMEGA-3 FATS: Results of a study of thirty-one nursing mothers found that those who consumed 100 grams of sardines two or three times a week had a significant increase in the omega-3 fat content of breast milk.

Tips on Using Sardines

SELECTION AND STORAGE:
- Buy fresh sardines from a fish market when available—they're delicious!
- Look for firm flesh and clear bright eyes.
- Rinse fresh sardines and place in a sealed container in a single layer

and covered with damp paper towels. Store the container in the refrigerator.
- For canned sardines, look for a sell-by date and use within that time.

PREPARATION AND SERVING SUGGESTIONS:
- For grilling fresh sardines, have the sardines scaled and gutted but leave the bones in.
- Drain the oil from canned sardines before using.
- Add sardines to your toast, cover with grated Swiss cheese, and place in a hot oven.
- In a skillet, heat olive oil, onion, garlic, and sardines that are canned in tomato sauce, until they are heated through, and add to your favorite cooked pasta.

Sardine Breakfast Toast
Adapted from www.cooks.com
Servings: 2 • Prep and cooking time: 15 minutes.

This recipe contains five powerhouse foods.

INGREDIENTS:

1 teaspoon canola-based mayonnaise

2 slices whole grain toast

6 sardines, olive oil–packed, drained

2 teaspoons capers, drained

¼ teaspoon freshly ground black pepper

1 clove garlic, minced

2 teaspoons chopped red onion

Wedge of fresh lemon

DIRECTIONS:
Spread mayonnaise on one side of each slice of toast. Mash 3 sardines onto each slice. Sprinkle on capers, chopped onion, lemon juice, pepper, and garlic. Toast until browned under broiler or in toaster oven.

BREAK IT DOWN . . .
Calories: 159; Total fat: 7g; Saturated fat: 1g; Cholesterol: 52mg; Sodium: 407mg; Total carbs: 15g; Fiber: 2g; Sugar: 2g; Protein: 12g.

Sesame *(Sesamun indicum)*

What's the Story?

Sesame seeds are flat, oval seeds that come from the sesame plant and in a variety of colors such as yellow, white, red, and black. Sesame seeds are used to make sesame oil, which is very resistant to rancidity.

A Serving of Food Lore...

Sesame seeds first originated in India and then made their way to the Middle East, Africa, and Asia. Sesame seeds were one of the earliest condiments and processed crops for oil. In the seventeenth century, they made their way from Africa to the United States.

Where Are Sesame Seeds Grown?

The largest commercial producers of sesame seeds are China, India, and Mexico.

Why Should I Eat Sesame Seeds?

Sesame seeds are a rich source of lignans that may fight many hormonally driven cancers, particularly breast and prostate. Sesame seed and wheat germ are ranked highest in phytosterols. Pistachios and sesame seeds are the richest nut and seed sources of phytosterols, thought to fight heart disease and help reduce benign prostatic hyperplasia (swollen prostate).

Home Remedies

ACHES AND PAINS: Mix the juice of grated fresh ginger with an equal amount of sesame oil, dip a cotton linen into the mix, and briskly rub into the skin of the affected area.

CONSTIPATION: To a mug of hot water add one tablespoon of honey and a dash of sesame oil, stir, and repeat every morning before breakfast.

CONGESTION: Add 15 grams of sesame seeds to 250 milliliters of water, add 1 tablespoon of linseed, a pinch of salt, and some honey. Consume this every day to help remove phlegm from the bronchial tubes.

Throw Me a Lifesaver!

CANCER: A study using human lymphoid leukemia cells found that treatment with a sesame extract, sesamolin, led to growth inhibition by inducing cell apoptosis.

HYPERTENSION AND STROKE: A study using hypertensive rats found that ingestion of sesamin, a phytochemical in sesame seeds, reduced both elevation in blood pressure, oxidative stress, and blood-clotting activity. Using sesame oil as the sole cooking oil for sixty days lowered patients' blood pressure levels.

MELANOMAS: A cell study using human malignant melanocytes found that sesame oil selectively inhibited malignant melanoma growth.

Tips on Using Sesame

SELECTION AND STORAGE:
- If purchasing from the bulk section, inspect for bugs and webbing.
- Sesame seeds come in whole or "hulled" forms.
- Sesame oil comes plain and "toasted."
- Unhulled seeds can be stored in an airtight container in a dry, cool, dark place.
- Once hulled, store in the refrigerator or freezer.

PREPARATION AND SERVING SUGGESTIONS:

- Toast your own sesame seeds by placing them on a cookie sheet and baking in the oven at 350 degrees for 10 to 15 minutes or until slightly brown.
- Baked goods: Add sesame seeds to your homemade bread, cookies, or muffin batter.
- Add sesame seeds to steamed broccoli and sprinkle with lemon juice.
- Salad dressing: Mix sesame seeds, tamari, rice vinegar, and crushed garlic.

Sesame Mushroom Beef
by Chef J. Hugh McEvoy
Servings: 5 (6 ounces) • Prep and cooking time: 20 minutes

For a vegetarian version, substitute "beef"-flavored seitan—a meat replacer made from wheat gluten—for beef. This recipe contains seven powerhouse foods.

INGREDIENTS:

2 ounces roasted and toasted whole sesame seeds
4 ounces beef sirloin strip or 4 ounces "beef" seitan
4 ounces shiitake mushrooms
4 ounces fresh portobella mushrooms, sliced
4 ounces fresh white mushrooms, sliced

8 ounces snow peas, whole
2 ounces fresh green onion bulbs and tops, chopped
4 ounces organic fat-free beef broth or vegetable broth
1 tablespoon canola oil
1 tablespoon organic s esame oil
1 tablespoon hoisin sauce

DIRECTIONS:

Cut beef or seitan into very thin slices across the grain. Coat the slices with the sesame oil. Spread sesame seeds on large plate. Coat with sesame seeds. Preheat a heavy, large, nonstick skillet over high heat. Add canola oil. Add mushrooms; stir-fry until golden brown on edges. Add green onions; stir-fry 1 minute. Add snow peas; stir-fry until crisp-tender, about 1 minute. Add beef; stir-fry until brown, about 1 to 2 minutes. Add broth and hoisin sauce. Reduce heat to low. Mix until evenly blended. Cook only until sauce comes to a boil. Season with salt and pepper to taste. Serve over white or brown rice or over steamed Asian noodles.

BREAK IT DOWN . . .
Calories: 200; Total fat: 14g; Saturated fat: 2g; Cholesterol: 12mg; Sodium: 100mg; Total carbs: 10g; Fiber: 4g; Sugar: 3g; Protein: 8g.

Sorghum *(Sorghum bicolor)*

I'LL DRINK TO THAT!
Did you know . . . that sorghum is a key ingredient in Guinness beer?

What's the Story?

Sorghum, like wheat and spelt, is actually a grass. There are many varieties and hybrids of sorghum but in the United States, sorghum is classified as a single species: *Sorghum bicolor.* There are two main types of sorghum: the grain (nonsaccharine), and the sweet (saccharine) sorghum. Sorghum is commonly used for fodder; foods, such as couscous, flour, porridge, syrup, and sugar; and the production of alcoholic beverages. It has become a popular grain worldwide as it is inexpensive and easy to grow in many areas of the world, making it an ideal tool in fighting world hunger! Like corn, sorghum can be used to produce ethanol to fuel cars. Currently, twelve percent of sorghum produced in the United States is used to make ethanol and that amount is expected to increase in light of the energy crisis.

A Serving of Food Lore . . .

Sorghum may have originated in northeast Africa some 2,000 years ago. Some believe that wild sorghum has been growing in the Middle East as far back as 8,000 years ago. Sorghum was brought to America during the Colonial period; settlers used to refer to sorghum as "chicken corn." Sweet sorghum (sorgo) was introduced to America from China in 1850; the place of origin of sorgo is thought to be Egypt. In the United States, sorghum is primarily used as livestock feed. In China, sorghum is important in producing many beverages, including Maotai and kaoliang. In many parts of India, bhakri (unleavened bread) made from sorghum is a staple in the diet.

Where Is Sorghum Grown?

Sixty million tons of sorghum are grown annually and the main producer is Africa, followed by North America and Asia. Most sorghum syrup production occurs in the south-central and southeastern United States.

Why Should I Eat Sorghum?

Sorghum is a good source of vitamins and minerals such as niacin, riboflavin, thiamine, calcium, iron, phosphorus, and potassium. Sorghum has in its bran layers high levels of phytochemicals, including proanthocyanidins, 3-deoxyanthocyanins, phenolic acids, phytosterols, and policosanols, known for fighting heart disease. Sorghum is high in fiber, and depending on the type of sorghum, fiber content can range anywhere from 9 to 11 grams per serving.

Throw Me a Lifesaver!

HEART HEALTH: Sorghum is a good source of phytochemicals that may help fight heart disease and lower cholesterol, such as phenolic compounds, plant sterols, and policosanols. In a study of male hamsters who had sorghum added to their diet for a four-week period, decreases in LDL cholesterol levels and reduced cholesterol absorption were observed.

CELIAC DISEASE: Sorghum lacks gluten-containing proteins typically found in wheat, rye, and barley, and is therefore considered safe for those diagnosed with celiac disease or gluten intolerance.

Tips for Using Sorghum

SELECTION AND STORAGE:
• Sorghum can be purchased in grain, flour, syrup, and sugar form. Sorghum can also be found in certain types of cereals.

- Store sorghum flour in an airtight container. It can be kept in the refrigerator for months.

PREPARATION AND SERVING SUGGESTIONS:
- Sorghum may be roughly ground and used as a mush or porridge or made into flour for mixing with wheat flour for breads.
- Add to recipes to increase fiber content without affecting the taste or look of the product. Because sorghum has little taste, it can be added to virtually any recipe.

Sorghum & Orange Marmalade Muffins with Cranberries
Adapted from *Gluten-Free 101* by Carol Fenster
Servings: 12 muffins • Prep and baking time: 60 minutes

This recipe contains six powerhouse ingredients.

INGREDIENTS:

1 cup sorghum flour

1 cup potato starch

⅓ cup tapioca flour

½ cup granulated sugar

1 tablespoon baking powder

1½ teaspoons xanthan gum

1 teaspoon salt

2 large eggs

¾ cup skim milk

¼ cup canola oil

¾ cup applesauce

½ cup fruit-only orange
   marmalade

1 teaspoon vanilla extract

½ cup dried cranberries

¼ cup finely chopped walnuts

DIRECTIONS:
Preheat oven to 375 degrees. Prepare muffin pan with nonstick cooking spray. In a large mixing bowl, combine all ingredients except cranberries. Mix on low to blend ingredients slowly, then increase speed to medium and beat until thoroughly blended. Stir in cranberries and nuts. Transfer batter to muffin pan. Bake 20 minutes or until muffins are nicely browned and firm to the touch. Remove from oven and cool muffins 5 minutes in pan. Transfer muffins to wire rack to finish cooling.

BREAK IT DOWN . . .
Calories: 230; Total fat: 6g; Saturated fat: .5g; Cholesterol: 30mg; Sodium: 340mg; Total carbs: 44g; Fiber: 1g; Sugar: 22g; Protein: 2g.

Soy *(Glycine max)*

GONE SOUR
Did you know . . . fermented soy foods like miso and tempeh have healthy bacteria like that found in yogurt?

What's the Story?

Soybeans are legumes that grow in pods and have edible seeds. The seeds can come in a variety of colors such as green, brown, yellow, or black. Soy is very versatile and is consumed in a variety of different ways: as young green soybeans (edamame), dried, soy milk, soy nuts, tempeh, soy flour, tofu, and many more.

A Serving of Food Lore . . .

The soybean is thought to have originated in China. Records dating back to the eleventh century B.C. showed early cultivation in northern China. The soybean was revered as one of the five sacred grains essential to existence. In the first century A.D., soybeans spread to central and southern China and Korea. In the seventh century, soybeans made their way to Japan and throughout Asia. It wasn't until the seventeenth century that European visitors to the East were introduced to soybeans. Soy sauce was the first soy product brought to the United States, in the late seventeenth century. Benjamin Franklin sent seeds from London to a botanist friend in North America in 1770 and ever since, the United States has been a leader in soybean farming.

Where Are Soybeans Grown?

The main producer of soybeans is the United States, followed by Brazil and Argentina.

Why Should I Eat Soybeans?

Soy is the richest source of protein of any legume. In whole bean form, soy is very rich in fiber but many processed soy foods are not. Soy can be an excellent source of calcium, ranging anywhere between 80 and 750 mg per serving, depending on the type of soy food. Although soy foods are high in both oxalates and phytate, two compounds that can inhibit calcium absorption, the calcium from soy foods is very well absorbed. Fermented soy foods, like tempeh and miso, are a good source of iron. Soy foods are rich in copper and magnesium and are also rich in B vitamins, particularly niacin, pyridoxine, and folacin. Soybeans are rich in phytochemicals known as isoflavones which may help prevent certain types of cancer, fight heart disease, and improve bone density.

Home Remedies

The Chinese have used fermented soybean curds to treat skin infections for over 3,000 years. Soy has also been used to alleviate hot flashes.

Throw Me a Lifesaver!

BONE HEALTH: A Chinese three-year study of approximately 24,403 women showed a reduced risk of fracture for those women who consumed soy, especially for those women in the early part of menopause.

PROSTATE CANCER: In vitro studies have shown that genistein, a soy isoflavone, inhibits prostate cancer cell growth. Most animal studies have shown that soy isoflavones inhibit prostate tumor development.

BREAST CANCER: The bulk of the literature suggests that including soy in the diet may have a protective effect for breast cancer, attributed in part to soybean's isoflavone content. However, the role of soy for those diagnosed with breast cancer remains controversial because data from in vitro and animal studies suggest that isoflavones found in soy, especially genistein, may stimulate the growth of estrogen-sensitive tumors. Unfortunately there are limited human data that directly confirm this concern. Most soy and health experts agree that moderate soy intake is safe for the general population. If you have breast cancer, consult with your doctor or registered dietitian to see if soy can fit into your diet.

CARDIOVASCULAR DISEASE: Over fifty trials, including human intervention trials, have shown that consumption of soy products improves cholesterol ratios, and reduces total cholesterol and LDL cholesterol, especially in individuals with elevated cholesterol.

Tips on Using Soy

SELECTION AND STORAGE:

- Dried soybeans can be purchased in prepackaged containers and bulk bins.
- Edamame can be purchased frozen or precooked. Edamame should be deep green and firm with no bruised pods. Fresh edamame may be available seasonally in natural food and specialty markets.
- Tofu comes in soft, firm, and extra-firm varieties. It is available in specialty Japanese markets in grilled or broiled form, which are handy for soups or stews. You can find many varieties and brands in the refrigerated section of the store but it is also available in aseptic packaging that does not require refrigeration until opened.
- Dried soybeans will last about one year if stored in a cool, dry place.
- Cooked soybeans should be stored in the refrigerator where they will last for about three days.
- Fresh edamame should be kept in the refrigerator and will last for about two days. Frozen edamame will last for a few months.

PREPARATION AND SERVING SUGGESTIONS:

- Check dried soybeans for small stones and then rinse under cold water. Presoak to shorten cooking time.
- Cook on the stove top or in a pressure cooker.
- Add unpasteurized miso at the end of cooking to preserve beneficial bacteria.
- Substitute soy milk in place of cow's milk.
- Increase the protein content of your baked goods by replacing some of the flour with soybean flour.
- Try edamame for a simple appetizer or snack.
- Use whipped tofu as a base for creamy soups, mousse, and puddings.
- Grill tempeh as a great meat alternative.

Crustless BOCA Sausage Quiche with Spring Vegetables
by Chef Nick Spinelli
Servings: 6 • Prep and cooking time: 60 minutes

This recipe contains six powerhouse foods.

INGREDIENTS:

2 cups cholesterol-free egg product

4 links BOCA Meatless Breakfast
    Links, cut into ½-inch pieces

¾ cup peas, frozen

¼ cup red bell pepper, diced

¾ cup low-fat cottage cheese

⅓ cup 2%-milk shredded reduced-
    fat mild cheddar cheese

¼ cup red onion, diced small

1 tablespoon Dijon mustard

2 tablespoons parsley,
    chopped fine

2 tablespoons sweet basil,
    chopped fine

1 9-inch pie tin

DIRECTIONS:

Preheat oven to 350 degrees. Spray 9-inch pie plate with cooking spray. Combine all ingredients until well blended. Pour into prepared pie plate—make sure ingredients are evenly distributed throughout the pan. Bake 45 minutes or until center is puffy and top is golden brown.

BREAK IT DOWN . . .
Calories: 150; Total fat: 6g; Saturated fat: 2.5g; Cholesterol: 80mg; Sodium: 340mg; Total carbs: 5g; Fiber: less than 1g; Sugar: 1g; Protein: 17g.

Spelt *(Triticum spelta)*

ELITE WHEAT?
Did you know . . . that spelt has more protein, complex carbohydrates, and B-complex vitamins than wheat?

What's the Story?

The use of spelt has long been popular in Europe, where it is also known as "Farro" in Italy and "Dinkle" in Germany. It is closely related to wheat

(*T. aestivum*) and has many of the same properties and taste similarities to wheat; however, many who have wheat sensitivities are able to enjoy spelt. It has a nutlike flavor and is a very nutritious grain. Ground spelt is used primarily as an alternative feed grain to oats and barley.

A Serving of Food Lore . . .

Spelt is one of the oldest cultivated grains, dating back over 7,000 years, with origins tracing back to early Mesopotamia. Native to Iran and southeastern Europe, spelt is one of the first known grains to be grown by farmers, as long ago as 5000 B.C. Spelt was one of the first grains to be used to make bread, and its use is mentioned in the Bible.

Throughout early European history, spelt became a popular grain, especially in Germany, Switzerland, and Austria. Spelt was introduced to the United States in the 1890s and was cultivated on a moderate level until the early twentieth century, when farmers turned their efforts to the cultivation of wheat, which was much easier to process than spelt.

Where Is Spelt Grown?

Germany and Switzerland are the main growers of spelt. In the United States, Ohio is the leading producer of spelt.

Why Should I Include Spelt?

Spelt is an excellent source of the B vitamins riboflavin, niacin, thiamine, and also a good source of iron, manganese, copper, and the amino acid tryptophan. Spelt is also a great source of dietary fiber and a great source of protein, compared to wheat.

Home Remedies

Over 800 years ago, a Benedictine nun by the name of Hildegard von Bingen (St. Hildegard) wrote of spelt's healing powers: "It is rich and nourishing and milder than other grain. It produces a strong body and healthy blood to those who eat it and it makes the spirit of man light and cheerful. If someone is ill boil some spelt, mix it with egg and this will heal them like a fine ointment." Ancient Greeks and Romans offered spelt as a gift to the pagan gods of agriculture to encourage harvest and fertility.

Throw Me a Lifesaver!

HEART HEALTH: A study in the *American Heart Journal* found that women who had coronary artery disease and ate at least six servings of whole grains per week, including spelt, showed a slowed progression of atherosclerosis.

GALLSTONE PREVENTION: Eating foods high in insoluble fiber, such as spelt, can help women avoid gallstones, according to a study in the *American Journal of Gastroenterology.*

Tips on Using Spelt

SELECTION AND STORAGE:
- Spelt is available in whole grain, flour, bread, and pasta forms.
- Store spelt grains in an airtight container in a cool, dry, and dark place.
- Spelt flour should be kept in the refrigerator.

PREPARATION AND SERVING SUGGESTIONS:
- Soak berries in water for eight hours or overnight. Drain, rinse well, and then add three parts water to each part spelt berries used; bring the water to a boil and simmer for about one hour.
- In Germany, the unripe spelt grains are dried and eaten as grunkern, which literally means "green seed."
- Cook spelt berries and use them as a side dish instead of rice or potatoes.
- Use spelt flour in bread, muffin, and waffle recipes.

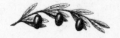

Spelt Burgers
Adapted from www.purityfoods.com
Servings: 6 burgers • Prep and cooking time: 40 minutes

This recipe contains eight powerhouse foods.

INGREDIENTS:

I cup Vita-Spelt kernels

I tablespoon canola margarine

¼ cup chopped onion

¼ cup chopped celery

¼ cup chopped carrots

I clove garlic, minced

2 cups vegetable stock

2 tablespoons ketchup

I tablespoon mild mustard

I egg (optional)

¼ cup olive oil

DIRECTIONS:

Preheat the oven to 350 degrees. Place the spelt kernels in a blender, and process at medium speed for 2 minutes, or until the kernels are half the size of a grain of rice. Set aside. Place the margarine in a 3-quart saucepan, and melt over medium heat. Add the onion, celery, carrots, and garlic, and cook, stirring often, until the vegetables are tender but firm. Add the stock and the ground kernels, and mix well. Increase the heat to high, and bring the mixture to a boil. Pour the vegetable mixture into a 2-quart casserole dish, and cover with aluminum foil. Bake for 20 minutes, or until the mixture is sticky and has the consistency of cooked white rice. Cool the mixture to room temperature. Add ketchup and mustard to taste, and stir to mix. Add egg and mix well. Using wet hands, form the mixture into 6 patties. Place the oil in a nonstick 10-inch skillet, and cook the patties over medium heat for 5 to 7 minutes on each side, or until browned and crisp. Transfer the patties to paper towels, and allow to drain. Garnish with your favorite toppings and serve on a spelt bun.

BREAK IT DOWN . . .

Calories: 190; Total fat: 8g; Saturated fat: 1.5g; Cholesterol: 45mg; Sodium: 460mg; Total carbs: 27g; Fiber: 4g; Sugar: 3g; Protein: 6g.

Spinach *(Spinacia oleracea)*

". . . I EATS ME SPINACH . . ."

Did you know . . . spinach capital Crystal City, Texas, erected a statue in 1937 to honor both cartoonist E. C. Segar and his character, Popeye, for their influence on America's consumption of spinach? Popeye was credited with a whopping thirty-three percent increase in sales and was given recognition for single-handedly saving the spinach industry!

What's the Story?

Spinach belongs to the same family as beets and chard. There are three main types of spinach including smooth leaf, savoy, and semi-savoy. All are delicious and rich in nutrients.

A Serving of Food Lore . . .

It is thought that spinach originated in ancient Persia. In the seventh century, the king of Nepal sent it to China as a gift and it became known as the "herb of Persia." In the eleventh century it was introduced to Spain by the Moors and was known in England as the "Spanish vegetable." In the sixteenth Century, Catherine de Medici brought her own cooks with her when she left Florence, Italy, to marry the king of France, because they could prepare spinach just the way she liked. This is why dishes prepared on a bed of spinach are described as "à la Florentine."

Where Is Spinach Grown?

The largest commercial producers of spinach are the United States and the Netherlands.

Why Should I Eat Spinach?

Spinach is an excellent source of fiber and vitamin K. It is a rich source of minerals such as calcium, iron, magnesium, and manganese. It is also rich in folate, a water-soluble B vitamin which is important for good cognitive function. Spinach is especially high in vitamin A and related compounds such as beta-carotene, zeaxanthin, and lutein, carotenoids that act as protection for the eye. Spinach is one of the richest sources of lutein, containing nearly 30,000 micrograms per cup of frozen spinach. Spinach is also rich in glycolipids, powerful phytochemicals known to have cancer cell growth suppression and antiproliferation qualities.

Home Remedies

Eating some cooked spinach every day is supposed to be helpful in relieving depression and neuritis, an inflammation of the nerves, because of spinach's high B-vitamin content.

Throw Me a Lifesaver!

AGE-RELATED MACULAR DEGENERATION: A case-control study involving 356 subjects with advanced macular degeneration found that higher intake of spinach resulted in a significantly lower risk for age-related macular degeneration.

LIVER CANCER: An in vitro study using human liver cancer cells found that spinach had the highest antiproliferative effect as compared to other vegetables.

GALLBLADDER CANCER: A case-control study involving 153 patients with gallbladder cancer found a significant inverse relationship between spinach consumption and the risk of gallbladder cancer.

COLON AND BREAST CANCER: An in vitro study using red spinach (*Amaranthus gangeticus*) extract on colon and breast cancer cells found significant antiproliferative effects.

PROSTATE CANCER: A study found that a natural antioxidant in spinach leaves slowed prostate cancer in both animal and human prostate cancer cell lines.

CERVICAL CANCER: Retinoids in spinach were found to have chemotherapeutic and chemopreventive potential in the uterine cervix.

NON-HODGKIN'S LYMPHOMA (NHL): A National Cancer Institute study found that higher intakes of vegetables that contain lutein and zea-xanthin, such as spinach, are associated with a lower NHL risk.

CATARACTS: A cohort study of 36,644 United States male health professionals found that spinach intake was correlated with a lower risk of developing cataracts.

NEUROPROTECTIVE: Rats who had suffered brain damage and were fed a spinach diet showed a reduction in damaged tissue and increased brain function.

Tips on Using Spinach

SELECTION AND STORAGE:
- Buy it FRESH! Between travel and storage at warmer temperatures, much of the nutrient content might already be gone. If it's wilted, take a pass.
- Choose spinach with stems that have no signs of yellowing and vibrant, deep green leaves.
- Unwashed spinach should be packed loosely in a plastic bag and placed in the refrigerator crisper where it will remain fresh and retain its nutrient content for about four days.
- Use cooked spinach the next day.
- Frozen spinach retains more of its nutrients because it is flash-frozen.

PREPARATION AND SERVING SUGGESTIONS:
- Trim and wash spinach very well as the leaves and stems tend to collect soil and sand.
- Remove any noticeably thick stems to allow more even cooking.
- Dry spinach leaves by patting them with a paper towel or using a salad spinner.
- Steaming is best. Keep cooking to a minimum. Vitamins C and B-complex can be destroyed by water, heat, or light.
- Replace iceberg lettuce with spinach.
- Add spinach to your lasagna, pasta, or pizza.

Sautéed Spinach
by Christine M. Palumbo
Servings: 4 • Prep and cooking time: 15 minutes

Simple but so good! We like to add a dash of crushed red pepper for excitement—be careful! Drizzle some basil-infused olive oil over the spinach for a taste you won't believe. This recipe contains four powerhouse foods.

INGREDIENTS:

10 ounces raw spinach, trimmed　　*Juice of ½ lemon*
1 garlic clove, sliced thinly　　　　*Salt, pepper, and red pepper flakes*
1 tablespoon extra-virgin olive oil　　　*to taste*

DIRECTIONS:

Wash the spinach well (even if it's bagged and washed, as there is some evidence that even prewashed greens need washing at home). Place in a colander. Heat the olive oil in a large pot and add the garlic, cooking a few minutes just until it is softened. Add the spinach, leaving the little bit of water that may be clinging to its leaves. Cover the pot and cook on medium-high heat, about 3 to 4 minutes, stirring occasionally. Turn off the heat while the spinach is still bright green, squeeze the lemon juice on it, and serve.

BREAK IT DOWN . . .
Calories: 50; Total fat: 4g; Saturated fat: .5g; Sodium: 243mg; Total carbs: 3g; Fiber: 2g; Sugar: 0g; Protein: 2g.

Strawberries (*Fragaria*)

WILL YOU BERRY ME?
Did you know . . . as the legend goes, if you break a double strawberry in half to share with someone of the opposite sex, you will fall in love with each other?

What's the Story?

Strawberries are a member of the rose family and are one of the most popular berries in the world. They are unique in that they are the only fruit to wear their seeds on the outside rather than the inside. Over six hundred different varieties exist.

A Serving of Food Lore . . .

During the Middle Ages in Europe, strawberries were used for medicinal purposes. In 1714, a French engineer found strawberries in Chile and Peru that were much larger than the ones grown in Europe. He brought plants back to France that were planted next to a North American variety and the hybrid that resulted was large, sweet, and juicy.

Where Are Strawberries Grown?

The largest producers of strawberries are Canada, France, the United States, Italy, Australia, Japan, and New Zealand.

Why Should I Eat Strawberries?

A serving of eight strawberries contains more vitamin C than an orange. Strawberries are also rich in folate, potassium, and fiber. They are second only to plums as the richest fruit in phenolics and antioxidants, being especially high in cancer- and heart disease–fighting flavonoids, anthocyanins, ellagic acid, quercetin, catechin, and kaempferol.

Home Remedies

A New York dentist believes that you can lighten your smile by combining a strawberry and baking soda to make a paste and spreading it on your teeth. After about 5 minutes, brush thoroughly with toothpaste to remove the strawberry mix. The ancient Romans believed that the berries alleviated symptoms of melancholy, fainting, all inflammations, fevers, throat infections, kidney stones, halitosis, attacks of gout, and diseases of the blood, liver, and spleen.

Throw Me a Lifesaver!

CANCER: Harvard researchers found strawberries to have protective qualities for a variety of cancers. An in vitro cell study using an extract from strawberry leaves on leukemia cells found significant cancer-killing activity. A cell study found that strawberry extracts significantly inhibited the growth of both colon and breast cancer cells. Organically cultivated strawberries had a significantly higher antiproliferative effect than the conventionally grown due to their higher antioxidant levels. Strawberries may play a role in reducing estrogen-driven cancer as they are rich in ellagic acid, which may function as an estrogen blocker. Freeze-dried strawberries inhibited growth of two types of cervical cancer cells grown in culture. A study using rats with esophageal cancer found that freeze-dried strawberries inhibited tumor growth and tumor initiation.

ANTI-INFLAMMATORY: Strawberries block enzymes (COX-2) responsible for promoting inflammation.

OBESITY: Ongoing research is investigating the role of strawberries in weight management.

DIABETES: Phytochemicals in strawberries were found to control type 2 diabetes by reducing blood glucose levels after a starchy meal.

COGNITIVE FUNCTION: Tufts University researchers found that strawberry extract slowed down the loss of cognitive function in rats.

HEART HEALTH: Eating eight strawberries a day for eight weeks lowered a leading risk factor of heart disease, homocysteine. In a similar study, the same researcher found that subjects who ate a serving of strawberries a day for four weeks had higher folate levels.

ANTITHROMBOSIS: An animal study found that strawberries had a powerful antithrombotic effect by promoting antiplatelet activity.

Tips on Using Strawberries

SELECTION AND STORAGE:
- Medium-size are more flavorful than large-size.
- Strawberries should be firm and dry to the touch. Avoid bruised and moldy ones. They should be plump with green caps attached, deep red in color, and you should be able to smell "strawberry" when you hold them up to your nose.
- Remove damaged or molded berries.
- They will stay fresh for a couple of days in the refrigerator if kept in their original container.

PREPARATION AND SERVING SUGGESTIONS:
- Wash them right before they will be used.
- Do not remove the caps before they are washed to prevent them from absorbing excess water, degrading their flavor and texture.
- Topping—add sliced strawberries to a salad, breakfast cereal, or yogurt.
- Blend into your favorite smoothie.

Strawberry Shortcake
by Heather Jose

Servings: 12 • Prep and cooking time: 25 minutes

Native Americans crushed strawberries and mixed them with cornmeal which they baked into a bread. Colonists loved it so much that they eventually developed their own version and "Strawberry Shortcake" was born! This recipe contains four powerhouse foods.

INGREDIENTS FOR STRAWBERRY TOPPING:

*1 quart fresh strawberries, washed   ¼ cup agave nectar
  and halved*

INGREDIENTS FOR SHORTCAKE:

2 cups Hodgson Mills Insta-Bake
   Baking Mix
2 tablespoons butter

⅔ cup soy milk (plain or vanilla)
2 tablespoons agave nectar
   (optional)

DIRECTIONS FOR THE SHORTCAKE:

Heat oven to 425 degrees. In medium bowl, combine Insta-Bake and butter until crumbly. Add soy milk and agave and stir to make a soft dough. Mix until dough pulls away from the bowl. Spread into a sprayed or nonstick 8- or 9-inch cake pan or drop by spoonfuls onto a sprayed baking sheet. Bake for 10 to 12 minutes or until golden brown; may be longer for cake pan. Yields 10 to 12 individual short-cakes or 8 pieces.

DIRECTIONS FOR THE STRAWBERRY TOPPING:

Pour the washed and halved strawberries into a medium bowl and add the agave nectar. Using a potato masher, smash the strawber-ries to desired consistency. Place a piece of shortcake into a bowl and ladle the strawberry topping over the top.

BREAK IT DOWN . . .

Calories: 170; Total fat: 3g; Saturated fat: 1.5g; Cholesterol: 5mg; Sodium: 180mg; Total carbs: 33g; Fiber: 3g; Sugar: 14g; Protein: 3g.

Sunflower Seeds (Helianthus Annuus L.)

THAT'S WHY THEY CALL IT A "SUN" FLOWER!

Did you know . . . when the sunflower plant is budding, it tracks the movement of the sun? Once the flower opens, exposing its beautiful yellow petals, its head is always facing east.

What's the Story?

Sunflower seeds are black or grayish-green in a shell that is black with white stripes. The seed has a mild nutty taste and tender texture. Sunflower seeds are one of the main sources for producing polyunsaturated oil.

A Serving of Food Lore . . .

Sunflowers are believed to have originated in Peru and Mexico. From the Americas, sunflowers made their way to Europe via Spanish explorers sometime around 1500. The plant traveled throughout Western Europe but mainly as an ornamental plant with a few limited medicinal uses. The English were the first to commercially produce oil from sunflower seed. The Russian Orthodox Church forbid most oil foods from being consumed during Lent; however, sunflower was not on the prohibited list and therefore gained immediate popularity as a food. By the early nineteenth century, Russian farmers were growing over two million acres of sunflower. By the late nineteenth century, Russian sunflower seeds found their way back into the United States.

Where Are Sunflower Seeds Grown?

Sunflower seeds are produced in Peru, Argentina, the Russian Federation, France, Spain, and China.

Home Remedies

Eating raw, shelled, and unsalted sunflower seeds promotes regularity. Sunflower seeds are a good source of thiamine and vitamin B1, and have been shown to relieve menstrual cramps.

Why Should I Eat Sunflower Seeds?

Sunflower seeds are a good source of vitamin E, folate, magnesium, selenium, and copper. A study that reviewed twenty-seven varieties of nuts and seeds found that the sunflower kernel was one of the richest in phytosterols, substances known to fight heart disease and prostate cancer.

Throw Me a Lifesaver!

CANCER: An in vivo study using mice with stage-two skin cancer found that sunflower oil reduced papillomas in the mice by twenty to forty percent.

CHOLESTEROL: A double-blind, randomized, controlled human study found that those given diets containing mid-oleic sunflower oil had a decrease in both total and low-density lipoprotein (LDL or "bad") cholesterol. Another human study involved men and women who were placed randomly into two groups: One was given a diet high in saturated fat and the other a monounsaturated fatty acid diet. The researchers found that high-oleic-acid sunflower oil lowered both LDL cholesterol and triglyceride levels.

Tips on Using Sunflower Seeds

SELECTION AND STORAGE:
- Sunflower seeds can be purchased shelled or unshelled, in the raw, roasted, salted, and unsalted.
- Avoid shelled seeds that are yellowish in color.
- Sunflower seeds are high in fat and can turn rancid if not stored in an airtight container in the refrigerator or freezer.

PREPARATION AND SERVING SUGGESTIONS:
- Sunflower seeds can be shelled by hand or by using a seed mill.
- Seeds can also be shelled by placing them in a bowl and using an electric mixer. Pulse on and off until the shells separate, and plunge into cold water.
- Sunflower seeds make a great addition to your chicken or tuna salad recipe.
- Add sunflower seeds to your mixed green salad, granola, and hot/cold cereals.

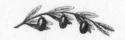

Sunny Sunflower Mini-Scones
by Sharon Grotto
Yield: Three dozen

Serving size: 1 scone • Prep and baking time: 25 minutes

This recipe contains six powerhouse foods.

INGREDIENTS:

¾ cup sugar

4 tablespoons margarine

4 tablespoons butter

1 teaspoon vanilla

⅔ cup all-purpose flour

⅔ cup whole wheat flour

¾ cup old-fashioned oats

½ teaspoon baking powder

¼ teaspoon salt

½ cup sunflower seeds, unsalted

½ cup dried cherries, chopped

1 egg

½ teaspoon almond extract

DIRECTIONS:

Heat oven to 350 degrees. Beat sugar, margarine, butter, vanilla, almond extract, and egg in a large bowl. Stir in flour, oats, baking powder, and salt. Stir in sunflower seeds and cherries. Drop dough by rounded tablespoon onto ungreased cookie sheet, two inches apart. Bake 12 to 14 minutes or until golden brown.

BREAK IT DOWN . . .

Calories: 80; Total fat: 3.5g; Saturated fat: 1g; Cholesterol: 10mg; Sodium: 35mg; Total carbs: 10g; Fiber: less than 1g; Sugar: 5g; Protein: 1g.

Sweet Potatoes *(Ipomoea batatas)*

I YAM WHAT I YAM

Did you know . . . at the beginning of the twentieth century in the United States, orange-fleshed sweet potatoes were given the name "yam" to set them apart from the white-fleshed sweet potato that was popular at that time?

What's the Story?

Maybe it's best to start off with what sweet potatoes are not. First of all, they're not even potatoes! All potatoes belong to the *Solanaceae* family and sweet potatoes belong to the *Convolvulaceae* family—which is a group of plants that have trumpet-shaped flowers. They're not yams either. The word "yam" comes from the African word *nyami* which describes huge root vegetables found in Africa (*Dioscoreae* family) that are starchier with a slick texture and a stronger, much less sweet taste than the garden variety sweet potato. To help avoid confusion that consumers might have, the United States Department of Agriculture requires "yams" to also have the term "sweet potato" on the label. There are about 400 different varieties, with skins varying in color from purple to red to orange to yellow to even white. And inside, the "flesh" may be white, orange, or yellow with textures ranging from firm, dry, and mealy to soft and moist.

A Serving of Food Lore . . .

Sweet potatoes, thought to be native to Central America, may be the oldest vegetable known to humans. Remnants have been found in Peruvian caves that date back 10,000 years. Sweet potatoes were first brought to Europe by Christopher Columbus after his first voyage to the New World. Portuguese explorers brought them to Africa, India, Indonesia, and southern Asia. Spanish explorers brought them to the Philippines by the sixteenth century and they were also being cultivated in the southern United States at about this same time.

Where Are Sweet Potatoes Grown?

Uganda, India, Vietnam, Japan, China, and Indonesia are the main producers of sweet potatoes. In 2004, world production was 127,000,000 tons according to the Food and Drug Organization, with the majority coming from China.

Why Should I Eat Sweet Potatoes?

They are an excellent source of vitamin A and beta-carotene, and a good source of vitamin C, B6, manganese, potassium, and fiber. The red variety of sweet potato is an excellent source of the phytochemical lycopene—which may help fight heart disease and breast and prostate cancer. Purple-flesh types are high in anthocyanins, potent antioxidants which protect the body against degenerative diseases.

Throw Me a Lifesaver!

LONGEVITY: A major source of nutrition for the Okinawans is the Okinawan sweet potato, a white-skinned, purple-fleshed version which may be a contributing factor to their long life expectancies.

DIABETES: Rats who ate white-fleshed sweet potatoes had marked improvement in pancreatic cell function, lipid levels, glucose management, and reduced insulin resistance within eight weeks. A human study also showed improved insulin resistance when sweet potatoes were included in the diet.

MEMORY ENHANCEMENT: Rats who ate purple-fleshed sweet potatoes showed significant improvement in cognitive function, which may be attributed to the anthocyanins present in the potato.

CANCER: A cell study showed that sweet potatoes have unique cancer-fighting properties.

BREAST CANCER: A case-control study found that those women who consumed more beta-carotene–rich foods had lower rates of breast cancer. Sweet potatoes are an excellent source of beta-carotene.

COLORECTAL CANCER: A study using male rats found that the development of colon lesions were inhibited when purple sweet potatoes were added to their diet.

GALLBLADDER CANCER: A case-control study involving diagnosed cases of gallbladder cancer found that sweet potatoes were among the vegetables that offered the greatest protective benefit.

KIDNEY CANCER: A Japanese cohort study that followed 47,997 males and 66,520 females for about 10 years found that consumption of sweet potatoes was linked to a decreased risk of kidney cancer.

Tips on Using Sweet Potatoes

SELECTION AND STORAGE:
- Choose firm sweet potatoes free of bruises, soft spots, and cracks.
- If selecting for carotene content, choose darker varieties.
- Sweet potatoes will stay fresh for about ten days if placed in a dark, cool, and ventilated location.
- Do not put uncooked sweet potatoes in the refrigerator.

PREPARATION AND SERVING SUGGESTIONS:
- To prevent them from darkening due to contact with the air, cook them promptly after cutting or peeling, or place them in a bowl and cover them with water until it is time to cook them.
- Poke holes in them before baking in the oven or in the microwave.
- Kids' favorites include sweet potato pie and pudding.
- Spread mashed sweet potatoes on a piece of whole wheat bread, top with a layer of peanut butter and sliced apples.
- Baked sweet potatoes are delicious even when served cold and therefore make a great food to pack in to-go lunches.

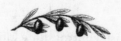

Sweet Potato Chips

by Dawn Jackson Blatner

Servings: 12 • Prep and cooking time: 30 minutes

Dawn's chips are so simple to make and are a healthier alternative to regular potato chips. You can jazz them up with additional ingredients like chopped garlic and onion and replace regular salt with flavored salt. Use the fresh-squeezed lime juice. . . . It really makes a difference. This recipe contains two powerhouse foods.

INGREDIENTS:

3 large sweet potatoes
3 limes, zest and juice

1 teaspoon salt (regular or
flavored)
Cooking spray

DIRECTIONS:

Preheat oven to 350 degrees. Slice potatoes into chips (use mandolin for thin and uniform chips). Lightly spray cookie sheets with oil. Place a single layer of potatoes on cookie sheets. Spray tops of potatoes with oil and top with salt and lime zest. Bake until browned, turning once (about 20 to 30 minutes). Sprinkle browned sweet potato chips with lime juice. Serve and enjoy!

BREAK IT DOWN . . .

Calories: 57; Total fat: 1g; Saturated fat: 0g; Cholesterol: 0mg; Sodium: 210mg; Total carbs: 12g; Fiber: 2g; Sugar: 4g; Protein: 1g.

Tea *(Camellia sinensis)*

BAG IT!

Did you know . . . tea that comes in the form of tea bags may be healthier than loose varieties? The tea in tea bags tends to be ground finer, providing more surface area to extract more health-promoting polyphenols (antioxidants) when submerged in hot water.

What's the Story?

"Tea" can refer to any number of beverages including herbals like mint or chamomile. But *true* tea is made from the leaves, stems, and buds of the *Camellia sinensis* plant. Whether your preference is black, green, white, or oolong, all varieties come from the exact same bush—*Camellia sinensis.* The difference between the teas is in how they are processed. "Green tea" is made from leaves that are dried right after harvesting, and the leaves used to make black tea are fermented after harvesting. Oolong tea leaves are fermented for a short time. White tea leaves do not undergo any oxidation and are shielded from the sun and are not allowed to produce any chlorophyll.

A Serving of Food Lore . . .

Camellia sinensis is thought to have originated in the northern part of China some 5,000 years ago. From there, tea made its way through northeast India to southwest China. Tea was brought to Japan from China around 805. Russia was introduced to tea in 1618 after a Ming emperor of China offered it as a gift to Czar Michael I. Tea was then introduced to England, where it was a sign of status and wealth, in 1650. Tea was brought to North America by the colonists, and in 1904 iced tea was introduced at the St. Louis World's Fair and has been a popular drink ever since.

Where Is Tea Grown?

The main tea growers throughout the world are India, China, Kenya, Sri Lanka, Indonesia, Turkey, Taiwan, Japan, Nepal, and Bangladesh.

Why Should I Drink Tea?

Tea is a good source of flavonoids called catechins, which are important antioxidants that can help prevent certain types of diseases. The major catechins, found mostly in green tea, include: epigallocatechin-3-gallate (EGCG), epigallocatechin (EGC), epicatechin-3-gallate (ECG), and epicatechin (EC). EGCG is the most abundant and widely studied tea polyphenol, and EGCG and ECG have the highest radical-scavenging activity. Caffeine levels tend to be higher in tea bag forms (the finer grind releases more caffeine) but typically range between 20 and 90 milligrams of caffeine per 8-ounce cup compared with brewed coffee's 60 to 120 milligrams.

Home Remedies

Ancient medical texts in China and Japan discuss tea's medicinal qualities, which include stimulant properties, curing blotchiness, quenching thirst, aiding indigestion, curing beriberi, preventing fatigue, and improving urinary and brain function.

Throw Me a Lifesaver!

CANCER PREVENTION: Polyphenols in tea are important antioxidants that help prevent certain types of cancer, such as oral, skin, digestive, ovarian, and lung.

HEART HEALTH: Though several studies suggest that the consumption of both green and black teas may help in reducing the risk of heart disease by improving endothelial function (keeping the lining of the arteries open to allow more blood flow), lowering blood pressure, reducing total cholesterol, and preventing LDL cholesterol from turning into a more harmful form, the Food and Drug Administration has not yet granted a functional food claim for green or black tea. That may be just a matter of time as further extensive research may provide good reason to drink tea literally to your heart's content.

OBESITY: There have been a handful of studies, mostly conducted in Japan, that have shown promising results in reducing body fat when green tea or green tea catechins were consumed. However, the amount of catechins used in these studies would be equivalent to more than 10 cups of green tea per day! Green tea may be a useful tool for achieving a healthy weight, but it is certainly not the entire solution.

OSTEOPOROSIS: Though too much caffeine is a concern for bone health, a study found that older women who drank tea had greater bone density than those who didn't.

BOOSTS INSULIN ACTIVITY: A study conducted by researchers from the U.S. Department of Agriculture found that black, green, and oolong teas increased insulin activity by about fifteen-fold in tests using fat cells obtained from rats.

Tips on Using Tea

SELECTION AND STORAGE:
- All varieties of *Camellia sinensis* come in either loose or tea bag forms.
- Out of all the forms of tea, instant tea has the least amount of catechins.
- Bottled teas start off with low levels of flavonoids, and tend to lose potency over time.
- Decaffeinated tea is a good option, though it has about ten percent fewer phytochemicals than tea with caffeine.
- Store tea in a cool, dark cabinet in an air- and moisture-tight container such as a glass jar.

PREPARATION AND SERVING SUGGESTIONS:
- Green and white teas are best brewed at a lower temperature (around 80 degrees Fahrenheit). If the water is too hot the tea leaves will burn, leaving a bitter taste.
- Black teas should be brewed at a higher temperature, around 100 degrees Fahrenheit.
- Black tea should not be allowed to steep for less than 30 seconds or more than about five minutes for the best flavor. Eighty percent of catechins are released by the five-minute mark.
- Honey, lemon, sugar, or jams may be added to tea for additional sweetness and flavor.

- Milk in your tea? The protein component in milk called casein may reduce the absorption of catechins.

Honey-Apricot Tea Biscotti
Adapted from www.Lipton.com
Servings: 36 biscotti • Prep and baking time: 1 hour, 20 minutes

This recipe contains five powerhouse foods.

INGREDIENTS:

¾ cup light soy milk

4 tea bags Lipton Honey & Lemon Flavored Black Tea bags

1¾ cups whole wheat flour

1 cup all-purpose flour

1¼ cups sugar

¾ teaspoon baking soda

¾ teaspoon baking powder

½ teaspoon salt

2 egg yolks

⅓ cup whole almonds, lightly toasted

⅓ cup coarsely chopped dried apricots

DIRECTIONS:

Preheat oven to 350 degrees. In small saucepan, bring milk to the boiling point. Remove from heat and add Lipton Honey & Lemon Flavored Black Tea bags; cover and brew 5 minutes. Remove tea bags and squeeze; cool. In large bowl, combine flours, sugar, baking soda, baking powder, and salt. With electric mixer, beat in tea mixture and egg yolks to form a dough. Stir in almonds and apricots. Turn dough onto lightly floured surface, then knead lightly. Divide in half. On greased and floured baking sheet, with floured hands, shape dough into two 12 × 2-inch logs. Bake 35 minutes or until pale golden. Remove from oven; let cool 10 minutes. With serrated knife, cut on the diagonal into ¾-inch-wide slices. Arrange slices, cut side down, on baking sheet. Bake 10 minutes or until crisp and golden, turning once. Cool completely on wire rack.

BREAK IT DOWN . . .
Calories: 80; Total fat: 1g; Saturated fat: 0g; Cholesterol: 10mg; Sodium: 70mg; Total carbs: 16g; Fiber: 1g; Sugar: 8g; Protein: 2g.

Teff *(Eragrostis teff)*

TEFF LUCK!

Did you know . . . "teff" means "lost," because if you drop it on the ground you won't find it? And in fact, it is the smallest grain in the world, measuring a mere $1/32$ of an inch!

What's the Story?

Teff is an annual grass from Ethiopia with very tiny seeds that have a mildly nutty flavor. There are three main types of teff: white, red, and brown.

- White teff has a chestnutlike taste and can only be grown in the Central Highlands region of Ethiopia—it is considered a status symbol there. White teff flour is used to make the staple bread *injera,* a flat sourish fermented pancake, and is a favorite in Ethiopian cuisine.
- Red teff is the least expensive and least preferred but it is becoming more popular in Ethiopia due to its high iron content. In the populations where red teff has been consumed, there has been an increase in hemoglobin levels, with a decreased risk of anemia.
- Brown teff has a taste similar to hazelnuts, makes a delicious breakfast porridge, and is commonly used in Ethiopia as an ingredient in home-brewed alcoholic drinks.

A Serving of Food Lore . . .

Teff is thought to have originated in Ethiopia between 4000 B.C. and 1000 B.C. Teff seeds were discovered in a brick of the Dassur Egyptian pyramid built in 3359 B.C. Today, teff straw is still used to make adobe in Ethiopia and it is cultivated for its hay in Kenya and Australia.

Where Is Teff Grown?

Ethiopia is the major grower of teff, which makes up about thirty-one percent of all grain that is grown in that country, followed by seventeen percent corn and thirteen percent wheat. It is also grown in other countries, including Eritrea, Uganda, Australia, Canada, the United States, and Kenya. In the United States, teff is typically grown in Idaho, and on a smaller scale in South Dakota.

Why Should I Eat Teff?

Teff is an excellent source of essential amino acids, especially lysine, and contains all eight essential amino acids needed in the human diet. Teff also contains high levels of trace minerals. Ounce for ounce, it supplies more fiber (15.3 grams of fiber per 4 ounces of flour) than any other grain. Teff is gluten-free, so it is appropriate for those with celiac disease. The Ethiopian pancake made from teff called *injera* goes through a fermentation process that enhances its amino acid and nutrient content.

Home Remedies

Darker varieties of teff were reserved for soldiers, servants, and peasants. Reportedly, they were the healthiest and outlived the wealthy.

Throw Me a Lifesaver!

ESOPHAGEAL CANCER: A human observation study showed that out of those subjects who ate teff (which were by far the majority of the subjects), fewer cases of esophageal cancer were observed compared with those who ate wheat.

Tips on Using Teff

SELECTION AND STORAGE:
- Teff can be purchased in flour or grain form. It may be purchased at a local health food store, online, or at an ethnic supermarket.
- Store teff flour and grain in an airtight container and place in a dry area. Teff can be refrigerated for longer storage.
- Cooked teff should be used within a few days.

PREPARATION AND SERVING SUGGESTIONS:
- For leavened bread, use wheat flour with up to twenty percent teff flour added.

- To cook teff, place 2 cups water and ½ cup teff (¼ teaspoon sea salt optional) in a saucepan. Bring to a boil, reduce heat, and simmer, covered, for 15 to 20 minutes or until the water is absorbed. Remove from heat and let stand covered for 5 minutes.
- Teff makes a good thickener for gravy, pudding, soup, or stew.
- Use teff in stir-fry dishes, casseroles, baked goods, and pancakes.
- Cooked teff can be mixed with herbs, seeds, beans or tofu, garlic, and onions to make "burgers."

Traditional Ethiopian Injera Bread
Adapted from www.BobsRedMill.com
Servings: 10 to 12 injeras • Prep time: 2 to 3 days
Cooking time: 2 to 3 minutes

This recipe contains one powerhouse food.

INGREDIENTS:

¾ cup Bob's Red Mill teff flour
3½ cups water
Pinch of salt

1 tablespoon sunflower, peanut, or
canola oil

DIRECTIONS:
Mix ground teff with water and let stand in a bowl covered with a dish towel, at room temperature, until it bubbles and has turned sour. This may take as long as 3 days. The mixture should be the consistency of pancake batter. Stir in salt, a little at a time, until you can just detect the taste. Lightly oil an 8- or 9-inch skillet. Heat over medium heat. Pour in enough batter to cover the bottom of the skillet—about ¼ cup will make a thin pancake. Spread the batter around the bottom of the pan by turning and rotating the skillet. This is the classic French method for very thin crepes. Injera is not supposed to be paper-thin, so you should use a bit more batter than you would for crepes, but less than you would for a flapjack. Cook briefly, until holes form in the injera and the edges lift from the pan. Remove and let cool.

BREAK IT DOWN . . .
Calories: 70; Total fat: 1.5g; Saturated fat: 0g; Cholesterol: 0mg; Sodium: 100mg; Total carbs: 14g; Fiber: 1g; Sugar: 0g; Protein: 2g.

Tomatoes *(Lycopersicon lycopersicum)*

FOOD FIGHT!
Did you know . . . in Buñol, Valencia, Spain, there's an annual tradition of pelting thy fellow neighbor with tomatoes, called "La Tomatina"?

What's the Story?

Tomatoes come from the *Solanaceae* family, which also include peppers, potatoes, and eggplant. There are over a thousand varieties of tomatoes that differ in size, shape, and color ranging from red, yellow, and orange to green and brown.

A Serving of Food Lore . . .

Tomatoes are thought to be native to South America, but they were first cultivated in Mexico. It was Spanish explorers who brought tomato seeds back to Europe. The tomato was introduced to Italy in the sixteenth century but Italians were fearful of eating them because tomatoes belonged to the nightshade family and were believed to be poisonous. The colonists who settled in Virginia brought the tomatoes with them but it wasn't until the nineteenth century that the tomato gained popularity.

Where Are Tomatoes Grown?

The main producers of tomatoes are the United States, Italy, Russia, Spain, Turkey, and China.

Why Should I Eat Tomatoes?

Tomatoes are rich in vitamin C and potassium. They are a good source of plant chemicals such as phytosterols, beta-carotene, and lycopene, a potent antioxidant that becomes more abundant when tomatoes are cooked. Epidemiological studies have demonstrated that lycopene reduces the risk of prostate cancer and also has cardioprotective, antimutagenic, anticarcinogenic, and anti-inflammatory properties. Tomatoes also contain polyphenols which have been shown effective in halting growth against liver and prostate cancer in cell line studies.

Home Remedies

Drinking tomato juice, and taking a bath in it, have been advocated for eczema and other skin disorders. Some find gargling tomato juice 3 to 4 times a day provides relief from mouth ulcers. A concoction of two teaspoons of tomato juice and ¼ cup buttermilk, applied to burned areas and left on for about a half hour and then rinsed, has provided relief.

Throw Me a Lifesaver!

CARDIOVASCULAR DISEASE: To date, the majority of research suggests that tomato products may be more cardioprotective than lycopene alone. An animal study in which subjects were given either tomato juice or a lycopene supplement, and then had heart damage introduced, found that both reduced lipid peroxidation; however, only tomato juice reduced heart cell death and damage to the heart and improved heart function. An in vitro study using tomato extract found that tomatoes contain compounds that reduced platelet aggregation (blood stickiness).

CANCER: A UC Davis study found that tomato products had a synergistic effect between lycopene and other naturally occurring nutrients in tomatoes that produced better results than lycopene supplementation alone in lowering biomarkers of oxidative stress and carcinogenesis.

COLORECTAL CANCER: A case-control study involving 1,953 cases found that tomato intake had a significant protective effect against colorectal cancer.

OVARIAN CANCER: A prospective study of seventy-one women diagnosed with ovarian cancer showed a significantly reduced risk of ovarian cancer with higher tomato consumption.

PROSTATE CANCER: Subjects who consumed tomato sauce daily for three weeks before their prostatectomy had a significant decrease in DNA damage in prostate tissues and an increase in prostate cancer cell death. A case-control study found a significant inverse association between higher plasma lycopene derived from plant sources such as tomatoes and lower risk of prostate cancer.

Tips on Using Tomatoes

SELECTION AND STORAGE:
- Choose red, plump, heavy tomatoes with smooth skin.
- They should have a mild fragrance (no fragrance means that the tomato was picked before it was ripe and will never ripen).
- Place them in a paper bag stem side up with a banana or apple to speed up ripening.
- Store at room temperature.
- Fully ripe tomatoes will last for a day or two.

PREPARATION AND SERVING SUGGESTIONS:
- Do not cook tomatoes with aluminum cookware because their acid will interact with the metal and may cause the aluminum to leech into the food.
- Add sliced tomatoes to your sandwiches and salads.
- Make salsa, soups, or add tomato juice to rice to make Spanish rice.

Noni's Marinara Sauce
by Arthur Grotto

Servings: 8 four-ounce servings • Prep time: 20 minutes
Cooking time: At least 1 hour. Longer for a thicker sauce.

My dad says you have to let a pasta sauce cook for at least an hour so the sauce clings to the pasta. This recipe contains seven power-house foods.

INGREDIENTS:

2 tablespoons olive oil

2 tablespoons parsley, rinsed and dried well, chopped fine

2 tablespoons celery leaves, rinsed and dried well, chopped fine

2 tablespoons yellow onion, rinsed and dried well, chopped fine

1 large clove garlic, quartered

1 teaspoon tomato paste

42 ounces Italian-style whole canned tomatoes

16 ounces tomato sauce

½ cup dry white wine

½ teaspoon baking soda

Pinch of cayenne or black pepper

Salt to taste

DIRECTIONS:

Pour whole tomatoes in a colander. Squeeze juice from tomatoes by hand until somewhat dry. Do not discard juice. Chop tomatoes to coarse texture, or finer if you desire. Once tomatoes are chopped, add back into reserved juice. Heat large and deep skillet for 1½ minutes. Add olive oil to pan. Immediately after, add onions, garlic, parsley, and celery leaves and sauté until onions are transparent, stirring occasionally. Add wine, stir, and cook until wine is reduced. Add pinch of cayenne pepper and raise heat to medium. Add in tomatoes with juice, tomato sauce, and tomato paste; raise heat to high and bring to near boil. Reduce heat and simmer until garlic is soft, approximately fifty minutes to an hour—test periodically by pressing garlic pieces against side of pan. When garlic is soft, remove and chop fine. Add back into sauce. Continue to simmer for another fifteen minutes. Taste sauce as it is cooking—add salt, if needed. Stir in baking soda at the end of cooking, until dissolved, to reduce the acidity of the sauce. Serve.

BREAK IT DOWN . . .

Calories: 78; Total fat: 4g; Saturated fat: 0g; Cholesterol: 0mg; Sodium: 498mg; Total carbs: 7g; Fiber: 1g; Sugar: 4g; Protein: 2g.

Turmeric *(Curcuma longa)*

TO DYE FOR

Did you know . . . turmeric is often used as a yellow dye for fabrics, and when it is mixed with lime juice, it becomes the red dye that Buddhists and Hindus use to mark their foreheads?

What's the Story?

Turmeric, often spelled tumeric (incorrectly), is a member of the ginger family. Turmeric is also known as Indian Saffron and is the ingredient that is responsible for making curry and mustard yellow-orange in color. Rhizomes, rootlike extensions from the stem of the plant, are the parts used to make turmeric powder, and are also used in making mustard, coloring butter or cheese, and flavoring various foods.

A Serving of Food Lore . . .

Turmeric is thought to have originated in western India and has been used there for at least 2,500 years. Turmeric reached China by 700 A.D. and then traveled throughout Africa. In the thirteenth century, Marco Polo wrote of this spice, marveling at a vegetable which exhibited qualities so similar to saffron. The use of turmeric as a coloring agent for food and fabric dates as far back as 600 B.C. In medieval Europe, turmeric was used as an inexpensive substitute for saffron. Turmeric was introduced to Jamaica in the eighteenth century and from there made its way into North America shortly after.

Where Is Turmeric Grown?

Ninety-four percent of the world's supply is produced in India. Turmeric is also grown in parts of China as well as the tropical region of Peru.

Why Should I Include Turmeric?

Turmeric contains important vitamins and minerals such as iron, manganese, potassium, vitamin B6, and vitamin C. Curcumin is a phytochemical found in turmeric that has strong antioxidant properties and which has been well researched for its cancer-fighting and anti-inflammatory properties.

Home Remedies

As early as 4,000 years ago, records from traditional healers of India and China mention turmeric benefiting many conditions. Traditionally, turmeric has been used for relieving menstrual cramps, respiratory conditions, intestinal worms, liver obstruction, ulcers, and inflammation. Turmeric is one of Okinawa's favorite herbs and claims many health benefits. Local folklore says that the herb strengthens the immune system, relieves inflammation, and improves digestion, among other conditions.

Throw Me a Lifesaver!

BRAIN INJURY: In a rat study, supplementation with curcumin was found to counteract the oxidative damage and cognitive impairment encountered in the injured brain.

DEMENTIA AND ALZHEIMER'S: One mouse study confirmed that curcumin significantly lowers oxidized proteins and inflammatory cytokines associated with Alzheimer's. Elderly people who ate curry at least once a month scored better on tests to measure cognitive function than those who reported they ate curry less frequently.

SKIN CANCER: In an animal study, turmeric was shown to reduce skin tumor size by thirty percent and skin tumor occurrence by eighty-seven percent compared to the control group.

A study out of the University of Texas M. D. Anderson Cancer Center in Houston treated three melanoma cell lines with curcumin. Cell growth was inhibited and increased tumor cell death was observed.

BREAST CANCER: Researchers found that curcumin inhibited metastasis to the lungs of mice with breast cancer. The researchers also found that curcumin helps make taxol, a chemotherapeutic drug for breast cancer, less toxic and even more effective.

Rats given large doses of turmeric each day over a five-day period had significant inhibition of breast tumors.

PROSTATE: In vivo and in vitro studies have shown that curcumin reduces the expression of prostate cancer genes, tumor volume and quantity of nodules in treated groups.

COLON CANCER: In a small study, patients who had precancerous polyps were treated with curcumin for six months. The average number of polyps dropped sixty percent, and the average size dropped by fifty percent.

HEART HEALTH: Rats who were fed higher doses of curcumin in their diet had significantly lower liver triacylglycerols and very-low-density lipoprotein (VLDL) cholesterol.

Tips on Using Turmeric

SELECTION AND STORAGE:

- Choose fresh turmeric roots that have a spicy fragrance and hearty rhizomes.
- When buying in powdered form, buy in small quantities and from fresh sources.
- Tightly wrap and refrigerate unpeeled turmeric for up to three weeks.
- Keep turmeric powder in sealable plastic bags or bottles.

PREPARATION AND SERVING SUGGESTIONS:

- Turmeric is usually steamed and then dried and ground into powder.
- Be careful when preparing turmeric—it will stain your hands and clothing.
- Use ground turmeric in stews, soups, rice, and fish dishes to add flavor and color.
- Turmeric is used in the production of some packaged goods to protect them from sunlight.

Penne Rigate with Broccoli and Turmeric
by Chef Nick Spinelli
Servings: 6 • Prep and cooking time: 30 minutes

This recipe contains five powerhouse foods.

INGREDIENTS:

3 cups broccoli, stems and florets, raw, trimmed

1 pound penne rigate pasta, raw

2 tablespoons extra-virgin olive oil

1 teaspoon turmeric, ground

½ teaspoon black pepper, cracked and ground

1 tablespoon garlic, fresh, minced

1 teaspoon ginger, fresh, minced

½ cup chicken or vegetable stock

¼ cup white wine, Chardonnay

¾ teaspoon salt

DIRECTIONS:

Fill a 4-quart pot with cold water and bring to a boil. Add broccoli and cook until tender. Once broccoli is cooked, take out of water and place into a strainer in the sink. Do not rinse. If necessary, add more water to pot to cook pasta and return to the stove. Bring water to boil and then add pasta. Cook until al dente. Strain pasta but do not rinse. Rinse pot and return to stove. Place olive oil into pot and heat on medium-high for ½ minute. Add turmeric, black pepper, garlic, and ginger to the oil and stir constantly until you can smell the garlic. Add chicken stock and white wine to pot and let mixture come to a boil. Add salt and stir twice. Add pasta to the seasoning mixture and fold into the sauce to completely cover noodles. Turn off heat and add broccoli to pasta and fold until completely coated.

BREAK IT DOWN . . .
Calories: 350; Total fat: 6g; Saturated fat: 1g; Cholesterol: 0mg; Sodium: 55mg; Total carbs: 61g; Fiber: 5g; Sugar: 5g; Protein: 13g.

Walnuts *(Juglans)*

NIGHTY NIGHT!
Did you know . . . walnuts contain a good amount of melatonin, a hormone that protects cells from oxidative damage and aids in normal sleep patterns?

What's the Story?

The three main types of walnuts are the white walnut or butternut (*Juglans cinerea*), the black walnut (*Juglans nigra*), and the English walnut (*Juglans regia*), which is the main type consumed in the United States.

A Serving of Food Lore . . .

Petrified walnut shells had been found in southwestern France dating back more than eight thousand years. What's more amazing—they were even roasted! Inscriptions found on clay tablets spoke of walnut groves in Mesopotamia as far back as 2000 B.C. The English walnut originated in India in areas that surrounded the Caspian Sea. In the fourth century A.D., the Romans introduced the walnut to Europe. The walnut made its way to the United States by English merchant ships. The white and black walnuts are native to North America, mainly in the Appalachian and the Central Mississippi Valley area.

Where Are Walnuts Grown?

The main producers of walnuts are China, the United States, Turkey, Romania, Iran, and France. Ninety-nine percent of English walnuts are grown in California.

Why Should I Eat Walnuts?

Walnuts have the highest level of omega-3 fats compared to any other nut. A one-ounce serving contains 2.6 grams of omega-3 fatty acid, providing two hundred percent of the recommended daily value. They are also a good source of B vitamins, especially thiamine, B6, folic acid, and minerals such as phosphorus, magnesium, and copper. They are an excellent source of gamma-tocopherol, a type of vitamin E which may help in fighting breast, prostate, and colon cancer. Walnuts are rich in ellagitannins, a type of polyphenol having antioxidant and anticarcinogenic properties.

Home Remedies

Because walnuts resemble a human brain, many cultures have used it as a "brain food." In Asia, students are known to munch on walnuts before exams in hopes of improving test results. One home remedy suggests consuming 20 grams of walnuts daily for amnesia. Walnut leaves were once used to treat pain and thought to benefit good digestion.

Throw Me a Lifesaver!

HEART HEALTH: According to the USDA, "Supportive but not conclusive research shows that eating 1.5 ounces of walnuts per day, as part of a low-saturated-fat and low-cholesterol diet and not resulting in increased caloric intake, may reduce the risk of coronary heart disease." A clinical intervention trial involving about 200 subjects found that consuming walnuts lowers cholesterol and decreases the risk of coronary heart disease. A cross-sectional study conducted in France involving 793 subjects found that walnut consumption increased blood HDL cholesterol (healthy type). A case-controlled study involving fifty-two subjects fed twenty grams per day of walnuts for eight weeks found significant increases in their HDL cholesterol and decreases in their triglycerides.

CANCER: Gamma-tocopherol, a form of vitamin E that is abundant in walnuts, may help fight breast, prostate, and lung cancer.

DIABETES: Walnuts may improve insulin resistance in those with type 2 diabetes.

WEIGHT MANAGEMENT: Walnuts have been found to reduce overeating by affecting hunger and satiety. Though they are high in fat (like most nuts), walnuts have not been found to cause weight gain when replacing commonly eaten foods.

SLEEP: Walnuts contain the powerful antioxidant melatonin, which promotes restful sleep. University of Texas researcher Russel Reiter found that adding walnuts to the diet increased blood levels of melatonin threefold!

Tips on Using Walnuts

SELECTION AND STORAGE:
- Shake the nut; if it rattles or feels light it may be withered out.
- Nuts should not be limp or rubbery or smell rancid or musty.
- Shelled walnuts will stay fresh for up to three weeks if refrigerated in a tightly covered container. They will keep up to six months if frozen.
- In-shell walnuts will stay fresh for up to a year as long as they are kept in a cool, dry place.

PREPARATION AND SERVING SUGGESTIONS:
- To toast walnuts, place the shelled nuts in a shallow baking pan and bake them at 350 degrees for about 10 minutes until they are golden. Stir on occasion.
- Walnuts are great additions to your favorite baked items such as muffins, pancakes, and banana or zucchini bread.

- Give your salad a boost by sprinkling some walnuts on top of your greens.
- Add walnuts to your homemade or store-bought granola and mix with nonfat yogurt.

Walnut & Cucumber Gazpacho
Courtesy of Chefs Duskie Estes and John Stewart
Servings: 8 (1 cup) • Prep time: 70 minutes

This recipe contains seven powerhouse foods.

INGREDIENTS:

4 English cucumbers, roughly chopped
½ bunch flat-leaf parsley
½ bunch mint
1 bunch scallions, roughly chopped
½ small red onion, peeled
½ cup extra-virgin olive oil

⅓ cup champagne vinegar
6 ounces plain yogurt
1 cup toasted California walnuts
1 cup ice
Salt and freshly cracked pepper, to taste
Optional: Meyer lemon olive oil to drizzle on top

DIRECTIONS:
Salt the cucumbers and let sit one hour. Drain off liquid. Combine all ingredients in a blender. Blend until smooth. Serve in a chilled bowl, and garnish, if desired, with Meyer lemon olive oil.

BREAK IT DOWN . . .
Calories: 275; Total fat: 23g; Saturated fat: 3g; Cholesterol: 1mg; Sodium: 30mg; Total carbs: 14g; Fiber: 3g; Sugar: 6g; Protein: 6g.

Watermelon *(Citrullis lanatus)*

DON'T SWALLOW THAT

Did you know . . . swallowing whole watermelon seeds won't cause a watermelon to grow in your stomach? Sure you did! In fact, many cultures outside of the United States consider watermelon seeds a delicacy.

What's the Story?

Watermelon is related to the cantaloupe, squash, pumpkin, and other plants that grow on vines on the ground. There are over 1,200 varieties of watermelon and about 200 to 300 varieties are grown in the United States and Mexico alone. There are about fifty varieties that are the most popular that fall into four general categories: Allsweet, Ice-Box, Seedless, and Yellow Flesh.

A Serving of Food Lore . . .

Watermelon is thought to have originated in the Kalahari Desert of Africa. The first reference to watermelons was discovered in ancient hieroglyphics on the walls of Egyptian buildings, occurring some 5,000 years ago. Watermelons were often placed in burial tombs of kings to nourish them in the afterlife. They made their way into countries along the Mediterranean Sea by way of merchant ships. By the tenth century, watermelon found its way to China, which is now the world's number one producer of watermelons. The thirteenth century found watermelon spread through the rest of Europe via the Moors. Watermelons made their way to the United States via slave ships.

Where Are Watermelons Grown?

Watermelons are grown commercially in over ninety-six countries. The top watermelon-producing countries are China, Turkey, Iran, and the United States. According to the National Agricultural Statistics Service, the top producing states for watermelons are Texas, Florida, California, and Georgia.

Why Should I Eat Watermelon?

The lycopene content of watermelon is comparable to what is found in raw tomatoes. A one-cup serving of watermelon contains about the same amount of lycopene as two medium-size tomatoes. Studies also suggest that the body's ability to absorb lycopene in fresh watermelon may be comparable to that in tomato juice, which has long been considered the optimal source of lycopene. Watermelon rind offers a natural source of citrulline, an amino acid that promotes nitric oxide production, improving blood flow through arteries. Watermelons are a good source of beta-carotene.

Home Remedies

Watermelon seed tea has been used as a diuretic and to lower blood pressure. Watermelon rind applied to the skin provides relief from itching caused by poison ivy and poison oak.

Throw Me a Lifesaver!

COLORECTAL CANCER: A human case-control study conducted in Korea found that men with a high intake of watermelon, along with other fruit, had a lower risk of colorectal cancer.

PROSTATE CANCER: Another human case-control study involving 130 patients with prostate cancer found that those who consumed watermelon, along with other foods high in carotenoids, had a lower risk of prostate cancer.

Tips on Using Watermelon

SELECTION AND STORAGE:
- Choose a firm watermelon that is free of bruises, cuts, and dents.
- Cover the cut surface of a melon with plastic wrap, and refrigerate.
- Whole melons will keep for 7 to 10 days at room temperature.

PREPARATION AND SERVING SUGGESTIONS:

- Try freezing watermelon juice in ice cube trays to add to lemonades and fruit punches for a flavorful addition to your drink.
- Wash the watermelon before cutting.
- The watermelon flesh can be cubed, sliced, or scooped into balls.
- Every part of a watermelon is edible, even the seeds and rinds.
- Salt can bring out the sweet taste in watermelon, though salt is not necessary to enjoy it.
- In Israel and Egypt, the sweet taste of watermelon is often paired with the salty taste of feta cheese.
- Make a cold soup by combining pureed cantaloupe, kiwi, and watermelon, and swirl in some plain yogurt.

Roasted Watermelon Salad

Adapted from *Homegrown Pure and Simple: Great Healthy Food from Garden to Table* by Michel Nischan and Mary Goodbody

Servings: 6 • Preparation and cooking time: 30 minutes

This recipe contains four powerhouse foods.

INGREDIENTS:

1 small watermelon sliced in 2" slices with rind removed	4 cups arugula or romaine leaves, loosely packed
Salt to taste	½ cup slivered almonds, lightly toasted
½ cup extra-virgin olive oil	
¼ cup balsamic vinegar	¼ cup sliced whole scallions
Fresh ground pepper to taste	12 red radishes

DIRECTIONS:

Wash watermelon and slice into 2" slices. Remove rind from all slices. Trim slices into triangular pieces that will fit nicely on a salad plate. Season each slice with salt. Brush one side of each slice with olive oil. Heat a large skillet over medium-high heat. When hot, place watermelon slices, oiled side down, on the hot skillet and grill until browned. With a large spatula or tongs, remove the slices and place heated side up on a chilled plate. Put the reserved watermelon in a sieve over a bowl and squeeze watermelon pieces with your hands, collecting juice in the bowl below. Measure out 1 cup of juice. In a saucepan, combine vinegar and watermelon juice and bring to a boil over medium heat. Reduce heat and simmer uncovered for about fifteen minutes or until reduced to about ¼ cup. Pour the reduced juice into a serving bowl and whisk in the remaining olive oil. Season to taste with salt and pepper. Add the arugula, almonds, scallions, and radishes and toss well. Gently mound the salad over melon slices and serve.

BREAK IT DOWN . . .
Calories: 270; Total fat: 24g; Saturated fat: 3g; Cholesterol: 0mg; Sodium: 210mg; Total carbs: 14g; Fiber: 3g; Sugar: 11g; Protein: 3g.

Wheat *(Triticum spp.)*

TELLING THE "WHOLE" TRUTH
Did you know . . . that Americans consume only ⅓ of the minimum amount of whole grains recommended in the dietary guidelines for Americans?

What's the Story?

Wheat is a grass that contains an edible kernel or "berry" and ranks as the second most produced grain in the world right behind corn. Some products derived from whole wheat include bulgur, cracked wheat, rolled wheat flakes, wheat berries, wheat germ, and wheat bran. To qualify as "whole wheat," the entire grain must be ground with all parts intact—the germ, endosperm, and bran. Before there were automated, mechanical grain mills, whole grains were ground between two large stones, resulting in flour that contained all three components of whole grain.

A Serving of Food Lore . . .

Wheat has been consumed for more than 12,000 years and is thought to have originated in southwestern Asia. Wheat gods and goddesses existed in Roman, Sumerian, and Greek mythology. Today, in parts of China, wheat is still considered sacred. It was introduced to the Western

Hemisphere in the fifteenth century when Columbus came to the New World. Wheat was not cultivated in the United States until the late nineteenth century. About one-third of the world's population is dependent on wheat for nourishment.

Along with modern technology, refinement of whole wheat blossomed. White bread became a status symbol among the Greeks and Romans. By 50 A.D., sifted flour was being produced on a large scale in most Mediterranean countries. Whole wheat bread became the food for peasants, slaves, and athletes. In Rome it became known as *panis sordidus* (dirty bread). In 1873, the roller miller was introduced at the World's Fair. Flour could now be refined better and more cheaply but some would argue that we have been "paying a price" ever since!

Where Is Wheat Grown?

The largest producers of wheat are the United States, the Russian Federation, China, France, Canada, and India.

Why Should I Eat Whole Wheat?

There is absolutely no comparison—whole wheat has significantly higher antioxidants than processed wheat, including phenolics and lectins, found in human case studies to resist digestion and bind to cancer cell membranes, inhibiting tumor growth and causing apoptosis (programmed cell death).

Home Remedies

Hippocrates recommended whole wheat flour to promote regulation of the bowel. Adding wheat germ to the diet has been used for treating acne. The vitamin E in wheat germ may relieve the frequency and severity of hot flashes. Using wheat grass juice as a mouthwash has been shown to diminish toothache pain.

Throw Me a Lifesaver!

LONGEVITY: Eating whole grains is associated with longevity and lower risk of many different types of disease in women.

HEART HEALTH: Several studies show reduction in cholesterol and triglycerides when whole grains, as opposed to refined grains, are part of the diet.

RHEUMATOID ARTHRITIS: A study of rheumatoid arthritis patients who were given a fermented wheat germ extract in addition to their steroid therapies found significant improvement compared to steroid use alone.

CANCER: A meta-analysis revealed that there is an inverse relationship between whole grain consumption and colorectal, gastric, and endometrial cancers.

DIABETES: People who consume at least three servings a day of whole grain foods are less likely to develop type 2 diabetes than those who consume less. In a study of nearly 3,000 middle-aged adults, whole grain consumption was associated with lower levels of total and LDL cholesterol, and improved insulin sensitivity. Fasting insulin was ten percent lower when whole grains were consumed versus when refined grains were eaten.

OBESITY: According to a study in the *American Journal of Clinical Nutrition,* people who consumed the most whole grain foods had a lower body mass index (BMI).

Tips on Using Wheat

SELECTION AND STORAGE:
- There are basically six classes of wheat to choose from:
  - Durum—Used to make semolina flour for pasta.
  - Hard Red Spring—High-protein wheat used for baked goods.
  - Hard Red Winter—High-protein wheat used for baked goods and as an adjunct in other flours to increase protein in pastry flour for pie crusts.
  - Soft Red Winter—Low-protein wheat used for cakes, pie crusts, biscuits, and muffins.
  - Hard White—Medium-protein wheat used for bread and beer-making.

- Soft White—Soft, very low-protein wheat used for pie crusts and pastries.
- Wheat berries should be kept in an airtight container in a dark, cool, dry place.
- Flour, bulgur, bran, and germ should be kept in an airtight container in the refrigerator to prevent them from becoming rancid.

PREPARATION AND SERVING SUGGESTIONS:
- Rinse wheat berries well under cold water before using.
- Choose whole wheat products when available, such as whole wheat bread, pasta, or crackers.
- Use sprouted wheat berries in vegetable salads.

Summer Garden Couscous Salad
by Sharon Grotto
Servings: 8 (1 cup) • Prep and cooking time: 20 minutes

This couscous salad is light, simple to make and tastes even better the next day. This recipe contains ten powerhouse foods.

INGREDIENTS:
3 cups prepared whole grain
   couscous
½ cup fresh basil, sliced
   chiffonade-style
½ teaspoon salt
½ teaspoon black pepper
½ cup green onions, chopped fine
½ cup red pepper, chopped

½ cup green pepper, chopped
2 garlic cloves, minced
1 large seeded tomato, chopped
1 small seeded cucumber, chopped
1 teaspoon fresh lemon juice
2 tablespoons extra-virgin
   olive oil
Optional: 8 black olives

DIRECTIONS:
Place cooked couscous in large bowl. Mix all other ingredients together, folding into couscous. Cover and refrigerate for at least one hour or preferably overnight. Fluff with fork and garnish with slices of black olives, if desired.

BREAK IT DOWN . . .
Calories: 120; Total fat: 4g; Saturated fat: .5g; Cholesterol: 0mg; Sodium: 150mg; Total carbs: 20g; Fiber: 4g; Sugar: 1g; Protein: 4g.

Whey

What's the Story?

Is it a food or a dietary supplement? Whey is a natural by-product of the cheese-making process but it typically comes in a powdered supplement form and can be found in most health food stores. The most common forms seen in dietary supplementation are whey protein concentrate and isolate. Whey protein isolate contains ninety percent or more protein and also contains little to no fat or lactose (making it tolerable by most that may be lactose-intolerant). Most who have "dairy protein allergies" often have sensitivity to the larger protein in milk called casein and are not usually allergic to whey protein.

A Serving of Food Lore . . .

For centuries, dairy farmers either sold whey or gave it away for use as feed or fertilizer. Now whey protein is revered and is one of the most popular foods around because of its multiple health benefits.

Why Should I Include Whey?

If Little Miss Muffet only knew! Whey protein contains the highest concentration of branched chain amino acids (BCAAs), which are the building blocks for muscle repair and development, compared with egg, milk, and soy protein. The non-denatured forms (uncooked) have high amounts of the amino acid cysteine, which, in turn, produces a cell protector called glutathione.

Home Remedies

Both Hippocrates and Galen valued whey protein and recommended it to their patients. "Whey cure" baths were the rage in Switzerland in the nineteenth and twentieth centuries and a popular society event. Spas across Europe offered the whey cure for a variety of ailments.

Throw Me a Lifesaver!

Many research studies have investigated the benefit of whey protein in the treatment of cancer, HIV, hepatitis B, cardiovascular disease, and osteoporosis, and as an antimicrobial agent.

CANCER: Whey helps lower resistance of cancer cells while enhancing the immune system. It also increases the activity of natural killer cells to help identify cancer cells.

COGNITIVE FUNCTION: Whey is high in the amino acid L-tryptophan, which may aid in improving cognitive function in stressed individuals and has also been associated with helping to decrease insomnia (sleep disturbances).

BONE DENSITY: Whey protein enhances the bioavailability (absorption) of calcium and is helpful in the prevention of osteoporosis.

IMMUNE ENHANCEMENT: Whey enhances a powerful cell protector called glutathione which neutralizes the harmful effects of free radicals.

HYPERTENSION: The whey portion of dairy products may be the beneficial part in controlling blood pressure. Studies show that low-fat dairy products are an essential part of a widely accepted optimal diet for lowering blood pressure called the Dietary Approaches to Stop Hypertension, or "DASH" diet for short.

OBESITY: Whey protein stimulates the body to produce cholecystokinin (CCK), the hormone that is released after eating to give a sense of satiation and that may aid in weight loss. Recent studies have linked low-fat dairy consumption with better weight management. And whey protein, out of all proteins, increases skeletal muscle growth best.

HUMAN IMMUNODEFICIENCY VIRUS (HIV): Impressive data exist demonstrating a positive role for whey protein in boosting immune function and aiding in muscle-mass preservation and improving strength in women diagnosed with HIV.

Tips for Using Whey

SELECTION AND STORAGE:
- Choose non-denatured, ion-exchanged, or microfiltered.
- Store container in a cool, dry place.

PREPARATION AND SERVING SUGGESTIONS:
- Many of the non-denatured forms of whey protein often create foam if mixed too rigorously. Suggestion: Make a rue or "paste" out of the whey powder. Mix a little of your favorite beverage with the powder until it becomes a paste. Then slowly beat in the remaining liquid with a fork until well mixed. Remember—slow but sure.
- Serving ideas: Try it in juice smoothies or as an ingredient in your favorite shake recipe using low-fat milk, soy, almond, or oat milk beverages.

My Daughters' Whey Protein Smoothie
by Chloe, Katie, and Madison Grotto
Servings: 2 • Prep time: 5 minutes

This recipe was a lifesaver for those times when my girls were being ultra-finicky about their food or if we were pressed for time and needed something quick and nutritious. This recipe contains five powerhouse foods.

INGREDIENTS:

1 teaspoon vanilla extract
8 ounces of nonfat, soy, rice, almond, or oat milk
1 packet frozen açaí pulp

½ cup frozen mango or mixed tropical fruit
1 scoop non-denatured whey protein
2 tablespoons agave nectar

DIRECTIONS:
Mix all ingredients together and blend until smooth. Garnish with
fruit chunks.

BREAK IT DOWN . . .
Calories: 220; Total fat: 3.5g; Saturated fat: 1g; Cholesterol: 0mg;
Sodium: 105mg; Total carbs: 35g; Fiber: 1g; Sugar: 29g; Protein: 16g.

Yogurt

YOGURT-FRESH BREATH!

**Did you know . . . a Japanese study found that volunteers who con-
sumed six ounces of unsweetened yogurt containing *Streptococcus
thermophilus* and *Lactobacillus bulgaricus* bacteria daily had a reduction in the odor-inducing bacteria?**

What's the Story?

According to the U.S. Food and Drug Administration, in order for a
product to be called "yogurt," it must be made from milk that has been
fermented by *Lactobacillus bulgaricus* and *Streptococcus thermophilus*,
specific bacteria that result in a thickened, semisolid product.

A Serving of Food Lore . . .

Yogurt may be one of the oldest foods in recorded history. It is believed to
date back as far as 10,000 years, with its place of origin being Turkey or
Iran. The first making of yogurt could very well have happened by acci-
dent—maybe even when milk was being stored in goatskin bags or urns
for later use. Later on, civilizations recognized yogurt's digestive health
benefits and spoke of yogurt's "cleansing" attributes and its contribution
to longevity. It was not until the turn of the twentieth century that the cultures used to make yogurt were isolated by Nobel Prize winner Elie
Metchnikoff from the Pasteur Institute.

Where Is Yogurt Made?

Yogurt is now made throughout the world. The largest yogurt manufacturing plant in the world is located in Minster, Ohio.

Why Should I Eat Yogurt?

Yogurt reigns supreme in calcium!

Top 5 Dairy Sources of Calcium

Food	Amount	Calcium (mg)
Yogurt, flavored	1 cup	389
Ricotta, part skim	½ cup	334
Skim milk	1 cup	302
Low-fat 1% milk	1 cup	300
Low-fat 2% milk	1 cup	297

Many people who are lactose-intolerant may be able to tolerate yogurt because of reduced lactose content. Similar to other dairy products, another key benefit of yogurt is that it is a good source of calcium, vitamins, and other minerals. Yogurt is considered a probiotic because it contains bacteria that produce lactic acid. The consumption of these bacteria is beneficial for boosting the immune system, enhancing intestinal tract health, lessening the symptoms of lactose intolerance, and reducing the risk of certain cancers.

Home Remedies

Eating yogurt that contains live cultures of *Lactobacillus acidophilus* on a daily basis will introduce good bacteria and help treat a yeast infection.

Throw Me a Lifesaver!

ARTHRITIS: A rat study found that arthritic rats fed yogurt containing *Lactobacillus GG* bacteria had only mild inflammation.

HEART HEALTH: A human study involved 33 female volunteers who consumed conventional yogurt for four weeks. Yogurt improved their LDL/HDL cholesterol ratios. Researchers found that yogurt was one of the foods that had an inverse relationship with serum homocysteine levels.

COLON CANCER: A study using mice induced with a colorectal carcinoma found that when yogurt was added to their diet there was an increase in apoptosis (cell death) induction and anticancer activity.

GUT HEALTH: An intervention study involving 59 human volunteers infected with *Helicobacter pylori* (*H. pylori*) who were given yogurt with *Lactobacillus* and *Bifidobacterium* twice daily for six weeks found that the *H. pylori* was effectively suppressed. A randomized study involving 160 subjects showed that those receiving antibiotic therapy who supplemented with *Lactobacillus*- and *Bifidobacterium*-containing yogurt had less *H. Pylori* infection.

Tips on Using Yogurt

SELECTION AND STORAGE:
- Choose yogurt that bears the "Live and Active Cultures" seal or states that it has "live active cultures" on the label.
- Check the expiration date to ensure freshness.
- Store yogurt in the refrigerator and, if unopened, it will last about a week after the expiration date.

PREPARATION AND SUGGESTED USES:
- Top yogurt with granola/cereal and fresh/dried fruit.
- Make a refreshing salad by adding dill weed and chopped cucumber to plain yogurt. Also great as a side with grilled chicken or lamb.

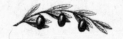

Chow Yogurt Granola Berry Parfait
by Mary Corlett
Servings: 8 • Prep and cooking time: 1 hour

This recipe contains eight powerhouse foods.

INGREDIENTS:
FOR THE GRANOLA:

1 ½ *cups honey*	¼ *cup walnut pieces*
¾ *cup pure maple syrup*	½ *cup sunflower seeds*
⅛ *teaspoon ground cinnamon*	½ *cup pecan pieces*
⅛ *teaspoon ground ginger*	½ *cup pistachios, shelled*
Pinch of nutmeg	1 ½ *cups almonds, slivered*
Pinch of ground cloves	1 ½ *cups coconut, flaked*
¼ *cup white sesame seeds*	3 *cups old-fashioned oats*

IN A SMALL BOWL COMBINE:

¼ *cup dried cherries*	¼ *cup dried apricots, chopped*
¼ *cup dried cranberries*	¼ *cup raisins*

GARNISH:

2 *cups fresh berries*

YOGURT:

2 *cups low-fat vanilla yogurt*

DIRECTIONS:
Preheat oven to 350 degrees. Add honey, maple syrup, cinnamon, ginger, nutmeg, and cloves to saucepan. Heat over medium heat on the stove top until honey and syrup thin to a pouring consistency; remove from heat. Toss remaining ingredients (except fruit mixture) together in a large bowl and pour honey mixture over the ingredients in the bowl. Stir with a wooden spoon until the honey-and-syrup mixture coats all the ingredients. Divide the contents of the bowl between two metal cookie or ½-sheet pans. Spread the mixture out to a thin layer and place into the oven. Bake 15 to 20 minutes or until the oats, nuts, and seeds are golden and toasted. Make sure to stir the mixture occasionally with a metal spatula for even coloring. Carefully scrape the hot granola back into the large bowl.

Add the dried fruits and stir well. Allow the granola to cool completely and break up with the wooden spoon. Alternate layers of granola and vanilla yogurt with fresh berries in a parfait glass and serve.

BREAK IT DOWN . . .
Calories: 190; Total fat: 8g; Saturated fat: 1.5g; Cholesterol: 0mg; Sodium: 20mg; Total carbs: 29g; Fiber: 3g; Sugar: 20g; Protein: 5g.

APPENDIX A

2,000-Calorie Meal Plan

SUNDAY

Breakfast:	Lunch:	Snack:	Dinner:	Snack:
2 Ina's Whole Wheat Oatmeal Pancakes (240) 1 cup skim milk (90) ½ banana (60) 1 cup of coffee (5)	1 cup Summer Garden Couscous Salad (120) 1 cup Black Bean Soup with Lime and Cumin (255) 2 persimmons (60)	Fun Fruit Kabobs (150)	3 Swiss Chard Tacos (360) 1 cup Mango Slaw (126) 1 cup Simple Southern Italian Onion, Tomato, and Basil Salad (110)	½ Berry and Almond Pizza (280) 1 cup soy milk (100)

1956 total calories

MONDAY

Breakfast:	Lunch:	Snack:	Dinner:	Snack:
2 whole grain toaster waffles with ⅓ cup Sharon's Simple Berry Sauce (305) 1 cup soy milk (100) 1 cup black tea (0)	1 cup Barley Orzo Salad (140) 1 cup Elisa's Cheesy Eggplant (370) Roasted Grapefruit Salad (110)	¼ cup Luxurious Guacomole (120) 12 corn chips (140)	6 Clove Tequila Shrimp (258) ½ cup Spicy Japanese Mint Noodles (180) ¾ cup Asparagus with Fresh Citrus Dressing (90)	½ cup Sweet Potato Chips (114) 1 cup skim milk (90)

2017 total calories

357

TUESDAY

Breakfast:	Lunch:	Snack:	Dinner:	Snack:
Brazilian-Style Açaí Bowl topped with ¼ cup Cinnamon-Walnut Granola (307) 1 cup of coffee (5)	Black Bean Soup with Lime and Cumin (221) Spelt Burger (190) 1 whole spelt hamburger bun (240)	¾ cup Apple Cranberry Fruit Salad (150)	1½ cups Roasted Watermelon Salad (270) 1 cup Moroccan Chicken with Figs (370) ¾ cup Art's Vesuvio Potatoes (180)	3 cups air-popped popcorn (80)

2013 total calories

WEDNESDAY

Breakfast:	Lunch:	Snack:	Dinner:	Snack:
1 slice Banana-Blueberry Bread (132) 6-oz cup fruited yogurt (180) Cheesy Asparagus and Mushroom Scramble (190) 1 cup of green tea (0)	1 cup Walnut & Cucumber Gazpacho (275) 1 slice crustless BOCA Sausage Quiche (150) 1 rye roll (202)	2 oz Sicilian Spread (80) Whole wheat pita triangles (140)	1 cup Fried Tofu in Curry Sauce (210) ¾ cup Kamut-Cranberry Salad (261)	½ cup Simple Blackberry Crisp (220)

2040 total calories

THURSDAY

Breakfast:	Lunch:	Snack:	Dinner:	Snack:
¾ cup Cherry Oatmeal Bake (210) ½ cup Breakfast Pudding (230) 1 cup coffee (5)	1 cup Romaine Sesame Stir-Fry (112) 1 cup Sesame Mushroom Beef (200) ⅔ cup brown rice (160)	¼ cup Red Pepper Hummus (210) ¼ Zahtar whole wheat pita (210)	1 Vegetarian Polish Cabbage Roll (360) ½ Steamed Artichoke with Cilantro Aioli (147) 1 slice Bursting Blueberry Bread Pudding (230)	¾ cup Apricot-Cranberry-Mango Ice (150)

2014 total calories

FRIDAY

Breakfast:	Lunch:	Snack:	Dinner:	Snack:
1 cup My Daughters' Whey Protein Smoothie (220)	Grapes of Wrap (190)	1 slice Carob Walnut Cake (160)	4 oz Grilled Salmon with Cranberry-Cherry Salsa (260)	¼ cup Red Pepper Hummus with ¼ pita (210)
Sorghum & Orange Marmalade Muffin (230)	1 cup Roasted Carrot Butternut Soup (80)	1 cup soy milk (100)	1 cup Wasabi Asian Noodles (275)	
1 cup black tea (0)	¾ cup Cranberry Pear Salad with Curried Hazelnuts (210)		1 cup Sautéed Spinach (100)	
	1 cup coffee (5)			

2040 total calories

SATURDAY

Breakfast:	Lunch:	Snack:	Dinner:	Snack:
1 slice Family Favorite Broccoli Frittata (200)	1 cup Easy Pasta Fagioli (273)	1 oz Aztec Cocoa Fire Peanuts (160)	6 oz Roasted Fish with Cumin Sweet Potatoes (300)	1 Banana-Cinnamon French Toast (155)
1 Raspberry-Peach Melba Tart (220)	¾ cup Caribbean Quinoa (190)	1 Sunny Sunflower Mini-Scones (80)	1 cup Comforting Kale and Lentil Soup (130)	
1 cup skim milk (90)	Strawberry Shortcake (170)			
1 cup coffee (5)				

1973 total calories

APPENDIX B

Phytochemicals and Nutrients
Commonly Found in the 101 Foods

Class/Components	Source*	Potential Benefit
Carotenoids		
Beta-carotene	Carrots, pumpkin, sweet potato	Neutralizes free radicals, which may damage cells; bolsters cellular antioxidant defenses; can be made into vitamin A in the body
Lutein, Zeaxanthin	Kale, spinach, corn, eggs, citrus	May contribute to maintenance of healthy vision
Lycopene	Tomatoes and processed tomato products, watermelon, red/pink grapefruit	May contribute to maintenance of prostate health
Dietary (functional and total) fiber		
Beta-glucan[†]	Oat bran, oatmeal, oat flour, barley, rye	May reduce risk of coronary heart disease (CHD)
Insoluble fiber	Wheat bran, corn bran, fruit skins	May contribute to maintenance of a healthy digestive tract; may reduce the risk of some types of cancer
Soluble fiber[†]	Peas, beans, apples, citrus fruit	May reduce risk of CHD and some types of cancer
Whole grains[†]	Cereal grains, whole wheat bread, oatmeal, brown rice	May reduce risk of CHD and some types of cancer; may contribute to maintenance of healthy blood glucose levels
Fatty acids		
Monounsaturated fatty acids (MUFAs)[†]	Tree nuts, olive oil, canola oil	May reduce risk of CHD

Class/Components	Source*	Potential Benefit
Polyunsaturated fatty acids (PUFAs)—omega-3 fatty acids—ALA	Walnuts, flax	May contribute to maintenance of heart health; may contribute to maintenance of mental and visual function
PUFAs—omega-3 fatty acids—DHA/EPA[†]	Salmon, tuna, marine, and other fish oils	May reduce risk of CHD; may contribute to maintenance of mental and visual function
Flavonoids		
Anthocyanins—cyanidin, delphinidin, malvidin	Berries, cherries, red grapes	Bolsters cellular antioxidant defenses; may contribute to maintenance of brain function
Flavonols—catechins, epicatechins, epigallocatechin, procyanidins	Tea, cocoa, apples, grapes	May contribute to maintenance of heart health
Flavanones—hesperetin, selenium	Citrus foods, fish, grains, garlic, eggs	Neutralize free radicals, which may damage cells; may contribute to healthy immune function
Phenolic acids		
Caffeic acid, ferulic acid	Apples, pears, citrus fruits, some vegetables, coffee	May bolster cellular antioxidant defenses; may contribute to maintenance of healthy vision and heart health
Plant stanols/sterols		
Free stanols/sterols[†]	Corn, soy, wheat, sunflower seeds	May reduce risk of CHD
Prebiotics		
Inulin, fructo-oligosaccharides (FOS), polydextrose	Whole grains, onions, some fruits, garlic, honey, leeks	May improve gastrointestinal health; may improve calcium absorption
Probiotics		
Yeast, *Lactobacilli, Bifidobacteria,* and other specific strains of beneficial bacteria	Yogurt and other cultured dairy, unpasteurized miso, sauerkraut	May improve gastrointestinal health and systemic immunity; benefits are strain-specific

Class/Components	Source*	Potential Benefit
Phytoestrogens		
Isoflavones—daidzein, genistein	Soybeans and soy-based foods	May contribute to maintenance of bone health, healthy brain and immune function; for women, may contribute to maintenance of menopausal health
Lignans	Flax, rye, some vegetables	May contribute to maintenance of heart health and healthy immune function
Sulfides/thiols		
Diallyl sulfide, allyl methyl trisulfide	Garlic, onions, leeks, scallions	May enhance detoxification of undesirable compounds; may contribute to maintenance of heart health and healthy immune function
Dithiolthiones	Cruciferous vegetables	May enhance detoxification of undesirable compounds; may contribute to maintenance of healthy immune function
Vitamins		
A[‡]	Milk, eggs, carrots, sweet potato, spinach	May contribute to maintenance of healthy vision, immune function, and bone health; may contribute to cell integrity
B1 (Thiamine)	Lentils, peas, long grain brown rice	May contribute to maintenance of mental function; helps regulate metabolism
B2 (Riboflavin)	Lean meats, eggs, green leafy vegetables	Helps support cell growth; helps regulate metabolism
B3 (Niacin)	Dairy products, poultry, fish, nuts, eggs	Helps support cell growth; helps regulate metabolism
B5 (Pantothenic acid)	Soybeans, lentils	Helps regulate metabolism and hormone synthesis
B6 (Pyridoxine)	Beans, nuts, legumes, fish, meat, whole grains	May contribute to maintenance of healthy immune function; helps regulate metabolism

Class/Components	Source*	Potential Benefit
B9 (Folate)†	Beans, legumes, citrus foods, green leafy vegetables, fortified breads and cereals	May reduce a woman's risk of having a child with a brain or spinal cord defect
B12 (Cobalamin)	Eggs, meat, poultry, milk	May contribute to maintenance of mental function; helps regulate metabolism and supports blood cell formation
Biotin	Salmon, dairy, eggs	Helps regulate metabolism and hormone synthesis
C	Guava, sweet red/green pepper, kiwi, citrus fruit, strawberries	Neutralizes free radicals, which may damage cells; may contribute to maintenance of bone health and immune function
D	Sunlight, fish, fortified milk and cereals	Helps regulate calcium and phosphorus; helps contribute to bone health; may contribute to healthy immune function; helps support cell growth
E	Sunflower seeds, almonds, hazelnuts, turnip greens	Neutralizes free radicals, which may damage cells; may contribute to healthy immune function and maintenance of heart health

*Examples are not an all-inclusive list.
†FDA-approved health claim established for component.
‡Preformed vitamin A is found in foods that come from animals. Provitamin A carotenoids are found in many darkly colored fruits and vegetables, and are a major source of vitamin A for vegetarians.

Adapted from the International Food Information Council Foundation

RECIPE CREDITS

I'd like to express my sincere gratitude to all of those individuals, organizations, and companies that contributed to the 101 recipes. Their time and talents surely helped make good-for-you foods taste spectacular!

Christine M. Palumbo, MBA, RD—www.christinepalumbo.com

Rick Bayless—author of many cookbooks and chef and owner of Frontera Grill and Topolobampo, Chicago, Illinois; www.rickbayless.com

Dave Hamlin—corporate executive chef for Price Chopper supermarkets; www.pricechopper.com

Cheryl Bell, MS, RD, LDN, CHE—executive chef and nutrition expert for Meijer Foods; www.meijer.com

Allen Susser—author of *The Great Mango Book* (Ten Speed Press, 2001); www.chefallens.com

Kyle Shadix, CCC, MS, RD—www.chefkyle.com

Steven Raichlen—author of *Healthy Latin Cooking* (Rodale, 1998) and host of *Barbeque University;* www.barbequebible.com

Mary Corlett—owner of Chow in Elmhurst, Illinois; www.chowtogo.com

Cynthia Sass, MPH, MA, RD, CSSD, LD/N—director of nutrition for *Prevention* magazine; www.prevention.com

Elisa Zied, MS, RD—author of *Feed Your Family Right!* (Wiley, 2007); www.elisazied.com

Lisa Dorfman, MS, RD—author of *The Tropical Diet* (Food Fitness International, 2004); www.runningnutritionist.com

Jane Reinhardt-Martin, RD, LD—author of *The Amazing Flax Cookbook* (TSA Press, 2004); www.FlaxRD.com

Ina Pinkney—www.breakfastqueen.com

Rosalie Gaziano—author of *Mothers Speak . . . for Love of Family* (Durban House, 2006)

Produce for Better Health Foundation—www.fruitsandveggiesmorematters.org

Georgia Pecan Commission—www.georgiapecans.org

Nick Spinelli—executive chef, Kraft Foods

Nicki Anderson—author, *Reality Fitness: Inspiration for Your Health and Well-Being* (New World Library, 2000); www.realityfitness.com

Royce Gracie—international star in the sport of jujitsu; www.roycegracie.tv

The Cranberry Marketing Committee—www.uscranberries.com

The Cherry Marketing Institute—www.choosecherries.com

The Cranberry Institute—www.cranberryinstitute.org

The Almond Board of California—www.almondsarein.com

The Hazelnut Council—www.hazelnutcouncil.org

www.cooks.com

www.purityfoods.com

Bob's Red Mill—www.BobsRedMill.com

Lipton Tea—www.liptontea.com

Folgers—www.folgers.com

Heather Jose—stage IV breast cancer survivor and author of *Letters to Sydney: Hope, Faith, and Cancer* (Author House, 2004); www.heatherjose.com

Arthur P. Grotto—"Noni"

Evelyn Tribole, MS, RD—author of *Stealth Health* (Viking, 2000); www.evelyntribole.com

Michel Nischan and Mary Goodbody, authors of *Homegrown Pure and Simple: Great Healthy Food from Garden to Table* (Chronicle Books, 2005); www.michelnischan.com

Duskie Estes and John Stewart—Zazu and Bovolo Restaurants in Sonoma County, California; www.zazurestaurant.com

Dawn Jackson Blatner, RD, LDN—national spokeswoman, American Dietetic Association; www.dawnjacksonblatner.com

Michel Stroot—author of *The Golden Door Cooks Light and Easy* (Gibbs Smith, 2003)

Carol Fenster, PhD—author of *Gluten-Free 101* (Savory Palate, 2006); www.savorypalate.com

Sandy Tomich—"Ma"

Giselle Ruecking—goddaughter extraordinaire

Treena and Graham Kerr—authors; www.grahamkerr.com

Michael Sena and Kirsten Straughan RD, LD—authors, *Lean Mom, Fit Family: The 6-Week Plan for a Slimmer You and a Healthier Family* (Rodale, 2005)

A very special thank-you to my good friend J. Hugh McEvoy, CRC, CEC—aka "Chef J," who graciously contributed 21 of the 101 delicious recipes; and to my wonderful wife, Sharon, who came up with a boatload of yummy dishes that kept our family well fed.

REFERENCES

The references provided below focus on the many research reports included within the "Throw Me a Lifesaver!" section under each food entry. This is not the complete list of all the studies and sources covered in this book. You will find all of the sources at www.101FoodsThatCouldSaveYourLife.com. I also include websites that I found especially helpful while researching the origin, history, and benefits of the 101 foods.

Açaí   www.acaifacts.com/main

Del Pozo-Insfran D, Percival SS, Talcott ST. J. Açaí (Euterpe oleracea Mart.) polyphenolics in their glycoside and aglycone forms induce apoptosis of HL-60 leukemia cells. *J Agric Food Chem.* 2006 Feb 22;54(4):1222–9.

Hong W, Cao G, Prior P. Oxygen radical absorbance capacity of anthocyanins. *J Agric Food Chem.* 45, 304–309, 1997.

Schauss AG et al. Antioxidant capacity and other bioactivities of the freeze-dried Amazonian palm berry, Euterpe oleraceae Mart. (Açaí). *J Agric Food Chem.* 2006 Nov 1;54(22):8604–8610.

Agave   www.succulent-plant.com/agave.html

Da Silva BP, De Sousa AC, Silva GM, Mendes TP, Parente JP. A new bioactive steroidal saponin from Agave attenuata. *Z Naturforsch.* 2002 May–Jun;57(5–6), 423–428.

Davidson JR, Ortiz de Montellano BR. The antibacterial properties of an Aztec wound remedy. *J Ethnopharmacol.* 1983 Aug;8(2):149–61.

Garcia MD, Quilez AM, Saenz MT, Martinez-Dominguez ME, de la Puerta R. Anti-inflammatory activity of Agave intermixta Trel. and Cissus sicyoides L., species used in the Caribbean traditional medicine. *J Ethnopharmacol.* 2000 Aug;71(3):395–400.

Ohtsuki T, Koyano T, Kowithayakorn T, Sakai S, Kawahara N, Goda Y, Yamaguchi N, Ishibahi M. New chlorogenin hexasaccharide isolated from Agave fourcroydes with cytotoxic and cell cycle inhibitory activities. *Bioorganic & Medicinal Chemistry.* 2004 Jul;12(14), 3841–3845.

Peana AT et al. Anti-inflammatory activity of aqueous extracts and steroidal sapogenins of Agave americana. *Planta Med.* 1997 Jun;63(3):199–202.

Saenz MT, Garcia MD, Quilez A, Ahumada MC. Cytotoxic activity of Agave intermixta L. (agavaceae) and Cissus sicyoides L. (vitaceae). *Pytother Res.* 2000 Nov;14(7), 552–554.

Verastegui MA, Sanchez CA, Heredia NL, Garcia-Alvarado JS. Antimicrobial activity of extracts of three major plants from the Chihuahuan desert. *J Ethnopharmacol.* 1996 Jul 5;52(3):175–177.

Yokosuka A, Mimaki Y, Kuroda M, Sashida Y. A new steroidal saponin from the leaves of Agave Americana. *Planta Med.* 2000 May;66(4), 393–396.

Almonds   www.almondsarein.com

Burton-Freeman B, Davis PA, Schneeman BO. Interaction of fat availability and sex on postprandial satiety and cholecystokinin after mixed-food meals. *Am J Clin Nutr.* 2004 Nov;80(5):1207–14.

Davis PA, Iwahashi CK. Whole almonds and almond fractions reduce aberrant crypt foci in a rat model of colon carcinogenesis. *Cancer Lett.* 2001 Apr 10;165(1): 27–33.

Ellis PR, Kendall CW, Ren Y, Parker C, Pacy JF, Waldron KW, Jenkins DJ. Role of cell walls in the bioaccessibility of lipids in almond seeds. *Am J Clin Nutr.* 2004 Sep;80(3):604–613.

Fraser GE, Bennett HW, Jaceldo KB, Sabate JM. Effect on body weight of a free 76 kilojoule (320 Calorie) daily supplement of almonds for six months. *Journal of the American College of Nutrition,* Vol. 21, No. 3, 275–283 (2002).

Jenkins DJ et al. Assessment of the longer-term effects of a dietary portfolio of cholesterol-lowering foods in hypercholesterolemia. *Am J Clin Nutr.* 2006 Mar;83(3): 582–91.

Jenkins DJ et al. Direct comparison of dietary portfolio vs statin on C-reactive protein. *Eur J Clin Nutr.* 2005 Jul;59(7):851–60.

Sabate J, Haddad E, Tanzman JS, Jambazian P, Rajaram S. Serum lipid response to a graded enrichment of a Step 1 diet with almonds: A randomized feeding trial. *American Journal of Clinical Nutrition* 2003; 77:1379–1384.

Wien MA, Sabate JM, Ikle DN, Cole SE, Kandeel FR. Almonds vs complex carbohydrates in a weight reduction program. *Int J Obes Relat Metab Disord.* 2003 Nov; 27(11):1365–1372.

Amaranth   www.jeffersoninstitute.org/pubs/amaranth.shtml

Gorenstein S, Katrich E, Trakhtenberg S, Lange E, Bartnikowska E, Leontowicz M, Leontowicz H, Czerwinski J. Oat (Avena sativa L.) and amaranth (Amaranthus hypochondriacus) meals positively affect plasma lipid profile in rats fed cholesterol-containing diets. *J Nutr Biochem.* 2004 Oct;15(10):622–629.

Kim HK, Kim MJ, Cho HY, Kim EK, Shin DH. Antioxidative and anti-diabetic effects of amaranth (Amaranthus esculantus) in streptozotocin-induced diabetic rats. *Cell Biochem Funct.* 2006 May–Jun;24(3):195–199.

Kim HK, Kim MJ, Shin DH. Improvement of lipid profile by amaranth (Amaranthus esculantus) supplementation in streptozotocin-induced diabetic rats. *Ann Nutr Metab.* 2006;50(3):277–281.

Shin DH, Heo HJ, Lee YJ, Kim HK. Amaranth squalene reduces serum and liver lipid levels in rats fed a cholesterol diet. *Br J Biomed Sci.* 2004;61(1):11–14.

Silvia-Sanchez C, González Castañeda J, de Léon-Rodríguez A, de la Rosa B. Functional and rheological properties of amaranth albumins extracted from two Mexican varieties. *Plant Foods Hum Nutr.* 2004 Fall;59(4):169–174.

Apples   US Apple Association: www.usapple.org

Conceicao M, Sichieri R, Sanchez Moura A. Weight loss associated with a daily intake of three apples or three pears among overweight women. *Nutrition.* 2003 Mar; 19(3):253–256.

Davis PA et al. Effect of apple extracts on NF-KB activation in human umbilical vein endothelial cells. *Experimental Biology and Medicine.* 2006;231:594–598.

Hertog MG, Feskens EJ, Hollman PC, Katan MB, Kromhout D. Dietary antioxidant flavinoids and risk of coronary heart disease: The Zutphen Elderly Study. *Lancet.* 1993 Oct 23; 342(8878):1007–1011.

Knekt P, Isotupa S, Rissanen H, Heliovaara M, Jarvinen R, Hakkinen S, Aromaa A, Reunanen A. Quercetin intake and the incidence of cerebrovascular disease. *Eur J Clin Nutr.* 2000 May;54(5):415–417.

Liu RH, Liu J, Chen B. Apples prevent mammary tumors in rats. *J Agric Food Chem.* 2005 Mar 23;53(6):2341–2343.

Marchand L, Murphy S, Hankin J, Wilkens L, Kolonel L. Intake of Flavonoids and Lung Cancer. *Journal of the National Cancer Institute.* 2000 Jan 19;92(2): 154–160.

Tchantchou F, Chan A, Kifle L, Ortiz D, Shea TB. Apple juice concentrate prevents oxidative damage and impaired maze performance in aged mice. *J Alzheimer's Dis.* 2005 Dec;8(3):283–287.

Tchantchou F, Graves M, Ortiz D, Rogers E, Shea TB. Dietary supplementation with apple juice concentrate alleviates the compensatory increase in glutathione synthase transcription and activity that accompanies dietary- and genetically-induced oxidative stress. *J Nutr Health Aging.* 2004;8(6):492–496.

Tirgoviste C, Poppa E, Sintu E, Mihalache N, Che D, Mincu I. Blood glucose and plasma insulin responses to various carbohydrates in type 2 (non-insulin dependent) diabetes. *Diabetologia.* 1983 Sept; 24(2):80–84.

Veeriah S, Kautenburger T, Habermann N, Sauer J, Dietrich H, Will F, Pool-Zobel BL. Apple flavonoids inhibit growth of HT29 human colon cancer cells and modulate expression of genes involved in the biotransformation of xenobiotics. *Mol Carcinog.* 2006 Mar;45(3):164–74.

Apricots   California Fresh Apricot Council: www.califapricot.com
American Cancer Society. Available at www.cancer.org. Accessed on May 16, 2006.

Hankinson SE, Stampfer MJ, Seddon JM, et al. Nutrient intake and cataract extraction in women: a prospective study. *BMJ* 1992;305(6849):335–339.

Jacques PF, Chylack LT. Epidemiologic evidence of a role for the antioxidant vitamins and carotenoids in cataract prevention. *Am J Clin Nutr.* 1991.

Otsuka T et al. Suppressive effects of fruit-juice concentrate of Prunus mume Sieb. et Zucc. (Japanese apricot, Ume) on Helicobacter pylori-induced glandular stomach lesions in Mongolian gerbils. *Asian Pac J Cancer Prev.* 2005;6(3):337–341.

Yusuf S et al. Effect of potentially modifiable risk factors associated with myocardial infarction in 52 countries (the INTERHEART study): case-control study. *Lancet.* 2004 Sep;364(9438):937–952.

Artichoke   California Artichoke Advisory Board: www.artichokes.org
Bundy R, Walker AF, Middleton RW, Marakis G, Booth J. Artichoke leaf extract reduces symptoms of irritable bowel syndrome and improves quality of life in otherwise healthy volunteers suffering from concomitant dyspepsia: a subset analysis. *J Altern Compl Med.* 2004 Aug; 10(4):667–669.

Emendorfer F, Emendorfer F, Bellato F, Noldin VF, Cechinel-Filho V, Yunes R, Delle Monache F, Cardozo A. Antispasmodic activity of fraction and cynaropicrin from Cynara scolymus on guinea-pig ileum. *Bil Pharm Bull.* 2005 May; 28(5):902–904.

Gebhardt R. Inhibition of Cholesterol Biosynthesis in Primary Cultured Rat Hepatocytes by Artichoke Extracts. *J Pharmacol Exp Ther.* 1998, Sept; (286):1122–1128.

Pittler MH, Thonpson CO, Ernst E. Artichoke leaf extract for treating hypercholesterolaemia. *Cochrane Database Syst Rev.* 2002; (3):CD003335.

Rossoni G, Grande S, Galli C, Visioli F. Wild artichoke prevents the age-associated loss of vasomotor function. *J Agric Food Chem.* 2005 Dec 28; 53(26):10291–10296.

Asparagus   Michigan Asparagus Advisory Board: www.asparagus.org; California Asparagus Commission: www.calasparagus.com
Clarke R, et al. Hyperhomocystenemia: an independent risk factor for. *New Eng J Med* 324 (1991):1149–55.

Mathews JN, Flatt PR, Abdel-Wahab YH. Asparagus adscendens (Shweta musali) stimulates insulin secretion, insulin action and inhibits starch digestion. *Br J Nutr.* 2006 Mar;95(3):576–581.

Avocado   California Avocado Commission: www.avocado.org; Chilean Avocado Importers Association: www.chileanavocados.org
Angermann, P. Avocado/soybean unsaponifiables in the treatment of knee and hip osteoarthritis. *Ugeskr Laeger.* 2005 Aug 15;167(33):3023–3025.

Kut-Lassere C, Miller CC, Ejeil AL, Gogly B, Dridi M, Piccardi N, Guillou B, Pellat B, Godeau G. Effect of avocado and soybean unsaponifiables on gelatinase A (MMP-2), stromelysin (MMP-3), and tissue inhibitors of matrix metalloproteinase (TIMP-1 and TIMP-2) secretion by human fibroblasts in culture. *J Periodontal.* 2001 Dec;72(12):1685–1694.

Lerman-Garber I et al. Effect of a high-monounsaturated fat diet enriched with avocado in NIDDM patients. *Diabetes Care.* 1994 Apr;17(4):311–315.

Lopez R, Frati AC, Hernandez BC, Cervantes S, Hernandez MH, Juarez C, Moran L. Monounsaturated fatty acid (avocado) rich diet for mild hypercholesterolemia. *Arch Med Res.* 1996 Winter;27(4):519–523.

Lu QY, Arteaga JR, Zhang Q, Huerta S, Go VL, Heber D. Inhibition of prostate cancer cell growth by an avocado extract: role of lipid-soluble bioactive substances. *J Nutr Biochem.* 2005 Jan;16(1):23–30.

Stucker M, Memmel U, Hoffmann M, Hartung J, Altmeyer P. Vitamin B(12) cream containing avocado oil in the therapy of plaque psoriasis. *Dermatology.* 2001; 203(2):141–147.

Bananas   www.banana.com
Emery EA, Ahmad S, Koethe JD, Skipper A, Perlmutter S, Paskin DL. Banana flakes control diarrhea in enterally fed patients. *Nutr Clin Pract.* 1997 Apr;12(2):72–75.

Rabbani GH et al. Clinical studies in persistent diarrhea: dietary management with green banana or pectin in Bangladeshi children. *Gastroenterology.* 2001 Sep;121(3):554–560.

Rabbani GH et al. Green banana and pectin improve small intestinal permeability and reduce fluid loss in Bangladeshi children with persistent diarrhea. *Dig Dis Sci.* 2004 Mar;49(3):475–484.

Rao NM. Protease inhibitors from ripened and unripened bananas. *Biochem Int.* 1991;24(1):13–22.

Rashidkhani B, Lindblad P, Wolk A. Fruits, vegetables and risk of renal cell carcinoma: a prospective study of Swedish women. *Int J Cancer.* 2005;113(3):451–455.

Barley   Barley Foods Council: www.barleyfoods.com
Behall KM, Scholfield DJ, Hallfrisch J. Diets containing barley significantly reduce lipids in mildly hypercholesterolemic men and women. *Am J Clin Nutr.* 2004 Nov;80(5):1185–1193.

Behall KM, Scholfield DJ, Hallfrisch J. Lipids significantly reduced by diets containing barley in moderately hypercholesterolemic men. *J Am Coll Nutr.* 2004 Feb;23(1): 55–62.

Kanauchi O, Hitomi Y, Agata K, Nakamura T, Fushiki T. Germinated barley foodstuff improves constipation induced by lopermide in rats. *Biosci Biotechnol Biochem.* 1998 Sep;62(9):1788–1790.

McIntosh GH, Jorgensen L, Royle P. The potential of an insoluble dietary fiber-rich source from barley to protect from DMH-induced intestinal tumors in rats. *Nutr Cancer.* 1993;19(2):213–221.

Pick M, Hawrysh Z, Gee M, Toth E. Barley bread products improve glycemic control of Type 2 subjects. *Int J Food Sci Nutr.* 1998; 49(1):71–78.

Yu YM, Wu CH, Tseng YH, Tsai CE, Chang WC. Antioxidative and hypolipemic effects of barley leaf essence in a rabbit model of atherosclerosis. *Jpn J Pharmacol.* 2002 Jun;89(2):142–148.

Basil   www.basil.com
Geetha RK, Vasudevan DM. Inhibition of lipid peroxidation by botanical extracts of Ociumem sanctum: in vivo and in vitro studies. *Life Sci.* 2004 Nov 19; 76(1):21–28.

Mediratta PK, Sharma KK, Singh S. Evaluation of immunomodulatory potential of Ocimum sanctum seed oil and its possible mechanism of action. *J Ethnopharmacol.* 2002 Apr; 80(1):15–20.

Opalchenova G, Obreshkova D. Comparative studies on the activity of basil—an essential oil from Ocimum basilicum L.—against multidrug resistant clinical isolates of the genera Staphylococcus, Enterocuccus and Pseudomonas by using different test methods. *J Microbiol Methods.* 2003 Jul;54(1):105–110.

Sharma M, Kishore K, Gupta SK, Joshi S, Arva DS. Cardioprotective potential of ocimum sanctum in isoproterenol induced myocardial infarction in rats. *Mol Cell Biochem.* 2001 Sep; 225(1):75–83.

Tohti I, Tursun M, Umar A, Turdi S, Imin H, Moore N. Aqueous extracts of Ocimum basilicum L. (sweet basil) decrease platelet aggregation induced by ADP and thrombin in vitro and rats arterio-venous shunt thrombosis in vivo. *Thromb Res.* 2006 Feb 7; 118(6):733–739.

Beans   www.americanbean.org; www.vegetablewithmore.com
Azevedo L, Gomes JC, Stringheta PC, Gontijo AM, Padovani CR, Ribeiro LR, Salvadori DM. Black bean (*Phaseolus vulgaris L.*) as a protective agent against DNA damage in mice. *Food Chem Toxicol.* 2003 Dec;41(12):1671–1676.

Bazzano LA, He J, Ogden LG, Loria CM, Whelton PK. Dietary fiber intake and reduced risk of coronary heart disease in US men and women: the National Health and Nutrition Examination Survey I Epidemiologic Follow-up Study. *Arch Intern Med.* 2003 Sep 8;163(16):1897–1904.

Darmadi-Blackberry et al. Legumes: the most important dietary predictor of survival in older people of different ethnicities. *Asia Pac J Clin Nutr.* 2004;13(2):217–220.

McIntosh M, Miller C. A diet containing food rich in soluble and insoluble fiber improves glycemic control and reduces hyperlipidemia among patients with type 2 diabetes mellitus. *Nutr Rev.* 2001;59(2):52–55.

Menotti A, Kromhout D, Blackburn H, et al. Food intake patterns and 25-year mortality from coronary heart disease: cross-cultural correlations in the Seven Countries Study. The Seven Countries Study Research Group. *Eur J Epidemiol* 1999 Jul;15(6):507–515.

Sacks FM. American Heart Association's annual meeting in Dallas, 2005.

Velie EM, Schairer C, Flood A, He JP, Khattree R, Schatzkin A. Empirically derived dietary patterns and risk of postmenopausal breast cancer in a large prospective cohort study. *Am J Clin Nutr.* 2005 Dec;82(6):1308–1319.

Blackberries   www.oregon-berries.com

Ding M et al. Cyanidin-3-glucoside, a natural product derived from blackberry, exhibits chemopreventive and chemotherapeutic activity. *J Biol Chem.* 2006 Jun 23;281(25):17359–17368.

Feng R, Bowman LL, Lu Y, Leonard SS, Shi X, Jiang BH, Castranova V, Vallyathan V, Ding M. Blackberry extracts inhibit activation protein 1 activation and cell transformation by perturbing mitogenic signaling pathway. *Nutr Cancer.* 2004;50(1):80–9.

Guerra MC, Galvano F, Bonsi L, Speroni E, Costa S, Renzulli C, Cervellati R. Cyanidin-3-O-beta-glucopyranoside, a natural free-radical scavenger against aflatoxin B1- and ochratoxin A-induced cell damage in a human hepatoma cell line and a human colonic adenocarcinoma cell line. *Br J Nutr.* 2005 Aug;94(2):211–220.

Stoner GD, Chen T, Kresty LA, Aziz RM, Reinemann T, Nines R. Protection against esophageal cancer in rodents with lyophilized berries: potential mechanisms. *Nutr Cancer.* 2006;54(1):33–46.

Blueberries   www.wildblueberries.com; www.blueberry.org

Goyarzu O et al. Blueberry supplemented diet: Effects on object recognition memory and nuclear factor-kappa B levels in aged rats. *Nutritional Neuroscience.* 2004;7:75–83.

Joseph JA et al. Blueberry supplementation enhances signaling and prevents behavioral deficits in an Alzheimer disease model. *Nutritional Neuroscience.* 6:153–162; 2003.

Joseph JA et al. Reversals of age-related declines in neuronal signal transduction, cognitive, and motor behavioral deficits with blueberry, spinach, or strawberry dietary supplementation. *Journal of Neuroscience.* September 15, 1999, 19(18); 8114–8121.

Kalea AZ et al. Wild blueberry (Vaccinium angustifolium) consumption affects the composition and structure of glycosaminoglycans in Sprague-Dawley rat aorta. *J Nutr Biochem.* 2006 Feb;17(2):109–116.

Schmidt BM et al. Effective separation of potent antiproliferation and antiadhesion components from wild blueberry (Vaccinium angustifolium Ait.) fruits. *J Agric Food Chem.* 2004 Oct 20;52(21):6433–6442.

Schmidt BM, Erdman JW Jr, Lila MA. Differential effects of blueberry proanthocyanidins on androgen sensitive and insensitive human prostate cancer cell lines. *Cancer Lett.* 2006 Jan 18;231(2):240–246.

Sweeney MI, Kalt W, MacKinnon SL, Ashby J, Gottschall-Pass KT. Feeding rats diets enriched in lowbush blueberries for six weeks decreases ischemia-induced brain damage. *Nutri Neuroscience.* 2002 Dec.; 5(6): 427–431.

United States National Institute of Health, National Institute on Aging. Available at: www.alzheimers.org/nianews23.html. Accessed on May 2, 2006.

Broccoli   www.answers.com/topic/broccoli

Fahey JW et al. Sulforaphane inhibits extracellular, intracellular, and antibiotic-resistant strains of Helicobacter pylori and prevents benzo[a]pyrene-induced stomach tumors. *Proc Natl Acad Sci USA.* 2002 May 28;99(11):7610–7615.

Fahey JW, Zhang Y, Talalay P. Broccoli sprouts: an exceptionally rich source of inducers of enzymes that protect against chemical carcinogens. *Proc Natl Acad Sci USA.* 1997 Sep 16;94(19):10367–10372.

Jackson SJ, Singletary KW. Sulforaphane inhibits human MCF-7 mammary cancer cell mitotic progression and tubulin polymerization. *J Nutr.* 2004 Sep;134(9):2229–2236.

Le HT, Schaldach CM, Firestone GL, Bjeldanes LF. Plant-derived 3,3'-Diindolylmethane is a strong androgen antagonist in human prostate cancer cells. *J Biol Chem.* 2003 Jun 6;278(23):21136–21145.

Matusheski NV, Juvik JA, Jeffery EH. Heating decreases epithiospecifier protein activity and increases sulforaphane formation in broccoli. *Phytochemistry.* 2004 May;65(9):1273–1281.

McGuire KP, Ngoubilly N, Neavyn M, Lanza-Jacoby S. 3,3'-diindolylmethane and paclitaxel act synergistically to promote apoptosis in HER2/Neu human breast cancer cells. *J Surg Res.* 2006 May 15;132(2):208–213.

Myzak MC, Hardin K, Wang R, Dashwood RH, Ho E. Sulforaphane inhibits histone deacetylase activity in BPH-1, LnCaP and PC-3 prostate epithelial cells. *Carcinogenesis.* 2006 Apr;27(4):811–819.

Tadi K, Chang Y, Ashok B, Chen Y, Moscatello A, Schaefer SD, Schantz SP, Policastro AJ, Geliebter J, Tiwari RK. 3,3'-Diindolylmethane, a cruciferous vegetable derived synthetic anti-proliferative compound in thyroid disease. *Biochem Biophys Res Commun.* 2005 Nov 25;337(3):1019–1025.

Takai M, Suido H, Tanaka T, Kotani M, Fujita A, Takeuchi A, Makino T, Sumikawa K, Origasa H, Tsuji K, Nakashima M. LDL-cholesterol-lowering effect of a mixed green vegetable and fruit beverage containing broccoli and cabbage in hypercholesterolemic subjects. *Rinsho Byori.* 2003 Nov;51(11):1073–1083.

Buckwheat   www.hort.purdue.edu/newcrop/crops/Buckwheat.html

Alvarez P, Alvarado C, De la Fuente M, Jimenez L, Puerto M, Schlumberger A. Improvement of leukocyte functions in prematurely aging mice after five weeks of diet supplementation with polyphenol-rich cereals. *Nutrition.* 2006 Jun 27.

Berti C, Brusamolino A, Porrini M, Riso P. Effect on appetite control of minor cereal and psuedocereal products. *Br J Nutr.* 2005 Nov;94(5):850–858.

Kato N, Kayashita J, Ohinata H, Tomotake H, Yamamoto N, Yamazaki R, Yanaka N. High protein buckwheat flour suppresses hypercholesterolemia in rats and gallstone formation in mice by hypercholesterolemic diet and body fat in rats because of its low protein digestibility. *Nutrition.* 2006 Feb;22(2):166–173.

Kawa JM, Przybylski R, Taylor CG. Buckwheat concentrate reduces serum glucose in streptozotocin-diabetic rats. *J Agric Food Chem.* 2003 Dec 3;51(25):7287–7291.

Cabbage   www.answers.com/topic/sauerkraut

Beecher C. Cancer preventive properties of varieties of Brassica oleracea: a review. *Am J Clin Nutr.* 1994;59:1166S–1170S.

Caragay AB. Cancer-preventative foods and ingredients. *Food Tech.* 1992;46(4):65–68.

Cheney G. Rapid healing of peptic ulcers in patients receiving fresh cabbage juice. *Cal Med.* 70 (1949):10–14.

Cohen JH, Kristal AR, et al. Fruit and vegetable intakes and prostate cancer risk. *J Natl Cancer Inst.* 2000;92(1):61–68.

Fowke JH, Chung FL, Jin F, Qi D, Cai Q, Conaway C, Cheng JR, Shu XO, Gao YT, Zheng W. Urinary isothiocyanate levels, brassica, and human breast cancer. *Cancer Res.* Jul 15;63(14):3980–3986.

Pathak DR et al. Joint association of high cabbage/sauerkraut intake at 12–13 years of age and adulthood with reduced breast cancer risk in Polish migrant women: results from the US component of the Polish women's health study. Abstract number 3697. Presented at the AACR 4th Annual Conference on Frontiers in Cancer Prevention Research, October 30–November 2, 2005, Baltimore, Maryland.

Qi M, Anderson AE, Chen DZ, Sun S, Auborn KJ. Indole-3-carbinol prevents PTEN loss in cervical cancer in vivo. *Mol Med.* 2005;11(1–12):59–63.

Cardamom   www.cardamom.com

al-Zuhair H, el-Sayeh B, Ameen HA, al-Shoora H. Pharmacological studies of cardamom oil in animals. *Pharmacol Res.* 1996 Jul–Aug;34(1–2):79–82.

Jamal A, Javed K, Aslam M, Jafri MA. Gastroprotective effect of cardamom, Elettaria cardamomum Maton. fruits in rats. *J Ethnopharmacol.* 2006 Jan 16;103(2):149–153.

Mahady GB et al. In vitro susceptibility of Helicobacter pylori to botanical extracts used traditionally for the treatment of gastrointestinal disorders. *Phytother Res.* 2005 Nov;19(11):988–991.

Sengupta A, Ghosh S, Bhattacharjee S. Dietary cardamom inhibits the formation of azoxymethane-induced aberrant crypt foci in mice and reduces COX-2 and iNOS expression in the colon. *Asian Pac J Cancer Prev.* 2005 Apr–Jun;6(2):118–122.

Suneetha WJ, Krishnakantha TP. Cardamom extract as inhibitor of human platelet aggregation. *Phytother Res.* 2005 May;19(5):437–440.

Carob   www.gilead.net/health/carob.html

Garcia AL, Gruendel S, Katz N, Koebnick C, Mueller C, Otto B, Speth M, Steinger J, Weickert MO. Carob pulp preparation rich in insoluble dietary fiber and polyphernols enhances lipid oxidation and lowers postprandial acylated ghrelin in humans. *J Nutr.* 2006 Jun; 136(6):1533–1538.

Graubaum HJ, Grunwald J, Haber B, Harde A, Koebnick C, Zunft HJ. Carob pulp preparation rich in insoluble fibre lowers total and LDL cholesterol in hypercholesterolemic patients. *Eur J Nutr.* 2003 Oct; 42(5):235–242.

Peng G, Tsai AC. Effects of locust bean gum on glucose tolerance, sugar digestion, and gastric motility in rats. *J Nutr.* 1981 Dec;111(12):2152–2156.

Carrots   http://plantanswers.tamu.edu/publications/vegetabletravelers/
carrot.html

Baybutt RC, Hu L, Molteni A. Vitamin A deficiency injures lung and liver parenchyma and impairs function of rat type II pneumocytes. *J Nutr.* 2000 May;130(5):1159–1165.

Gaziano JM, Manson JE, Branch LG, et al. A prospective study of consumption of carotenoids in fruits and vegetables and decreased cardiovascular mortality in the elderly. *Ann Epidemiol.* 1995; 5:255–260.

Gustafsson K, Asp NG, Hagander B, Nyman M, Schweizer T. Influence of processing and cooking of carrots in mixed meals on satiety, glucose and hormonal response. *Int J Food Sci Nutr.* 1995 Feb;46(1):3–12.

Kritchevsky SB. Beta-carotene, carotenoids and the prevention of coronary heart disease. *J Nutr.* 1999 Jan;129(1):5–8.

Michaud DS, Feskanich D, Rimm EB, et al. Intake of specific carotenoids and risk of lung cancer in 2 prospective US cohorts. *Am J Clin Nutr.* 2000;72(4):990–997.

ProteKobaek-Larsen M, Christensen LP, Vach W, Ritskes-Hoitinga J, Brandt K. Inhibitory effects of feeding with carrots or (-)-falcarinol on development of azoxymethane-induced preneoplastic lesions in the rat colon. *J Agric Food Chem.* 2005. Mar 9;53(5):1823–1827.

Suzuki K, Ito Y, Nakamura S et al. Relationship between serum carotenoids and hyperglycemia: a population-based cross-sectional study. *J Epidemiol.* 2002 Sep;12(5):357–366.

Wood R. *The Whole Foods Encyclopedia.* New York, NY: Prentice-Hall Press; 1988.

Ylonen K, Alfthan G, Groop, L et al. Dietary intakes and plasma concentrations of carotenoids and tocopherols in relation to glucose metabolism in subjects at high risk of type 2 diabetes: The Botnia Dietary Study. *Am J Clin Nutr.* 2003 Jun;77(6):1434–1441.

Cauliflower   www.dole5aday.com/ReferenceCenter/
Encyclopedia/Cauliflower

Anand R, Biedebach M, Jevning R. Cruciferous vegetables and human breast cancer: An important interdisciplinary hypothesis in the field of diet and cancer. *Family Economics and Nutrition Review.* 1999;12(2).

Brandi G et al. Mechanisms of action and antiproliferative properties of Brassica oleracea juice in human breast cancer cell lines. *J Nutr.* 2005 Jun;135(6):1503–1509.

Cerhan J, Criswell L, Merlino L, Mikuls T, Saag K. Antioxidant micronutrients and risk of rheumatoid arthritis in a cohort of older women. *Am J Epidemiol.* 2003; 157:345–354.

Fan S, Meng Q, Auborn K, Carter T, Rosen EM. BRCA1 and BRCA2 as molecular targets for phytochemicals indole-3-carbinol and genistein in breast and prostate cancer cells. *Br J Cancer.* 2006 Feb 13;94(3):407–426.

Herman-Antosiewicz A, Johnson DE, Singh SV. Sulforaphane causes autophagy to inhibit release of cytochrome C and apotosis in human prostate cancer cells. *Cancer Res.* 2006 Jun 1; 66(11):5828–5835.

Kuttan G, Thejass P. Antimetastatic activity of sulforaphane. *Life Sci.* 2006 May 22; 78(26):3043–3050.

Celery   www.michigancelery.com/celeryinfo.htm

Belanger JT. Perillyl alcohol: applications in oncology. *Altern Med Rev.* 1998 Dec; 3(6):448–457.

Sultana S, Ahmed S, Jahangir T, Sharma S. Inhibitory effect of celery seeds extract on chemically induced hepatocarcinogenesis: modulation of cell proliferation, metabolism and altered hepatic foci development. *Cancer Lett.* 2005 Apr 18;221(1):11–20.

Tsi D, Das NP, Tan BK. Effects of aqueous celery (Apium graveolens) extract on lipid parameters of rats fed a high fat diet. *Planta Med.* 1995 Feb;61(1):18–21.

Tsi D, Tan BK. The mechanism underlying the hypocholesterolaemic activity of aqueous celery extract, its butanol and aqueous fractions in genetically hypercholesterolaemic RICO rats. *Life Sci.* 2000;66(8):755–767.

Chard   http://food.oregonstate.edu/faq/uffva/swisschard2.html

Ayanoglu-Dulger G, Sacan O, Sener G, Yanardaq R. Effects of chard (Beta vulgaris L. var. cicla) extract on oxidative injury in the aorta and heart of streptozotocin-diabetic rats. *J Med Food.* 2002 Spring;5(1):37–42.

Bobek P, Galbavy S, Mariassyova M. The effect of red beet (Beta vulgaris var. rubra) fiber on alimentary hypercholesterolemia and chemically induced colon carcinogenesis in rats. *Nahrung* 2000 Jun;44(3):184–187.

Senner G et al. Effects of chard (Beta vulgaris L. var. cicla) extract on oxidative injury in the aorta and heart of streptozotocin-diabetic rats. *J Med Food.* 2002 Spring;5(1):37–42.

Yanardag R, Bolkent S, Ozsoy-Sacan O et al. The effects of chard (Beta vulgaris L. var. cicla) extract on the kidney tissue, serum urea and creatinine levels of diabetic rats. *Phytother Res* 2002 Dec;16(8):758–761.

Cherries   www.usacherries.com; www.calcherry.com

Bourquin LD, Kang SY, Nair MG, Seeram NP. Tart cherry anthocyanins inhibit tumor development in Apc (Min) mice and reduce proliferation of human colon cancer cells. *Cancer Lett.* 2003 May 8;194(1):13–19.

Carlson L, Connolly DA, McHugh MP, Padilla-Zakour OI, Sayers S. Efficacy of a tart cherry juice blend in preventing the symptoms of muscle damage. *Br J Sports Med.* 2006 Aug;40(8):679–683.

He YH et al. Antioxidant and anti-inflammatory effects of cyanidin from cherries on rat adjuvant-induced arthritis. *Zhongguo Zhong Yao Za Zhi.* 2005 Oct;30(20): 1602–1605.

Heo H, Kim D, Kim Y, Lee C, Yang H. Sweet and sour cherry phenolics and their protective effects on neuronal cells. *J Agric Food Chem.* 2005 Oct. 53(26).

Jacob RA, Kader AA, Kelley DS, Mackey BE, Rasooly R. Consumption of bing sweet cherries lowers circulating concentrations of inflammation markers in healthy men and women. *J Nutr.* 2006 Apr;136(4):981–986.

Jacob RA, Spinozzi GM, Simon VA, Kelley DS, Prior RL, Hess-Pierce B, Kader AA. Consumption of cherries lowers plasma urate in healthy women. *J Nutr.* 2003 Jun;133(6):1826–1829.

Kelley DS, Rasooly R, Jacob RA, Kader AA, Mackey BE. Consumption of bing sweet cherries lowers circulating concentrations of inflammation markers in healthy men and women. *J Nutr.* 136:981–986, April 2006.

Kim DO et al. Sweet and sour cherry phenolics and their protective effects on neuronal cells. *J Agric Food Chem.* 2005 Dec 28;53(26):9921–9927.

Meyer RA, Nair MG, Raja SN, Seeram NP, Tall JM, Zhao C. Tart cherry anthocyanins suppress inflammation-induced pain behavior in rats. *Behav Brain Res.* 2004 Aug 12;153(1):181–188.

Schlesinger N. Dietary factors and hyperuricaemia. *Curr Pharm Des.* 2005;11(32): 4133–4138.

Chocolate/Cocoa   www.icco.org

Buijsse B, Feskens EJ, Kok FJ, Kromhout D. Cocoa intake, blood pressure, and cardio-vascular mortality: the Zutphen Elderly Study. *Arch Intern Med.* 2006; 166: 411–417.

Engler MB et al. Flavonoid-rich dark chocolate improves endothelial function and increases plasma epicatechin concentrations in healthy adults. *J Am Coll Nutr.* 2004 Jun;23(3):197–204.

Grassi D et al. Cocoa reduces blood pressure and insulin resistance and improves endothelium-dependent vasodilation in hypertensives. *Hypertension.* 2005 Aug; 46(2):398–405.

Grassi D et al. Short-term administration of dark chocolate is followed by a significant increase in insulin sensitivity and a decrease in blood pressure in healthy persons. *Am J Clin Nutr.* 2005 Mar;81(3):611–614.

Heinrich U, Neukam K, Tronnier H, Sies H, Wilhelm S. Long-term ingestion of high flavanol cocoa provides photoprotection against UV-induced erythema and improves skin condition in women. *Journal of Nutrition.* 2006;136:1–5.

Noe V et al. Epicatechin and a cocoa polyphenolic extract modulate gene expression in human Caco-2 cells. *J Nutr.* 2004 Oct;134(10):2509–2516.

Schuier M, Sies H, Illek B, Fischer H. Cocoa-related flavonoids inhibit CFTR-mediated chloride transport across T84 human colon epithelia. *J Nutr.* 2005 Oct;135(10):2320–2325.

Taubert D, Berkels R, Roesen R, Klaus W. Chocolate and blood pressure in elderly individuals with isolated systolic hypertension. *JAMA.* 2003 Aug 27;290(8):1029–1030.

Usmani OS et al. Theobromine inhibits sensory nerve activation and cough. *FASEB J.* 2005 Feb;19(2):231–233.

Vlachopoulos C et al. Effect of dark chocolate on arterial function in healthy individuals. *Am J Hypertens.* 2005 Jun;18(6):785–791.

Cilantro/Coriander   http://whatscookingamerica.net/cilantro.htm

Chithra V, Leelamma S. Coriandrum sativum changes the levels of lipid peroxides and activity of antioxidant enzymes in experimental animals. *Indian J Biochem Biophys.* 1999 Feb;36(1):59–61.

Chithra V, Leelamma S. Hypolipidemic effect of coriander seeds (Coriandrum sativum): mechanism of action. *Plant Foods Hum Nutr.* 1997;51(2):167–172.

Delaquis PJ, Stanich K, Girard B et al. Antimicrobial activity of individual and mixed fractions of dill, cilantro, coriander and eucalyptus essential oils. *Int J Food Microbiol.* 2002 Mar 25;74(1–2):101–109.

Gray AM, Flatt PR. Insulin-releasing and insulin-like activity of the traditional anti-diabetic plant Coriandrum sativum (coriander). *Br J Nutr.* 1999 Mar;81(3):203–209.

Kubo I, Fujita K, Kubo A, Nihei K, Ogura T. Antibacterial activity of coriander volatile compounds against salmonella choleraesuis. *J Agric Food Chem.* 2004 Jun 2;52(11): 3329–3332.

Platel K, Rao A, Saraswathi G, Srinivasan K. Digestive stimulant action of three Indian spice mixes in experimental rats. Department of Biochemistry and Nutrition, Central Food Technological Research Institute, Mysore 570 013, India.

Cinnamon   www.ars.usda.gov/is/video/vnr/cinnamon.htm
Anderson R, Echard B, Polansky MM, Preuss HG. Whole cinnamon and aqueous ex-tracts ameliorate sucrose-induced blood pressure elevations in spontaneously hyper-tensive rats. *J Am Coll Nutr.* 2006 Apr; 25(2):144–150.

Hahn A, Kelb K, Lichtinghagen R, Mang B, Schmitt B, Stichtenoth DO, Wolters M. Effects of a cinnamon extract on plasma glucose, HbA, and serum lipids in diabetes mellitus type 2. *Eur J Clin Invest.* 2006 May;36(5): 340–344.

Kahn A et al. Cinnamon improves glucose and lipids of people with type 2 diabetes. *Diabetes Care.* 2003 Dec;26(12):3215–3218.

Kam SL, Li Y, Ooi LS, Ooi VE, Wang H, Wong EY. Antimicrobial activities of cinna-mon oil and cinnamaldehyde from the Chinese medicinal herb Cinnamomum cassia Blume. *Am J Chin Med.* 2006;34(3):511–522.

Kim W et al. Naphthalenemethyl ester derivative of dihydroxyhydrocinnamic acid, a component of cinnamon, increases glucose disposal by enhancing translocation of glucose transporter 4. *Diabetologia.* 2006 Aug 9.

Kong LD, Cai Y, Huang WW, Cheng CH, Tan RX. Inhibition of xanthine oxidase by some Chinese medicinal plants used to treat gout. *J Ethnopharmacol.* 2000 Nov;73(1–2):199–207.

Mang B et al. Effects of a cinnamon extract on plasma glucose, HbA, and serum lipids in diabetes mellitus type 2. *Eur J Clin Invest.* 2006 May;36(5):340–344.

Clove   www.intelihealth.com
Ahmad N, Alam MK, Bisht D, Hakim SR, Khan A, Mannan A, Owais M, Shehbaz A. Antimicrobial activity of clove oil and its potential in the treatment of vaginal can-didiasis. *J Drug Target.* 2005 Dec;13(10):555–561.

Algareer A, Alyhaya A, Andersson L. The effect of clove and benzocaine versus placebo as topical anesthetics. *J Dent.* 2006 Mar 10.

Banerjee S, Das S, Panda CK. Clove (Syzgium aromaticum L.), a potential chemopre-ventive agent for lung cancer. *Carcinogenesis.* 2006 Aug; 27(8):1645–1654.

Choi HK, Jung GW, Moon KH, et al. Clinical study of SS-cream in patients with life-long premature ejaculation. *Urology.* 2000;55(2):257–261.

Diwakr BT, Lokesh BR, Naidu KA, Raghavenra H. Eugenol—the active principle from cloves inhibits 5-lipoxygenase activity and leukotriene-C4 in human PMNL cells. *Prostaglandins Leukot Essent Fatty Acids*. 2006 Jan;74(1):23–27.

Coffee   www.ncausa.org

Andersen LF, Jacobs DR Jr, Carlsen MH, Blomhoff R. Consumption of coffee is associated with reduced risk of death attributed to inflammatory and cardiovascular diseases in the Iowa Women's Health Study. *Am J Clin Nutr*. 2006 May;83(5):1039–1046.

Ascherio A et al. Coffee consumption, gender, and Parkinson's disease mortality in the cancer prevention study II cohort: the modifying effects of estrogen. *Am J Epidemiol*. 2004 Nov 15;160(10):977–984.

Buijsse B, Giampaoli S, Kalmijn S, Kromhout D, Nissinen A, Tijhuis M, van Gelder BM. Coffee consumption is inversely associated with cognitive decline in elderly European men: the FINE study. *Eur J Clin Nutr*. 2006 Aug 16.

Folsom AR, Parker ED, Pereira MA. Coffee consumption and risk of type 2 diabetes mellitus: an 11-year prospective study of 28,812 postmenopausal women. *Arch Intern Med*. 2006 Jun 26;166(12):1311–1316.

Klatsky AL, Morton C, Udaltsova N, Friedman GD. Coffee, cirrhosis, and transaminase enzymes. *Arch Intern Med*. 2006 Jun 12;166(11):1190–1195.

Lee WJ, Zhu BT. Inhibition of DNA methylation by caffeic acid and chlorogenic acid, two common catechol-containing coffee polyphenols. *Carcinogenesis*. 2006 Feb; 27(2):269–277.

Paluska SA. Caffeine and exercise. *Curr Sports Med Rep*. 2003 Aug;2(4):213–219.

Van Dam RM, Hu FB. Coffee consumption and risk of type 2 diabetes: a systematic review. *JAMA*. 2005 Jul 6;294(1):97–104.

Corn   www.resistantstarch.com; www.urbanext.uiuc.edu/corn

Adom KK, Liu RH. Antioxidant activity of grains. *J Agric Food Chem*. 2002;50: 6182–6187.

Bauer-Marinovic M, Florian S, Muller-Schmehl K, Glatt H, Jacobasch G. Dietary resistant starch type 3 prevents tumor induction by 1,2-dimethylhydrazine and alters proliferation, apoptosis and dedifferentiation in rat colon. *Carcinogenesis*. 2006 Apr 20.

Bazzano LA, He J, Odgen LG et al. Dietary intake of folate and risk of stroke in US men and women:NHANES I Epidemiologic Follow-up Study. *Stroke*. 2002 May; 33(5):1183–1189.

Behall KM, Scholfield DJ, Hallfrisch JG, Liljeberg-Elmstahl HG. Consumption of both resistant starch and beta-glucan improves postprandial plasma glucose and insulin in women. *Diabetes Care*. 2006 May;29(5):976–981.

Erichsen-Brown C. *Medicinal and Other Uses of North American Plants*. Mineola, NY: Courier Dover Publications, 1989.

Hylla S, Gostner A, Dusel G, Anger H, Bartram H-P, Christl S, Kasper H, Scheppach W: Effects of resistant starch on the colon in healthy volunteers: possible implications for cancer prevention. *Am J Clin Nutr.* 1998, 67:136–142.

Maksimovic Z, Dobric S, Kovacevic N, Milovanovic Z. Diuretic activity of *Maydis stigma* extract in rats. *Pharmazie.* 2004;59:967–971.

Toden S, Bird AR, Topping DL, Conlon MA. Resistant starch prevents colonic DNA damage induced by high dietary cooked red meat or casein in rats. *Cancer Biol Ther.* 2006 Mar;5(3):267–272.

Velazquez DVO, Xavier HS, Batista JEM, de Castro-Chaves D. *Zea mays L* extracts modify glomerular function and potassium urinary excretion in conscious rats. *Phytomedicine* 2005; 12:363–369.

Yuan JM, Stram DO, Arakawa K, Lee HP, Yu MC. Dietary cryptoxanthin and reduced risk of lung cancer: the Singapore Chinese Health Study. *Cancer Epidemiol Biomarkers Prev.* 2003 Sep;12(9):890–898.

Cranberries   www.cranberryinstitute.com;
http://nccam.nih.gov/health/cranberry/
Antioxidant and antiproliferative activities of common fruits. *J Agric Food Chem.* 2002 Dec 4;50(25):7449–7454.

Crews WD et al. A double-blinded, placebo-controlled, randomized trial of the neuropsychologic efficacy of cranberry juice in a sample of cognitively intact older adults: pilot study findings. *J Altern Compl Med.* 2005 Apr;11(2):305–309.

Labrecque J, Bodet C, Chandad F, Grenier D. Effects of a high-molecular-weight cranberry fraction on growth, biofilm formation and adherence of Porphyromonas gingivalis. *J Antimicrob Chemother.* 2006 Aug;58(2):439–443.

Ruel G et al. Changes in plasma antioxidant capacity and oxidized low-density lipoprotein levels in men after short-term cranberry juice consumption. *Metabolism.* 2005 Jul;54(7):856–861.

Ruel G et al. Favourable impact of low-calorie cranberry juice consumption on plasma HDL-cholesterol concentrations in men. *Br J Nutr.* 2006 Aug;96(2):357–364.

Turner A. Inhibition of uropathogenic Escherichia coli by cranberry juice: a new anti-adherence assay. *J Agric Food Chem.* 2005 Nov 16;53(23):8940–8947.

Weiss EI et al. Inhibiting interspecies coaggregation of plaque bacteria with a cranberry juice constituent [published erratam appear in *J Am Dent Assoc.* 1999 Jan;130(1):36 and 1999 Mar;130(3):332] *J Am Dent Assoc.* 1998 Dec;129(12): 1719–1723.

Yan X, Murphy BT, Hammond GB, Vinson JA, Neto CC. Antioxidant activities and antitumor screening of extracts from cranberry fruit (Vaccinium macrocarpon). *J Agric Food Chem.* 2002 Oct 9;50(21):5844–5849.

Zhang L. Efficacy of cranberry juice on Helicobacter pylori infection: a double-blind, randomized placebo-controlled trial. *Helicobacter.* 2005 Apr;10(2):139–145.

Cumin   http://www.hort.purdue.edu/newcrop.med-aro/factsheets/ CUMIN.html

Ensminger AH, Esminger M et al. *Food for Health: A Nutrition Encyclopedia.* Clovis, California: Pegus Press, 1986.

Hypolipidemic effect of Cuminum cyminum L. on alloxan-induced diabetic rats. *Pharmacol Res.* 2002 Sep;46(3):251–255.

Lee HS. Cuminaldehyde: Aldose reductase and alpha-glucosidase inhibitor derived from Cuminum cyminum L. seeds. *J Agric Food Chem.* 2005; 53(7):2446–2450.

Martinez-Tome M, Jimenez AM, Ruggieri S, et al. Antioxidant properties of Mediterranean spices compared with common food additives. *J Food Prot.* 2001 Sep;64(9):1412–1419.

Nalini N, Manju V, Menon VP. Effect of spices on lipid metabolism in 1,2-dimethylhydrazine-induced rat colon carcinogenesis. *J Med Food.* 2006 Summer; 9(2):237–245.

O'Mahoney R et al. Bactericidal and anti-adhesive properties of culinary and medicinal plants against Helicobacter pylori. *World J Gastroenterol.* 2005 Dec 21;11(47):7499–7507.

Tekeoglu I, Dogan A, Demiralp L. Effects of thymoquinone (volatile oil of black cumin) on rheumatoid arthritis in rat models. *Phytother Res.* July 11, 2006.

Currants   http://asktheberryman.com

Carey AN, Fisher DR, Joseph JA. Fruit extracts antagonize A beta- or DA-induced deficits in Ca2+ flux in M1-transfected COS-7 cells. *J Alzheimer's Dis.* 2004 Aug; 6(4): 403–411.

Deferne JL, Leeds AR. Resting blood pressure and cardiovascular reactivity to mental arithmetic in mild hypertensive males supplemented with black currant seed oil. *J Hum Hypertens.* 1996 Aug; 10(8):531–537.

Konno O, Okubo T, Takata R, Yamamoto R, Yanai T. Immunostimulatory effects of a polysaccharide-rich substance with antitumor activity isolated from black currant (Ribes nigrum L.). *Biosci Biotechnol Biochem.* 2005 Nov; 69(11):2042–2050.

Eggplant   asiafood.org

Baek EJ, Chang EY, Chang JS, Friedman M, Han JS, Kozukue N, Lee KR, Park JH. Glycoalkaloids and metabolites inhibit the growth of human colon (HT29) and liver (HepG2) cancer cells. *J Agric Food Chem.* 2004 May 19; 52(10): 2832–2839.

Bragagnoio N, de Almeida E, Jorge PA, Neyra LC, Osaki RM. Effect of eggplant on plasma lipid levels, lipidic peroxidation and reversion of endothelial dysfunction in experimental hypercholesterolemia. *Arg Bras Cardiol.* 1998 Feb; 70(2): 87–91.

Kaneyuki T, Matsubara K, Miyake T, Mori M. Antiangiogenic activity of nasunin, an antioxidant anthocyanin, in eggplant peels. *J Agric Food Chem.* 2005 Aug 10; 53(16): 6272–6275.

Yeh CT, Yen GC. Effect of vegetables on human phenolsulfotransferases in relation to their antioxidant activity and total phenolics. *Free Radic Res.* 2005 Aug; 39(8):893–904.

Eggs   www.aeb.org
Blumberg JB, Jacques PF, Moeller SM. The potential role of dietary xanthophylls in cataract and age-related macular degeneration. *J Am Coll Nutr.* 2000 Oct; 19(5): 522S–527S.

Colditz G, Frazier L, Rockett H, Tomeo Ryan C, Willett W. Adolescent diet and risk of breast cancer. Available at: http://breast-cancer-research.com/content/5/2/R59. Accessed on: June 2, 2007.

Dhurandhar N, Jen C, Khosla P, Marth JM, Vander Wal J. Short-term effect of eggs on satiety in overweight and obese subjects. *Journal of the American College of Nutrition.* 2005;24(6):510–515.

Elderberry   http://plants.usda.gov/plantguide/pdf/cs_sanic5.pdf
Bobek P, Nosalova V, Cerna S. Influence of diet containing extract of black elder (sambucus nigra) on colitis in rats. *Biologia Bratislava.* 2001;56(6):643–648.

Zakay-Rones Z et al. Randomized study of the efficacy and safety of oral elderberry extract in the treatment of influenza A and B virus infections. *J Int Med Res.* 2004 Mar–Apr;32(2):132–140.

Fennel   www.hort.purdue.edu/newcrop/NewCropsNews/ 93-3-1/fennel.html
Alexandrovich I, Rakovitskaya O, Kolmo E et al. The effect of fennel (*Foeniculum vulgare*) seed oil emulsion in infantile colic: a randomized, placebo-controlled study. *Altern Ther Health Med.* 2003;9:58–61.

Chainy GB, Manna SK, Chaturvedi MM, Aggarwal BB. Anethole blocks both early and late cellular responses transduced by tumor necrosis factor: effect on NF-kappaB, AP-1, JNK, MAPKK and apoptosis. *Oncogene.* 2000 Jun 8;19(25):2943–2950.

Forster HB, Niklas H, Lutz S. Antispasmodic effects of some medicinal plants. *Plant Med.* 1980;40:303–319.

Tanira MOM, Shah AH, Mohsin A et al. Pharmacological and toxicological investigations on Foeniculum vulgare dried fruit extract in experimental animals. *Phytother Res.* 1996;10:33–36.

Figs   www.calfresh.figs.com; www.californiafigs.com; www.nafex.org/figs.htm
Brown L, Rosner B, Willet W, Sacks FM. Cholesterol lowering effects of dietary fiber: a meta-analysis. *Amer J Clin Nutr.* 1999;69:30–42.

Emenaker NJ. Short-chain fatty acids derived from dietary fiber may protect against invasive human colon cancer. *On-line.* 1999; 7(1):1, 4–9.

Ferguson LR, Chavan RR, Harris PJ. Changing concepts of dietary fiber: implications for carcinogenesis. *Nutr & Cancer.* 2001;39(2):155–169.

Hosein S. Immunomodulators: psoralens. CATIE. 1994;48. Accessed Online May 2006 at http://www.aegis.com/pubs/catie/1994/CATI4807.html

Lairon D, et al. Dietary fiber intake and risk factors for cardiovascular disease in French adults. *Amer J Clin Nutr.* 2005;82:1185–1194.

Lebwohl M. A clinician's paradigm in the treatment of psoriasis. *J Am Acad Dermatol.* 2005;53:S59–69.

Montonen J, et al. Whole-grain and fiber intake and the incidence of type 2 diabetes. *Amer J Clin Nutr.* 2003;77:622–629.

Rubnov S, Kashman Y, Rabinowitz R, Schlesinger M, Mechoulam R. Suppressors of cancer cell proliferation from fig (ficus carica) resin: isolation and structure elucidation. *J Nat Prod.* 64:993–996, 2001.

Slavin JL. Dietary fiber and body weight. *Nutrition.* 2005;21:411–418.

Streppel MT, et al. Dietary fiber and blood pressure. *Arch Intern Med.* 2005; 165:150–156.

Upton J. New roles for fiber focus on heart disease, diabetes, blood pressure. *Environmental Nutrition.* 2005;28(4):1, 6.

Flax   www.flaxcouncil.ca; www.flaxrd.com
Bloedon LT, Szapary PO. Flaxseed and cardiovascular risk. *Nutr Rev.* 2004;62:18–27.

Chen J, Hui E, Thompson L. Proceedings of the AACR, Volume 44, 2nd ed., July 2003. Department of Nutritional Sciences, University of Toronto, Toronto, ON.

Dwivedi C, Natarajan K, Matthees DP. Chemopreventive effects of dietary flaxseed oil on colon tumor development. *Drug News Perspect.* 2000;13(2):99.

Johnson PV. Flaxseed oil and cancer: alpha-linolenic acid and carcinogenesis, in *Flaxseed in Human Nutrition,* eds. S.C. Cunnane and L.U. Thompson. AOCS Press, Champaign, IL. 1995. pp 207–218.

Joshi K et al. Supplementation with flax oil and vitamin C improves the outcome of Attention Deficit Hyperactivity Disorder (ADHD). *Prostaglandins Leukot Essent Fatty Acids.* 2006 Jan;74(1):17–21.

Piller RA, Chang-Claude JB, Linseisen, Jakob AB. Plasma enterolactone and genistein and the risk of premenopausal breast cancer. *European Journal of Cancer Prevention.* 2006 (Vol. 15, pp. 225–232).

Prasad K, Mantha SV, Muir AD, Wstcott ND. Reduction of hypercholesterolemic athersclerosis by CDC-flaxseed with very low alpha linolenic acid. *Atherosclerosis.* 1998;136:367–375.

Prasad K. Secoisolariciresinol diglucoside from flaxseed delays the development of type 2 diabetes in Zucker rat. *J Lab Clin Med.* 2001 Jul;138(1):32–39.

Velasquez MT et al. Dietary flaxseed meal reduces proteinuria and ameliorates nephropathy in an animal model of type II diabetes mellitus. *Kidney Int.* 2003 Dec;64(6):2100–2107.

Garlic   http://anrcatalog.ucdavis.edu/pdf/7231.pdf
Garlic: Effects on Cardiovascular Risks and Disease, Proliferative Effects Against Cancer, and Clinical Adverse Effects. http://ahrq.gov/clinic/epcsums/garlicsum.htm. Accessed June 2, 2007.

Allium Vegetables and Organosulfur Compounds: Do They Help Prevent Cancer? http://ehpnet1.niehs.nih.gov/members/2001/109p893-902bianchini/bianchinifull.html. Accessed June 3, 2007.

Efendy, JL et al. The effect of the aged garlic extract, "Kyolic," on the development of experimental atherosclerosis. *Arterosclerosis*. 1997;132:37–42.

Fleischauer, AT, Arab L. Garlic and cancer: a critical review of the epidemiologic literature. *J Nutrition*. 2001;131:1032S–1040S.

Gonzalez C et al. Fruit and vegetable intake and the risk of stomach and oesophagus adenocarcinoma in the European Prospective Investigation into Cancer and Nutrition (EPIC-EURGAST). *Int J Cancer*. 2006 May 15;118(10):2559–2566.

Hsing AW, Chokkalingam AP, Gao YT, et al. Allium vegetables and risk of prostate cancer: a population-based study. *J Natl Cancer Inst*. 2002;94(21):1648–1651.

Jain AK. Can garlic reduce levels of serum lipids? A controlled clinical study. *American Journal of Medicine*. 1993;94: 632–635.

Johnston N. Garlic: A natural antibiotic. *Modern Drug Discovery*. 2002;(5):12.

Mader FH. Treatment of hyperlipidemia with garlic-powder tablets. *Arzneimittel-Forschung/Drug Research*. 1990;40:3–8.

Milner JA. (2001) Mechanisms by which garlic and allyl sulfur compounds suppress carcinogen bioactivation. Garlic and carcinogenesis. *Adv Exp Med Biol* 492: 69–81.

Milner, JA. A historical perspective on garlic and cancer. *J. Nutrition*. 2001. 131: 1027S–1031S.

Steiner M, Lin RS. Changes in platelet function and susceptibility of lipoproteins to oxidation associated with administration of aged garlic extract. *J Cardiovasc Pharmacol*. 1998;31:904–908.

Ginger   www.mayoclinic.com/health/ginger/NS_patient-ginger; www.umm.edu/altmed/consherbs/gingerch.html#overview
Altman RD and Marcussen KC. Effects of ginger extract on knee pain in patients with osteoarthritis. *Arthritis Rheum*. 2001;44(11):2461–2462.

American Association for Cancer Research 97th annual meeting, April 1–5, 2006, Washington, D.C. Study author J. Rebecca Liu, M.D., assistant professor of obstetrics and gynecology at the U-M Medical School and a member of the U-M Comprehensive Cancer Center.

Grontved A, Brask T, Kambskard J, Hentzer E. Ginger root against sea sickness: a controlled trial on the open sea. *Otorhinolaryngol Relat Spec*. 1986;48(5): 282–286.

Han-Chung L, et al. Effects of ginger on motion sickness and gastric slow-wave dysrythmias induced by circular vection. *Am J Physiol Gastrintest Liver Physiol*. 2003;283:G481–G489.

Manju V, Nalini N. Chemopreventive efficacy of ginger, a naturally occurring anticarcinogen during the initiation, post-initiation stages of 1,2 dimethylhydrazine-induced colon cancer. *Clin Chim Acta*. 2005 Aug;358(1–2):60–67.

Phase II randomized study of ginger in patients with cancer and chemotherapy-induced nausea and vomiting (CCUM-0201). http://www.cancer.gov/clinicaltrials/ft-CCUM-0201.

Phillips S, Ruggier R, Hutchinson SE. Zingiber officinale (ginger)1: an antiemetic for day case surgery. *Anaesthesia.* 1993;48(12):1118.

Smith C, et al. A randomized controlled trial of ginger to treat nausea and vomiting in pregnancy. *Obstets & Gynecol.* 2004;103:639–645.

Willets KE, Ekangaki A, Eden JA. Effect of ginger abstract on pregnancy-induced nausea: a randomized controlled trial. *Australian and New Zealand J Obstetrics & Gyn.* 2003;43:139–144.

Goji Berries   http://www.mbhs.org/healthgate/GetHGContent.aspx? token=9C315661-83b7-472d-a7ab-bc858217 1f86&chunkiid=146769
Breithaupt DE, Weller P, Wolters M, Hahn A. Comparison of plasma responses in human subjects after the ingestion of 3R,3R'-zeaxanthin dipalmitate from wolfberry (Lycium barbarum) and non-esterified 3R,3R'-zeaxanthin using chiral high-performance liquid chromatography. *Br J Nutr.* 2004 May;91(5):707–713.

Chao JC et al. Hot water-extracted Lycium barbarum and Rehmannia glutinosa inhibit proliferation and induce apoptosis of hepatocellular carcinoma cells. *World J Gastroenterol.* 2006 Jul 28;12(28):4478–4484.

Gan L, Wang J, Zhang S. Inhibition of the growth of human leukemia cells by Lycium barbarum polysaccharide. *Wei Sheng Yan Jiu.* 2001;30:333–335.

Gan L, Zhang SH, Liu Q, Xu HB. A polysaccharide-protein complex from Lycium barbarum upregulates cytokine expression in human peripheral blood mononuclear cells. *Eur J Pharmacol.* 2003;471:217–222.

Lu CX, Cheng BQ. Radiosensitizing effects of Lycium barbarum polysaccharide for Lewis lung cancer. *Zhong Xi Yi Jie He Za Zhi.* 1991;11:611–612, 582.

Luo Q et al. Hypoglycemic and hypolipidemic effects and antioxidant activity of fruit extracts from Lycium barbarum. *Life Sci.* 2004 Nov 26:76(2):137–149.

Wu X, Beecher GR, Holden JM, Haytowitz DB, Gebhardt SE, Prior RL. Lipophilic and hydrophilic antioxidant capacities of common foods in the United States. *Journal of Agricultural Food Chemistry.* 2004;52:4026–4037.

Zhao R, Li Q, Xiao B. Effect of Lycium barbarum polysaccharide on the improvement of insulin resistance in NIDDM rats. *Yakugaku Zasshi.* 2005 Dec;125(12):981–988.

Grapefruit   www.floridajuice.com
Fujioka K, Greenway F, Sheard J, Ying Y. The effects of grapefruit on weight and insulin resistance: relationship to the metabolic syndrome. *J Med Food.* 2006;9:49–54.

Gao K, Henning SM, Niu Y, Youssefian AA, Seeram NP, Xu A, Heber D. The citrus flavonoid naringenin stimulates DNA repair in prostate cancer cells. *J Nutr Biochem.* 2006;17:89–95.

Gorinstein S et al. Red grapefruit positively influences serum triglyceride level in patients suffering from coronary atherosclerosis: Studies in vitro and in humans. *J Agric Food Chem.* 2006;54:1887–1892.

Staudte H, Sigusch BW, Glockmann E. Grapefruit consumption improves vitamin C status in periodontitis patients. *British Dental Journal.* 2005;199: 213–217.

Vanamala J et al. Suppression of colon carcinogenesis by bioactive compounds in grapefruit. *Carcinogenesis.* 2006 Jun;27(6):1257–1265.

Grapes   www.tablegrape.com
Agarwal C, Singh RP, Agarwal R. (2002, November). Grape seed extract induces apoptotic death of human prostate carcinoma DU145 cells via caspases activation accompanied by dissipation of mitochondrial membrane potential and cytochrome c release. *Carcinogenesis.* 23(11), 1869–1876.

Albers AR et al. The antiinflammatory effects of purple grape juice consumption in subjects with stable coronary artery disease. *Arterioscler Thromb Vasc Biol.* 2004 Nov;24(11):e179–180.

Falchi M et al. Comparison of cardioprotective abilities between the flesh and skin of grapes. *J Agric Food Chem.* 2006 Sep 6;54(18):6613–6622.

Fuhrman B, Volkova N, Coleman R, Aviram M. (2006, August). Grape powder polyphenols attenuate atherosclerosis development in apolipoprotein E deficient (E0) mice and reduce macrophage atherogenicity. *J Nutr.* 136(8), 2272.

Jung KJ, Wallig MA, Singletary KW. (2006, February). Purple grape juice inhibits 7,12-dimethylbenz[a]anthracene (DMBA)-induced rat mammary tumorigenesis and in vivo DMBA-DNA adduct formation. *Cancer Letters.* 233(2), 279–288.

Kim, H. (2005, November). New nutrition, proteomics, and how both can enhance studies in cancer prevention and therapy. *J Nutr.* 135(11), 2715–2722.

Moreno DA, Ilic N, Poulev A, Brasaemle DL, Fried SK, Raskin I. (2003, October). Inhibitory effects of grape seed extract on lipases. *Nutrition.* 11(10), 876–879.

Shukitt-Hale B et al. Effects of Concord grape juice on cognitive and motor deficits in aging. *Nutrition.* 2006 Mar;22(3):295–302.

Guava   www.hort.purdue.edu/newcrop/morton/guava.html
Abdelrahim, S. I., et al. Antimicrobial activity of Psidium guajava L. *Fitoterapia.* 2002; 73(7–8): 713–715.

Arima H et al. Isolation of antimicrobial compounds from guava (*Psidium guajava* L.) and their structural elucidation. *Biosci Biotechnol Biochem.* 2002; 66(8):1727–1730.

Cheng JT et al. Hypoglycemic effect of guava juice in mice and human subjects. *Am. J. Clin. Med.* 1983; 11(1–4): 74–76.

Conde Garcia EA et al. Inotropic effects of extracts of *Psidium guajava* L. (guava) leaves on the guinea pig atrium. *Braz J of Med & Biol Res.* 2003; 36:661–668.

Lozoya X et al. Intestinal anti-spasmodic effect of a phytodrug of *Psidium guajava* folia in the treatment of acute diarrheic disease. *J Ethnopharmacol.* 2002; 83(1–2):19–24.

Lozoya X et al. Quercetin glycosides in *Psidium guajava* L. leaves and determination of a spasmolytic principle. *Arch Med Res.* 1994; 25(1):11–15.

Lutterodt GD. Inhibition of gastrointestinal release of acetylcholine by quercetin as a possible mode of action of *Psidium guajava* leaf extracts in the treatment of acute diarrhoeal disease. *J Ethnopharmcol.* 1989; 25(3):235–247.

Morales MA et al. Calcium-antagonist effect of quercetin and its relation with the spasmolytic properties of *Psidium guajava* L. *Arch Med Res.* 1994; 25(1):17–21.

Mukhtar HM et al. Effect of water extract of Psidium guajava leaves on alloxan-induced diabetic rats. *Pharmazie.* 2004 Sep;59(9):734–753.

Oh WK et al. Antidiabetic effects of extracts from Psidium guajava. *J Ethnopharmacol.* 2005 Jan 15;96(3):411–415.

Singh RB et al. Can guava fruit intake decrease blood pressure and blood lipids? *J Hum Hypertens.* 1993; 7(1):33–38.

Singh RB et al. Effects of guava intake on serum total and high-density lipoprotein cholesterol levels and on systemic blood pressure. *Am J Cardiol.* 1992; 70(15): 1287–1291.

Wei L et al. Clinical study on treatment of infantile rotaviral enteritis with *Psidium guajava* L. *Zhongguo Zhong Xi Yi Jie He Za Zhi* 2000; 20(12):893–895.

Yamashiro S et al. Cardioprotective effects of extracts from *Psidium guajava L.* and *Limonium wrigth* II, Okinawan medicinal plants, against ischemia-reperfusion injury in perfused rat hearts. *Pharmacology* 2003; 67(3):128–135.

Hazelnuts   www.hazelnutcouncil.org
Bayer A et al. Doxorubicin-induced cataract formation in rats and the inhibitory effects of hazelnut, a natural antioxidant: a histopathological study. *Med Sci Monit.* 2005 Aug;11(8):BR300–304.

Mercanligil SM, Arslan P, Alasalvar C, Okut E, Akgul E, Pinar A, Geyik PO, Tokgozoglu L, Shahidi F. (2006, September 13). Effects of hazelnut-enriched diet on plasma cholesterol and lipoprotein profiles in hypercholesterolemic adult men. *Eur J Clin Nutri.* (epub ahead of print).

Honey   www.honey.com
Al-Waili NS. (2004, Spring). Natural honey lowers plasma glucose, C-reactive protein, homocysteine, and blood lipids in healthy, diabetic, and hyperlipidemic subjects: comparison with dextrose and sucrose. *J Med Food.* 7(1), 100–107.

Mahgoub AA, el-Medany AH, Hagar HH, Sabah DM. (2002, April–June). Protective effect of natural honey against acetic acid-induced colitis in rats. *Trop Gastroenterol.* 23(2), 82–87.

Osuagwu RC, Oladejo OW, Imosemi IO, Aiku A, Ekpos OE, Salami AA, Oyedele OO, Akang EU. (2004, April–June). Enhanced wound contraction in fresh wounds dressed with honey in Wistar rats (Rattus Novergicus). *West Afr J Med.* 23(2), 114–118.

Simon A et al. Wound care with antibacterial honey (Medihoney) in pediatric hematology-oncology. *Support Care Cancer.* 2006 Jan;14(1):91–97.

Swellam T et al. Antineoplastic activity of honey in an experimental bladder cancer implantation model: in vivo and in vitro studies. *Int J Urol.* 2003 Apr;10(4):213–219.

Wilkinson JM, Cavanagh HM. (2005, Spring). Antibacterial activity of 13 honeys against Escherichia coli and Pseudomonas aeruginosa. *J Med Food,* 8(1), 100–103.

Worthington HV, Clarkson JE, Eden OB. Interventions for preventing oral mucositis for patients with cancer receiving treatment. *Cochrane Database Syst Rev.* 2006 Apr 19;(2):CD000978.

Horseradish/Wasabi   www.japan-guide.com/e/e2311.html;
www.horseradish.org

Fuke Y et al. Preventive effect of oral administration of 6-(methylsulfinyl)hexyl iso-thiocyanate derived from wasabi (Wasabia japonica Matsum) against pulmonary metastasis of B16-BL6 mouse melanoma cells. *Cancer Detect Prev.* 2006;30(2): 174–179.

Kinae N et al. Functional properties of wasabi and horseradish. *Biofactors.* 2000; 13(1–4):265–269.

Morimitsu Y et al. Antiplatelet and anticancer isothiocyanates in Japanese domestic horseradish, wasabi. *Biofactors.* 2000;13(1–4):271–276.

Nomurá T et al. Selective sensitivity to wasabi-derived 6-(methylsulfinyl)hexyl isoth-iocyanate of human breast cancer and melanoma cell lines studied in vitro. *Cancer Detect Prev.* 2005;29(2):155–160.

Ono H et al. 6-Methylsulfinylhexyl isothiocyanate and its homologues as food-originated compounds with antibacterial activity against Escherichia coli and Staphylococcus aureus. *Biosci Biotechnol Biochem.* 1998 Feb;62(2):363–365.

Shin IS, Masuda H, Naohide K. Bactericidal activity of wasabi (Wasabia japonica) against Helicobacter pylori. *Int J Food Microbiol.* 2004 Aug 1;94(3):255–261.

Weil MJ, Zhang Y, Nair MG. Colon cancer proliferating desulfosinigrin in wasabi (Wasabia japonica). *Nutr Cancer.* 2004;48(2):207–213.

Weil MJ, Zhang Y, Nair MG. Tumor cell proliferation and cyclooxygenase inhibitory constituents in horseradish (Armoracia rusticana) and Wasabi (Wasabia japonica). *J Agric Food Chem.* 2005 Mar 9;53(5):1440–1444.

Kale   http://plantanswers.tamu.edu/publications/vegetabletravelers/
kale.html

Brown L et al. A prospective study of carotenoid intake and risk of cataract extraction in US men. *Am J Clin Nutr.* 1999 Oct;70(4):517–524.

Kopsell DE et al. Kale carotenoids remain stable while flavor compounds respond to changes in sulfur fertility. *J Agric Food Chem.* 2003 Aug 27;51(18):5319–5325.

Radosavljevic V, Jankovic S, Marinkovic J, Dokic M. Diet and bladder cancer: a case-control study. *Int Urol Nephrol.* 2005;37(2):283–289.

Van Duyn MA, Pivonka E. Overview of the health benefits of fruit and vegetable consumption for the dietetics professional: Selected literature. *J Am Diet Assoc.* 2000;100:1511–1521.

Kiwi   www.kiwifruit.org; www.crfg.org/pubs/ff/kiwifruit.html
Collins BH, Horska A, Hotten PM, Riddoch C, Collins AR. Kiwifruit protects against oxidative DNA damage in human cells and in vitro. *Nutr Cancer.* 2001;(1):148–153.

Duttaroy AK, Jorgensen A. Effects of kiwi fruit consumption on platelet aggregation and plasma lipids in healthy human volunteers. *Platelets.* 2004 Aug;15(5):287–292.

Kopsell D, Kopsell D, Curran-Celentano J. Carotenoid variability among kale and spinach cultivars. *Hortscience.* 2004;(2):34.

Motohashi N et al. Cancer prevention and therapy with kiwifruit in Chinese folklore medicine: a study of kiwifruit extracts. *J Ethnopharmacol.* 2002 Aug;81(3):357–364.

Rinzler CA. *The New Complete Book of Food: A Nutritional, Medical, and Culinary Guide.* New York: Checkmark Books, 1999.

Lemons   www.hort.purdue.edu/newcrop/morton/lemon.html
Khaw KT, Day N, Symmons DP. Vitamin C and the risk of developing inflammatory polyarthritis: prospective nested case-control study. *Ann Rheum Dis.* 2004 Jul;63(7): 843–847.

Manners GD at al. Bioavailability of citrus limonoids in humans. *J Agric Food Chem.* 2003 Jul 2;51(14):4156–4161.

Pattison DJ, Silman AJ, Goodson NJ, Lunt M, Bunn D, Luben R, Welch A, Bingham S, Poulose SM, Harris ED, Patil BS. Citrus limonoids induce apoptosis in human neuroblastoma cells and have radical scavenging activity. *J Nutr.* 2005 Apr;135(4): 870–877.

Sun J, Chu YF, Wu X, Liu RH. Antioxidant and antiproliferative activities of common fruits. *J Agric Food Chem.* 2002 Dec 4;50(25):7449–7454.

Limes   www.fruitsandveggiesmatter.gov
Gharagozloo M, Ghaderi A. Immunomodulatory effect of concentrated lime juice extract on activated human mononuclear cells. *J Ethnopharmacol.* 2001;77(1):85–90.

Kawaii S, Tomono Y, Katase E et al. Antiproliferative effects of the readily extractable fractions prepared from various citrus juices on several cancer cell lines. *J Agric Food Chem.* 1999;47(7):2509–2512.

Rodrigues A, Brun H, Sandstrom A. Risk factors for cholera infection in the initial phase of an epidemic in Guinea-Bissau: protection by lime juice. *Am J Trop Med Hyg.* 1997;57(5):601–604.

Mango   www.crfg.org/pubs/ff/mango.html; www.freshmangos.com
Monterrey-Rodriguez J. Interaction between warfarin and mango fruit. *Ann Pharmacother.* 2002;36(5):940–941.

Percival SS, Talcott ST, Chin ST, Mallak AC, Lounds-Singleton A, Pettit-Moore J. Neoplastic transformation of BALB/3T3 cells and cell cycle of HL-60 cells are inhibited by mango (Mangifera indica L.) juice and mango juice extracts. *J Nutr.* 2006 May;136(5):1300–1304.

Pott I, Marx M, Neidhart S, Muhlbauer W, Carle R. Quantitative determination of beta-carotene stereoisomers in fresh, dried, and solar-dried mangoes. *J Agric Food Chem.* 2003; 51:4527–4531.

Van Duyn MAS, Pivonka E. Overview of the health benefits of fruit and vegetable consumption for the dietetics professional: Selected literature. *J Am Diet Assoc.* 2000;100:1511–1521.

Millet   http://www.hort.purdue.edu/newcrop/afcm/millet.html
Choi YY et al. Effects of dietary protein of Korean foxtail millet on plasma adiponectin, HDL-cholesterol, and insulin levels in genetically type 2 diabetic mice. *Biosci Biotechnol Biochem.* 2005 Jan;69(1):31–37.

Nishizawa N. Proso millet protein elevates plasma level of high-density lipoprotein: a new food function of proso millet. *Biomed Environ Sci.* 1996 Sep;9(2–3):209–212.

Shimanuki S, Nagasawa T, Nishizawa N. Plasma HDL subfraction levels increase in rats fed proso-millet protein concentrate. *Med Sci Monit.* 2006 Jul;12(7):BR221–6.

Mint   www.herbsociety-stu.org/mint.htm
Kozan E, Kupeli E, Yesilada E. Evaluation of some plants used in Turkish folk medicine against parasitic infections for their in vivo anthelmintic activity. *J Ethnopharmacol.* 2006 May 16; 108(2):211–216.

McKay DL, Blumberg JB. A review of the bioactivity and potential health benefits of peppermint tea (Mentha piperita L.). *Phytother Res.* 2006 Aug;20(8):619–633.

Moreira MR, Ponce AG, del Valle CE, Roura SI. Inhibitory parameters of essential oils to reduce a foodborne pathogen. *LWT.* 2005; 38:565–570.

Salleh MN, Runnie I, Roach PD, Mohamed S, Abeywardena MY. Inhibition of low-density lipoprotein oxidation and up-regulation of low-density lipoprotein receptor in HepG2 cells by tropical plant extracts. *J Agric Food Chem.* 2002;50:3693–3697.

Samarth RM, Panwar M, Kumar M, Kumar A. Protective effects of Mentha piperita Linn on benzo[a]pyrene-induced lung carcinogenicity and mutagenicity in Swiss albino mice. *Mutagenesis.* 2006 Jan;21(1):61–66.

Scheier L. Salicylic acid: One more reason to eat your fruits and vegetables. *J Am Diet Assoc.* 200; 101:1406–1408.

Spirling LI, Daniels IR. Botanical perspectives on health peppermint: more than just an after-dinner mint. *J R Soc Health.* 2001 Mar;121(1):62–63.

Mushrooms   www.mushroomcouncil.com
Aruoma OI, Spencer JP, Mahmood N. Protection against oxidative damage and cell death by the natural antioxidant ergothioneine. *Food Chem Toxicol.* 1999 Nov; 37(11):1043–1053.

Chen S, Phung S, Hur G, Kwok S, Ye J, and Oh SR. Breast cancer prevention with phytochemicals in mushrooms. *Proceedings of the American Association for Cancer Research,* vol. 46, Abs. 5186.

Duffield-Lillico AJ, Shureiqu I, Lippman SM. Can selenium prevent colorectal cancer? A signpost from epidemiology. *J Natl Cancer Inst.* 2004;92:1645–1647.

Lull C, Wichers HJ, Savelkoul HF. Anti-inflammatory and immunomodulating properties of fungal metabolites. *Mediators Inflamm.* 2005 Jun 9;2005(2):63–80.

Phung S., Ye Jingjing, Hur G., Kwok S., Lui K. and Chen S. White button mushrooms and prostate cancer prevention. *Proceedings of the American Association for Cancer Research;*46: Abs. 1580.

Wasser SP. Medicinal mushrooms as a source of antitumor and immunomodulating polysaccharides. *Appl Microbiol Biotechnol.* 2002 Nov;60(3):258–274.

Oats   www.namamillers.org

Pins JJ, Geleva D, Keenan JM, Frazel C, O'Connor PJ, Cherney LM. Do whole-grain oat cereals reduce the need for antihypertensive medications and improve blood pressure control? *J Fam Pract.* 2002;51:353–359.

Pomeroy S, Tupper R, Cehun-Anders, Nestel P. Oat beta-glucan lowers total and LDL-cholesterol. *Aust J Nut Diet.* 2001;58:51–54.

Queenan KL et al. Concentrated oat beta-glucan, a fermentable fiber, lowers serum cholesterol in hypercholesterolemic adults in a randomized controlled trial. *Nutr J.* 2007 Mar 26;6:6.

Reyna-Villasmil N et al. Oat-derived beta-glucan significantly improves HDLC and diminishes LDLC and non-HDL cholesterol in overweight individuals with mild hypercholesterolemia. *Am J Ther.* 2007 Mar–Apr;14(2):203–212.

Slavin JL, Jacobs D, Marquart L, Wiemer K. The role of whole grains in disease prevention. *J Am Diet Assoc.* 2001;101:780–785.

Olives   www.calolive.org

Bondia-Pons I et al. Moderate consumption of olive oil by healthy European men reduces systolic blood pressure in non-Mediterranean participants. *J Nutr.* 2007 Jan;137(1):84–87.

Covas MI et al. The effect of polyphenols in olive oil on heart disease risk factors: a randomized trial. *Ann Intern Med.* 2006 Sep 5;145(5):333–341.

Juan ME et al. Olive fruit extracts inhibit proliferation and induce apoptosis in HT-29 human colon cancer cells. *J Nutr.* 2006 Oct;136(10):2553–2557.

Lee A, Thurnham DI, Chopra C. Consumption of tomato products with olive oil but not sunflower oil increases the antioxidant activity of plasma. *Free Radical Biology & Medicine.* 29:1051–1055; 2000.

Owen RW et al. Olives and olive oil in cancer prevention. *Eur J Cancer Prev.* 2004 Aug;13(4):319–326.

Onions   www.onions-usa.org

Arai Y, Watanabe S, Kimira M, Shimoi K, Mochizuki R, Kinae N. Dietary intakes of flavonols, flavones and isoflavones by Japanese women and the inverse correlation between quercetin intake and plasma LDL cholesterol concentration. *J Nutr.* 2000 Sep;130(9):2243–2250.

Chu YF, Sun J, Wu X, Liu RH. Antioxidant and antiproliferative activities of common vegetables. *J Agric Food Chem.* 2002 Nov 6;50(23):6910–6916.

Craig WJ. Phytochemicals: Guardians of our health. *J Am Diet Assoc.* 1997;97: S199–S204.

Dole Nutrition Institute. "Onions Boost Bone Health." 2005. Available at: www.dolenutrition.com. Accessed 5/18/06.

Grant WB. A multicountry ecologic study of risk and risk reduction factors for prostate cancer mortality. *Eur Urol.* 2004 Mar;45(3):271–279.

Knekt P et al. Flavonoid intake and risk of chronic diseases. *Am J Clin Nutr.* 2002 Sep;76(3):560–568.

Le Marchand L, Murphy SP, Hankin JH, Wilkens LR, Kolonel LN. Intake of flavonoids and lung cancer. *J Natl Cancer Inst.* 2000 Jan 19;92(2):154–160.

Onion extract gel versus petrolatum emollient on new surgical scars: prospective double-blinded study. *Dermatol Surg.* 2006 Feb;32(2):193–197.

Osmont KS, Arnt CR, Goldman IL. Temporal aspects of onion-induced antiplatelet activity. *Plant Foods Hum Nutr.* 2003 Winter;58(1):27–40.

Yang J, Meyers KJ, van der Heide J, Liu RH. Varietal differences in phenolic content and antioxidant and antiproliferative activities of onions. *J Agric Food Chem.* 2004 Nov 3;52(22):6787–6793.

Oranges   www.hort.purdue.edu/newcrop/morton/orange.html
Daher CF, Abou-Khalil J, Baroody GM. Effect of acute and chronic grapefruit, orange, and pineapple juice intake on blood lipid profile in normolipidemic rat. *Med Sci Monit.* 2005 Dec;11(12):BR465–472.

Lehrner J, Marwinski G, Lehr S, Johren P, Deecke L. Ambient odors of orange and lavender reduce anxiety and improve mood in a dental office. *Physiol Behav.* 2005 Sep 15;86(1–2):92–95.

Nyyssönen et al. Vitamin C deficiency and risk of myocardial infarction: prospective population study of men from Eastern Finland. *Journal of American Dietetic Association*, March 1997.

Rolls, Barbara. *The Volumetrics Weight-Control Plan*, HarperCollins, New York, 2005.

Tiwary, C.M., Ward, J.A., Jackson, B.A. Effect of pectin on satiety in healthy US Army adults. *JACN.* 1997;16(5):423–428.

Vitali F et al. Effect of a standardized extract of red orange juice on proliferation of human prostate cells in vitro. *Fitoterapia.* 2006 Apr;77(3):151–5. Epub 2006 Feb 23.

Oregano   www.answers.com/topic/oregano
Burt SA, Reinders RD. Antibacterial activity of selected plant essential oils against Escherichia coli O157:H. *Soc for Applied Microbio.* 2003;36:162–167.

Lin YT, Kwon YI, Labbe RG, Shetty K. Inhibition of Helicobacter pylori and associated urease by oregano and cranberry phytochemical synergies. *Appl Environ Microbiol.* 2005 Dec;71(12):8558–8564.

Oussalah M, Caillet S, Lacroix M. Mechanism of action of Spanish oregano, Chinese cinnamon, and savory essential oils against cell membranes and walls of Escherichia coli O157:H7 and Listeria monocytogenes. *J Food Prot.* 2006 May;69(5):1046–1055.

Rao BS et al. Antioxidant, anticlastogenic and radioprotective effect of Coleus aromaticus on Chinese hamster fibroblast cells (V79) exposed to gamma radiation. *Mutagenesis.* 2006 May 30.

Shan B, Cai YZ, Sun M, and Corke H. Antioxidant capacity of 26 spice extracts and characterization of their phenolic constitutes. *J Agric Food Chem.* 2005;53:7749–7759.

Talpur N, Echard B, Ingram C, Bagchi D, and Preuss H. Effects of a novel formulation of essential oils on glucose-insulin metabolism in diabetic and hypertensive rats: A pilot study. *Doi.* 2005;7:193–199.

Papaya   www.crfg.org/pubs/ff/papaya.html
The General Practitioner. "The power of papaya could speed burn healing." *GP.* 2005;83.

Giuliano AR et al. Dietary intake and risk of persistent human papillomavirus (HPV) infection: The Ludwig-McGill HPV natural history study. *JID.* 2003;188:1508–1506.

Leclerc D et al. Proteasome-independent major histocompatibility complex class I cross-presentation mediated by papaya mosaic virus-like particles leads to expansion of specific human T cells. *J Virol.* 2007 Feb;81(3):1319–1326. Epub 2006 Nov 22.

Mozaffarieh M, Sacu S, and Wedrich A. The role of the carotenoids, lutein and zeaxanthin, in protecting against age-related macular degeneration. *Nutr J.* 2003;2:20–28.

Parsley   www.health-topic.com/Dictionary-P.aspx
Bolkent S, Yanardag R, Ozsoy-Sacan O, Karabulut-Bulan O. Effects of parsley (Petroselinum crispum) on the liver of diabetic rats: a morphological and biochemical study. *Phytother Res.* 2004 Dec;18(12):996–999.

Ozsoy-Sacan O, Yanardag R, Orak H, Ozgey Y, Yarat A, Tunali T. Effects of parsley (Petroselinum crispum) extract versus glibornuride on the liver of streptozotocin-induced diabetic rats. *J Ethnopharmacol.* 2006 Mar 8;104(1–2):175–81.

Yoshikawa M et al. Medicinal foodstuffs. XVIII. Phytoestrogens from the aerial part of Petroselinum crispum MIll. (Parsley) and structures of 6"-acetylapiin and a new monoterpene glycoside, petroside. *Chem Pharm Bull* (Tokyo). 2000 Jul;48(7): 1039–1044.

Zheng GQ, Kenney PM, Zhang J, Lam LK. Inhibition of benzo[a]pyrene-induced tumorigenesis by myristicin, a volatile aroma constituent of parsley leaf oil. *Carcinogenesis.* 1992 Oct;13(10):1921–1923.

Passion fruit   www.crfg.org/pubs/ff/passionfruit.html
Chau CF, Huang YL. Effects of the insoluble fiber derived from Passiflora edulis seed on plasma and hepatic lipids and fecal output. *Mol Nutr Food Res.* 2005 Aug;49(8): 786–790.

Ichimura T et al. Antihypertensive effect of an extract of Passiflora edulis rind in spontaneously hypertensive rats. *Biosci Biotechnol Biochem.* 2006 Mar;70(3):718–721.

Talcott ST, Percival SS, Pittet-Moore J, Celoria C. Phytochemical composition and antioxidant stability of fortified yellow passion fruit (Passiflora edulis). *J Agric Food Chem.* 2003 Feb 12;51(4):935–941.

Rowe CA, Nantz MP, Deniera C, Green K, Talcott ST, Percival SS. Inhibition of neoplastic transformation of benzo[alpha]pyrene-treated BALB/c 3T3 murine cells by a phytochemical extract of passionfruit juice. *J Med Food.* 2004 Winter;7(4):402–407.

Peanuts   www.peanut-institute.org; www.peanutusa.com
Awad AB, Chan KC, Downie AC, Fink CS. Peanuts as a source of B-sitosterol, a sterol with anticancer properties. *Nutrition and Cancer.* 2000;36(2):238–241.

Jiang R et al. Nut and peanut butter consumption and risk of type 2 diabetes in women. *JAMA.* 2002;288:2554–2560.

Kris-Etherton et al. Improved diet quality with peanut consumption. *JADA.* 2004;23(6):660–668.

Sanders TH, McMichael RW, Hendrix KW. Occurrence or resveratrol in edible peanuts. *Journal of Agricultural and Food Chemistry.* 2000;48(4):1243–1246. April 2003 AJCN.

Yeh CC, You SL, Chen CJ, Sung FC. Peanut consumption and reduced risk of colorectal cancer in women: a prospective study in Taiwan. *World J Gastroenterol.* 2006 Jan 14;12(2):222–227.

Pears   www.usapears.com; www.calpear.com
Butler LM, Koh WP, Lee HP, Yu MC, London SJ. Dietary fiber and reduced cough with phlegm: A cohort study in Singapore. *Am J Respir Crit Care Med.* 2004;170: 279–287.

Conceicao de Olivceira M, Sichieri R, and Moura AS. Weight loss associated with a daily intake of three apples or three pears among overweight women. *Nutrition.* 2003;19:253–256.

Mink PJ. Flavonoid intake and cardiovascular disease mortality: a prospective study in postmenopausal women. *Am J Clin Nutr.* 2007 Mar;85(3):895–909.

Pecans   www.georgiapecans.org; www.ilovepecans.org
Bes-Rastrollo M et al. Nut consumption and weight gain in a Mediterranean cohort: The SUN study. *Obesity* (Silver Spring). 2007 Jan;15(1):107–116.

Halvorsen BL et al. Content of redox-active compounds (ie, antioxidants) in foods consumed in the United States. *Am J Clin Nutr.* 2006 Jul;84(1):95–135.

Morgan et al. Pecans lower low-density lipoprotein cholesterol in people with normal lipid levels. *JADA.* 2000. 100: 312–318.

Rajaram et al. A monounsaturated fatty acid-rich pecan-enriched diet favorably alters the serum lipid profile of healthy men and women. *J Nutr.* 2001 Sep;131(9): 2275–2279.

Xianli W et al. Lipophilic and hydrophilic antioxidant capacities of common foods in the United States. *Journal of Agricultural and Food Chemistry,* 2004, 52: 4026–4037.

Peppers   www.fruitsandveggiesmatter.gov

Belza A, Frandsen E, Kondrup J. Body fat loss achieved by stimulation of thermogenesis by a combination of bioactive food ingredients: a placebo-controlled, double-blind 8-week intervention in obese subjects. *Int J Obes* (Lond). 2006 Apr 25.

Diepvens K, Westerterp KR, Westerterp-Plantenga MS. Obesity and thermogenesis related to the consumption of caffeine, ephedrine, capsaicin and green tea. *Am J Physiol Regul Integr Comp Physiol.* 2007 Jan;292(1):R77–85.

Macho A et al. Non-pungent capsaicinoids from sweet pepper synthesis and evaluation of the chemopreventive and anticancer potential. *Eur J Nutr.* 2003 Jan;42(1):2–9.

Mori A et al. Capsaicin, a component of red peppers, inhibits the growth of androgen-independent, p53 mutant prostate cancer cells. *Cancer Res.* 2006 Mar 15; 66(6):3222–3229.

Sancho R et al. Immunosuppressive activity of capsaicinoids: capsiate derived from sweet peppers inhibits NF-kappaB activation and is a potent antiinflammatory compound in vivo. *Eur J Immunol.* 2002 Jun;32(6):1753–1763.

Tandan R et al. Topical capsaicin in painful diabetic neuropathy. Controlled study with long-term follow-up. *Diabetes Care.* 1992 Jan;15(1):8–14.

Zhang W et al. Eular evidence based recommendations for the management of hand osteoarthritis—report of a task force of the Eular Standing Committee for International Clinical Studies Including Therapeutics (ESCISIT). *Ann Rheum Dis.* 2006 Oct 17.

Persimmons   www.crfg.org/pubs/ff/persimmon.html

Achiwa Y, Hibasami H, Katsuzaki H, Imai K, Komiya T. Inhibitory effects of persimmon (Diospyros kaki) extract and related polyphenol compounds on growth of human lymphoid leukemia cells. *Biosci Biotechnol Biochem.* 1997 Jul;61(7): 1099–1101.

Goreinstein S et al. Comparative contents of dietary fiber, total phenolics, and minerals in persimmons and apples. *J Agric Food Chem.* 2001 Feb;49(2):952–957.

Gorinstein S, Bartnikowska E, Kulasek G, Zemser M, Trakhtenberg S. Dietary persimmon improves lipid metabolism in rats fed diets containing cholesterol. *J Nutr.* 1998, 128:2023–2027.

Hibasami H, Achiwa Y, Fujikawa T, Komiya T. Induction of programmed cell death (apoptosis) in human lymphoid leukemia cells by catechin compounds. *Anticancer Res.* 1996 Jul–Aug;16(4A):1943–1946.

Pineapple   www.howtocutapineapple.com;
www.crfg.org/pubs/ff/pineapple.html

Glaser D, Hilberg T. The influence of bromelain on platelet count and platelet activity in vitro. *Platelets.* 2006 Feb;17(1):37–41.

Helser MA, Hotchkiss JH, Roe DA. Influence of fruit and vegetable juices on the endogenous formation of N-nitrosoproline and N-nitrosothiazolidine-4-carboxylic acid in humans on controlled diets. *Carcinogenesis.* 1992 Dec;13(12):2277–2280.

Taussig SJ, Batkin S. Bromelain, the enzyme complex of pineapple (Ananas comosus) and its clinical application. An update. *J Ethnopharmacol.* 1988 Feb-Mar;22(2):191–203.

Pistachios   www.pistachios.org
Awad AB, Chinnam M, Fink CS, Bradford PG. beta-Sitosterol activates Fas signaling in human breast cancer cells. *Phytomedicine.* 2007 Mar 9 [Epub ahead of print].

Kocyigit A, Koylu AA, Keles H. Effects of pistachio nuts consumption on plasma lipid profile and oxidative status in healthy volunteers. *Nutr Metab Cardiovasc Dis.* 2006 Apr;16(3):202–209.

Plums (prunes)   www.californiadriedplums.org
Aggarwal BB, Shishodia S. Molecular targets of dietary agents for prevention and therapy of cancer. *Biochemical Pharmacology.* 2007 May;71(10):1397–1421.

Arjmandi BH et al. Dried plums improve indices of bone formation in postmenopausal women. *J Womens Health Gend Based Med.* 2002 Jan–Feb;11(1):61–68.

Franklin M, Bu SY, Lerner MR, Lancaster EA, Bellmer D, Marlow D, Lightfoot SA, Arjmandi BH, Brackett DJ, Lucas EA, Smith BJ. Dried plum prevents bone loss in a male osteoporosis model via IGF-I and the RANK pathway. *Bone.* 2006 October.

Kayano S, Kikuzaki H, Yamada NK, Aoki A, Kasamatsu K, Yamasaki Y, Ikami T, Suzuki T, Mitani T, Nakatani N. Antioxidant properties of prunes (Prunus domestica L.) and their constituents. *Biofactors.* 2004;21(1–4):309–313.

Muller-Lissner S, Kaatz, V, Brandt W, Keller J, Layer P. The perceived effect of various foods and beverages on stool consistency. *Eur J Gastro Hep.* 2005 Jan;17(1): 109–112.

Mühlbauer RC, Lozano A, Reinli A, Wetli H. Various selected vegetables, fruits, mushrooms and red wine residue inhibit bone resorption in rats. *J of Nutr.* 2003 Nov; 133(11):3592–3597.

Piga A, Del Caro A, Corda G. From plums to prunes: influence of drying parameters on polyphenols and antioxidant activity. *J Agric Food Chem.* 2003 June;51(12): 3675–3681.

Tinker LF, Schneeman BO, Davis PA, Gallaher DD, Waggoner CR. Consumption of prunes as a source of dietary fiber in men with mild hypercholesterolemia. *Am J Clin Nutr.* 1991 May;53(5):1259–1265.

Yuqing Y, Gallaher DD. Effect of dried plums on colon cancer risk factors in rats. *Nutr Cancer.* 2005;53(1):117–125.

Pomegranate   www.pomegranates.org
Adams LS, Seeram NP, Aggarwal BB, Takada Y, Sand D, Heber D. Pomegranate juice, total pomegranate ellagitannins, and punicalagin suppress inflammatory cell signaling in colon cancer cells. *J Agric Food Chem.* 2006 Feb 8;54(3):980–985.

Aviram M, Dornfeld L. Pomegranate juice consumption inhibits serum angiotensin converting enzyme activity and reduces systolic blood pressure. *Atherosclerosis*. 2001 Sep;158(1):195–198.

Aviram M, Dornfeld L, Kaplan M, Coleman R, Gaitini D, Nitecki S, Hofman A, Rosenblat M, Volkova N, Presser D, Attias J, Hayek T, Fuhrman B. Pomegranate juice flavonoids inhibit low-density lipoprotein oxidation and cardiovascular diseases: studies in atherosclerotic mice and in humans. *Drugs Exp Clin Res*. 2002;28(2–3):49–62.

Azadzoi KM, Schulman RN, Aviram M, Siroky MB. Oxidative stress in arteriogenic erectile dysfunction: prophylactic role of antioxidants. *J Urol*. 2005 Jul;174(1): 386–393.

De M, Krishna De A, Banerjee AB. Antimicrobial screening of some Indian spices. *Phytother Res*. 1999 Nov;13(7):616–623.

Jeune MA, Kumi-Diaka J, Brown J. Anticancer activities of pomegranate extracts and genistein in human breast cancer cells. *J Med Food*. 2005;8(4):469–475.

Loren DJ, Seeram NP, Schulman RN, Holtzman DM. Maternal dietary supplementation with pomegranate juice is neuroprotective in an animal model of neonatal hypoxic-ischemic brain injury. *Pediatr Res*. 2005 June;57(6):858–864.

Malik A, Afaq F, Sarfaraz S, Adhami VM, Syed DN, Hukhtar H. Pomegranate fruit juice for chemoprevention and chemotherapy of prostate cancer. *Proc Natl Acad Sci USA*. 2005 Oct 11;102(41):14813–14818.

Mori-Okamoto J, Otawara-Hamamoto Y, Yamato H, Yoshimura H. Pomegranate extract improves a depressive state and bone properties in menopausal syndrome model ovariectomized mice. *J Ethnopharmacol*. 2004 May;92(1):93–101.

Pantuck AJ, Leppert JT, Zomorodian N, Aronson W, Hong J, Barnard RJ, Seeram N, Liker H, Wang H, Elashoff R, Heber D, Aviram M, Ignarro L, Belldegrun A. Phase II study of pomegranate juice for men with rising prostate-specific antigen following surgery or radiation for prostate cancer. *Clin Cancer Res*. 2006 Jul 1;12(13):4018–4026.

Sumner MD, Elliott-Eller M, Weidner G, Daubenmier JJ, Chew MH, Marlin R, Raisin CJ, Ornish D. Effects of pomegranate juice consumption on myocardial perfusion in patients with coronary heart disease. *Am J Cardiol*. 2005 Sep 15;96(6):810–813.

Potatoes   www.healthypotato.com
Albert, NM. We are what we eat: women and diet for cardiovascular health. *J of Cardiovas Nurs*. 2005;20(6):451–460.

Betturer K. Better than a banana. *Health*. 1997 Apr;11(3):38.

De Mejía EG, Prisecaru V. Lectins as bioactive plant proteins: a potential in cancer treatment. *Critical Reviews in Food Science & Nutrition*. 2005 Nov;45(6):425–445.

Ruano-Ravina A, Figueiras A, Dosil-Diaz O, Barreiro-Carracedo A, Barros-Dios JM. A population-based case-control study on fruit and vegetable intake and lung cancer: a paradox effect? *Nutrition and Cancer*. 2002;43(1):47–51.

Russo P, Barba G, Venezia A, Siani A. Dietary potassium in cardiovascular prevention: nutritional and clinical implications. *Current Medicinal Chemistry—Immunology, Endocrine & Metabolic Agents*. 2005 Jan;5(1):23–31.

Singh N, Kamath V, Rajini PS. Protective effect of potato peel powder in ameliorating oxidative stress in streptozotocin diabetic rats. *Plant Foods Hum Nutr.* 2005 Jun;60(2):49–54.

Pumpkin   www.urbanext.uiuc.edu/pumpkins/history.html
Binns CW, Jian L. & Lee, AH. The relationship between dietary carotenoids and prostate cancer risk in Southeast Chinese men. *Asia Pac J Clin Nutr.* 2004;13:S117.

Huang XE, Hirose K, Wakai K, Matsuo K, Ito H, Xiang J, Takezaki T, Tajima K. Comparison of lifestyle risk factors by family history of gastric, breast, lung and colo-rectal cancer. *Asian Pac J Cancer Prev.* 2004 Oct;5(4):419–427.

Jaber R. Respiratory and allergic diseases: from upper respiratory tract infections to asthma. *Prim Care.* 2002 June;29(2):231–261.

Schleich S, Papaioannou M, Baniahmad A, Matusch R. Extracts from Pygeum africanum and other ethnobotanical species with antiandrogenic activity. *Planta Med.* 2006 Jul;72(9):807–13.

Suzuki K, Ito Y, Nakamura S, Ochiai J, Aoki K. Relationship between serum carotenoids and hyperglycemia: a population-based cross-sectional study. *J Epidemiol.* 2002 Sep;12(5):357–366.

Zuhair HA, Abd El-Fattah AA, El-Sayed MI. Pumpkin-seed oil modulates the effect of felodipine and captropril in spontaneously hypertensive rats. *Pharmacol Res.* 2000 May;41(5):555–563.

Quinoa   www.quinoa.net
Berti C, Riso P, Brusamolino A, Porrini M. Effect on appetite control of minor cereal and pseudocereal products. *Br J Nutr.* 2005 Nov;94(5):850–858.

Estrada A, Li B, Laarveld B. Adjuvant action of Chenopodium quinoa saponins on the induction of antibody responses to intragastric and intranasal administered antigens in mice. *Comp Immunol Microbiol Infect Dis.* 1998 Jul;21(3):225–36.

Raspberries   www.raspberries.us; www.raspberryblackberry.com
Casto, BC et al. Chemoprevention of oral cancer by black raspberries. *Anticancer Res.* 2002 Nov–Dec;22(6C):4005–4015.

Chen T, Hwang H, Rose ME, Nines RG, Stoner GD. Chemopreventive properties of black raspberries in *N*-nitrosomethylbenzylamine-induced rat esophageal tumorigenesis: down-regulation of cyclooxygenase-2, inducible nitric oxide synthase, and c-*Jun. Cancer Res.* 2006 Mar;66(5):2853–2859.

Han C, Ding H, Casto B, Stoner GD, D'Ambrosio SM. Inhibition of the growth of pre-malignant and malignant human oral cell lines by extracts and components of black raspberries. *Nutr Cancer.* 2005:51(2):207–217.

Larrosa M, Tomas-Barberan FA, Espin JC. The dietary hydrolysable tannin punicala-gin releases ellagic acid that induces apoptosis in human colon adenocarcinoma Caco-2 cells by using the mitochondrial pathway. *J Nutri Biochem.* 2005 Oct (Epub ahead of print).

Liu M, Li XQ, Weber C, Lee CY, Brown J, Liu RH. Antioxidant and antiproliferative activities of raspberries. *J Agric Food Chem.* 2002 May;50(10):2926–2930.

McDougall GJ, Stewart D. The inhibitory effects of berry polyphenols on digestive enzymes. *Biofactors.* 2005;23(4), 189–195.

Morimoto C, Satoh Y, Hara M, Inoue S, Tsujita T, Okuda H. Anti-obese action of raspberry ketone. *Life Sciences.* 2005 May;77(2):194–204.

Rice, brown   www.usarice.com
Anderson JW, Hanna TJ, Peng X, Kryscio RJ. Whole grain foods and heart disease risk. *J Am Coll Nutr.* 2000 Jun;19(3 Suppl):291S–299S.

Jensen MK, Koh-Banerjee P, Hu FB, Franz M, Sampson L, Gronbaek M, Rimm EB. Intakes of whole grains, bran, and germ and the risk of coronary heart disease in men. *Am J Clin Nutr.* 2004;80(6):1492–1499.

Johnsen NF, Hausner H, Olsen A, Tetens I, Christensen J, Knudsen KE, Overvad K, Tjonneland A. Intake of whole grains and vegetables determines the plasma enterolactone concentration of Danish women. *J Nutr.* 2004 Oct;134(10):2691–2697.

Mamiya T et al. Effects of pre-germinated brown rice on beta-amyloid protein-induced learning and memory deficits in mice. *Biol Pharm Bull.* 2004 Jul; 27(7):1041–1045.

Most MM, Tulley R, Morales S, Lefevre M. Rice bran oil, not fiber, lowers cholesterol in humans. *Am J Clin Nutr.* 2005 Jan;81(1):64–68.

Romaine Lettuce   http://edis.ifas.ufl.edu/MV125
Ingster LM, Feinleib M. Could salicylates in food have contributed to the decline in cardiovascular disease mortality? A new hypothesis. *Am J Public Health.* 1997;87: 1554–1557.

Mozaffarieh M, Sacu S, Wedrich A. The role of carotenoids, lutein and zeaxanthin, in protecting against age-related macular degeneration: A review based on controversial evidence. *Nut J.* 2003;2:20–28.

Paterson JR, Lawrence JR. Salicylic acid: a link between aspirin, diet and the prevention of colorectal cancer. *QJM.* 2001;94:445–448.

Rolls BJ, Roe LS, Meengs JS. Salad and satiety: Energy density and portion size of a first-course salad affect energy intake at lunch. *J Am Diet Assoc.* 2004; 104: 1570–1576.

Scheier L. Salicylic Acid: One more reason to eat your fruits and vegetables. *J Am Diet Assoc.* 2001; 101:1406–1408.

Rosemary   www.botanical.com/botanical/mgmh/r/rosema17.html
Del Bano MJ, Castillo J, Benavente-Garcia O, Lorente J, Martin-Gil R, Acevedo C, Alcaraz M. Radioprotective-antimutagenic effects of rosemary phenolics against chromosomal damage induced in human lymphocytes by gamma-rays. *J Agric Food Chem.* 2006;54:2064–2068.

Inoue K et al. Effects of volatile constituents of rosemary extract on lung inflammation induced by diesel exhaust particles. *Basic Clin Pharmacol Toxicol.* 2006 Jul;99(1):52–57.

Moreira MR, Ponce AG, del Valle CE, Roura SI. Inhibitory parameters of essential oils to reduce a foodborne pathogen. *LWT.* 2005;38:565–570.

Sancheti G, Goyal P. Modulatory influence of Rosemarinus officinalis on DMBA-induced mouse skin tumorigenesis. *Asian Pac J Cancer Prev.* 2006 Apr–Jun;7(2): 331–335.

Sharaboni H. Cooperative antitumor effects of vitamin D3 derivatives and rosemary preparations in a mouse model of myeloid leukemia. *Int J Cancer.* 2006 Jun 15; 118(12):3012–3021.

Rye   www.wholegrainscouncil.org

Davies MJ, Bowey EA, Adlercreutz H, Rowland IR, Rumsby PC. Effects of soy or rye supplementation of high-fat diets on colon tumour development in azoxymethane-treated rats. *Carcinogenesis.* 1999 June;20(6):927–931.

Matscheski A, Richter DU, Hartmann AM, Effmert U, Jeschke U, Kupka MS, Abarzua S, Briese V, Ruth W, Kragl U, Piechulla B. Effects of phytoestrogen extracts isolated from rye, green and yellow pea seeds on hormone production and proliferation of trophoblast tumor cells Jeg3. *Horm Res.* 2006;65(6):276–288.

McIntosh GH et al. Whole-grain rye and wheat foods and markers of bowel health in overweight middle-aged men. *Am J Clin Nutr.* 2003 Apr;77(4):967–974.

Mozaffarian D, Kumanyika SK, Lemaitre RN, Olson JL, Burke GL, Siscovick DS. Cereal, fruit, and vegetable fiber intake and the risk of cardiovascular disease in elderly individuals. *JAMA.* 2003 Apr 2;289(13):1659–1666.

Pietinen P, Stumpf K, Mannisto S, Kataja V, Uusitupa M, Adlercreutz H. Serum enterolactone and risk of breast cancer: a case-control study in eastern Finland. *Cancer Epidemiol Biomarkers Prev.* 2001 Apr;10(4):339–344.

Wikstrom P et al. Rye bran diet increases epithelial cell apoptosis and decreases epithelial cell volume in TRAMP (transgenic adenocarcinoma of the mouse prostate) tumors. *Nutr Cancer.* 2005;53(1):111–116.

Zhang JX, Lundin E, Reuterving CO, Hallmans G, Stenling R, Westerlund E, Aman P. Effects of rye bran, oat bran and soya-bean fibre on bile composition, gallstone formation, gall-bladder morphology and serum cholesterol in Syrian golden hamsters (Mesocricetus auratus). *Br J Nutr.* 1994 Jun;71(6):861–870.

Salmon   www.great-salmon-recipes.com;
www.salmonoftheamericas.com

De Lorgeril M, et al. Mediterranean diet, traditional risk factors, and the rate of cardiovascular complications after myocardial infarction. *Circulation.* 1999; 99: 779–785.

Harris WS, Isley WL. Clinical trial evidence for the cardioprotective effects of omega-3 acids. *Curr Atheroscler Rep.* 2001; 3(2): 174–179.

Jho DH, Cole SM, Lee EM, Espat NJ. Role of omega-3 fatty acid supplementation in inflammation and malignancy. *Integr Cancer Ther.* 2004 Jun;3(2):98–111.

Kris-Etherton P, Harris WS, Appel LJ. Fish consumption, fish oil, omega-3 fatty acids, and cardiovascular disease. *Am Heart Assoc Sci Statement.* 2002; 2747–2757.

Marchioli R, Barzi F, Bomba E, et al. Early protection against sudden death by n-3 polyunsaturated fatty acids after myocardial infarction. *Circulation.* 2002;105: 1897–1903.

Singh RB, et al. Effect of an Indo-Mediterranean diet on progression of coronary artery disease in high risk patients. *Lancet.* 2002; 360:1455–1461.

Surette ME, Koumenis IL, Edens MB, Tramposch KM, Clayton B, Bowton D, Chilton FH. Inhibition of leukotriene biosynthesis by a novel dietary fatty acid formulation in patients with atopic asthma: a randomized, placebo-controlled, parallel-group, prospective trial. *Clin Ther Mar.* 2003; 25(3):972–979.

Suzuki S et al. Daily omega-3 fatty acid intake and depression in Japanese patients with newly diagnosed lung cancer. *Br J Cancer.* 2004 Feb;23:90(4):787–793.

Von Schacky C, Angerer P, Kothny W, Thiesen K, Mudra H. The effect of dietary n-3 fatty acids on coronary atherosclerosis. *Ann Intern Med.* 1999; 130: 554–562.

Sardines   www.oceansalive.org

Patent RV et al. The influence of sardine consumption on the omega-3 fatty acid content of mature human milk. *J Pediatr (Rio J).* 2006 Jan–Feb;82(1):63–69.

Sanchez-Muniz FJ, Garcia-Linares MC, Garcia-Arias MT, Bastida S, Viejo J. Fat and protein from olive oil-fried sardines interact to normalize serum lipoproteins and reduce liver lipids in hypercholesterolemic rats. *J Nutr.* 2003 Jul;133(7):2302–2308.

Sesame   www.hort.purdue.edu/newcrop/afcm/sesame.html

Liu Z, Saarinen NM, Thompson LU. Sesamin is one of the major precursors of mammalian lignans in sesame seed (Sesamum indicum) as observed in vitro and in rats. *J Nutr.* 2006 Apr;136(4):906–912.

Miyahara Y, Hibasami H, Katsuzaki H, Imai K, Komiya T. Sesamolin from sesame seed inhibits proliferation by inducing apoptosis in human lymphoid leukemia Molt 4B cells. *Int J Mol Med.* 2001 Apr;7(4):369–371.

Noguchi T, Ikeda K, Sasaki Y, Yamamoto J, Yamori Y. Effects of vitamin E and sesamin on hypertension and cerebral thrombogenesis in stroke-prone spontaneously hypertensive rats. *Clin Exp Pharmacol Physiol.* 2004 Dec;31 Suppl 2:S24–S26.

Smith DE, Salerno JW. Selective growth inhibition of a human malignant melanoma cell line by sesame oil in vitro. *Prostaglandins Leukot Essent Fatty Acids.* 1992 Jun; 46(2), 145–150.

Sorghum   www.sorghumgrowers.com; www.wholegrainscouncil.org/recipesSorghum.htm

Awika JM, McDonough CM, Rooney LW. Decorticating sorghum to concentrate healthy phytochemicals. *J Agric Food Chem.* 2005;53:6230–6234.

Carr TP, Weller CL. Schlegel VL, Cuppett SL. Grain sorghum lipid extract reduces cholesterol absorption and plasma non-HDL cholesterol concentration in hamsters 1,2. *J Nutr.* 2005;135:2236–2240.

Soy   www.soybean.org; www.thesoyfoodscouncil.com
Hermansen K, Dinesen B, Hoie LH, Morgenstern E, Gruenwald J. (2003, January–February). Effects of soy and other natural products on LDL: HDL ratio and other lipid parameters: a literature review. *Adv Ther.* 20(1), 50–78.

Jin Z, MacDonald RS. Soy isoflavones increase latency of spontaneous mammary tumors in mice. *J Nutr.* 2002 Oct;132(10):3186–3190.

Messina M, McCaskill-Stevens W, Lampe JW. Addressing the soy and breast cancer relationship: review, commentary, and workshop proceedings. *J Natl Cancer Inst.* 2006 Sep 20;98(18):1275–1284.

Messina, M.J. Emerging evidence on the role of soy in reducing prostate cancer risk. *Nutr Rev.* 2004 Apr 6;61(4):117–131.

Reinwald S, Weaver CM. Soy isoflavones and bone health: a double edged sword? *J Nat Prod.* 2006 Mar;69(3):450–459.

Totta P, Acconcia F, Virgili F, Cassidy A, Weinberg PD, Rimback G, Marino M. Daidzein-sulfate metabolites affect transcriptional and antiproliferative activities of estrogen receptor-beta in cultured human cancer cells. *J Nutr.* 2005 Nov;135(11): 2687–2693.

Zhang X, Shu XO, Li H, Yang G, Li Q, Gao YT, Zheng W. Prospective cohort study of soy food consumption and risk of bone fracture among postmenopausal women. *Arch Intern Med.* 2005 Sep;165(16):1890–1895.

Spelt   www.agmrc.org/agmrc/commodity/grainsoilseeds/spelt/
Erkkila AT, Herrington DM, Mozaffarian D, Lichtenstein AH. Cereal fiber and wholegrain intake are associated with reduced progression of coronary-artery atherosclerosis in postmenopausal women with coronary artery disease. *Am Heart J.* 2005; 150:94–101.

Ruibal-Mendieta NL et al. Spelt (Triticum aestivum ssp. spelta) as a source of breadmaking flours and bran naturally enriched in oleic acid and minerals but not phytic acid. *J Agric Food Chem.* 2005 Apr 6;53(7):2751–2759.

Ruibal-Mendieta NL et al. Spelt (Triticum spelta L.) and winter wheat (Triticum aestivum L.) wholemeals have similar sterol profiles, as determined by quantitative liquid chromatography and mass spectrometry analysis. *J Agric Food Chem.* 2004 Jul 28;52(15):4802–4807.

Spinach   www.uga.edu/vegetable/spinach.html
Abu J, Batuwangala M, Herbert K, Symonds P. Retinoic acid and retinoid receptors: potential chemopreventive and therapeutic role in cervical cancer. *Lancet Oncol.* 2005 Sep;6(9):712–720.

Brown L, Rimm EB, Seddon JM, Giovannucci EL, Chasan-Taber L, Spiegelman D, Willett WC, Hankinson SE. A prospective study of carotenoid intake and risk of cataract extraction in US men. *Am J Clin Nutr.* 1999 Oct;70(4):431–432.

Chu YF, Sun J, Wu X, Liu RH. Antioxidant and antiproliferative activities of common vegetables. *J Agric Food Chem.* 2002 Nov 6;50(23):6910–6916.

Kelemen et al. Vegetables, fruit, and antioxidant-related nutrients and risk of non-Hodgkin lymphoma: a National Cancer Institute—surveillance, epidemiology, and end results population-based case-control study. *Am J Clin Nutr.* 2006 Jun;83(6):1401–1410.

Kuriyama I et al. Inhibitory effects of glycolipids fraction from spinach on mammalian DNA polymerase activity and human cancer cell proliferation. *Journal of Nutritional Biochemistry.* 2005 Oct;16(10):594–601.

Nyska A et al. Slowing tumorigenic progression in TRAMP mice and prostatic carcinoma cell lines using natural anti-oxidant from spinach, NAO—A comparative study of three anti-oxidants. *Toxicologic Pathology.* 2003 Jan/Feb;31(1):39–51.

Rai A, Mohapatra SC, Shukla HS. Correlates between vegetable consumption and gallbladder cancer. *Eur J Cancer Prev.* 2006 Apr;15(2):134–137.

Sani HA, Rahmat A, Ismail M, Rosli R, Endrini S. Potential anticancer effect of red spinach (Amaranthus gangeticus) extract. *Asia Pacific Journal of Clinical Nutrition.* 2004;13(4):396–400.

Seddon JM et al. Dietary carotenoids, vitamins A, C, and E, and advanced age-related macular degeneration. Eye disease case-control study group. *JAMA.* 1994 Nov 9; 272(18):1413–1420.

Wang Y, Chang C, Chou J, Chen H, Deng X, Harvey B, Cadet JL, Bickford PC. Dietary supplementation with blueberries, spinach, or spirulina reduces ischemic brain damage. *Experimental Neurology.* 2005 May;193(1):75–84.

Strawberries   www.calstrawberry.com;
www.urbanext.uiuc.edu/strawberries/

Hannum SM. Potential impact of strawberries on human health: a review of the science. *Crit Rev Food Sci Nutr.* 2004;44(1):1–17.

McDougall GJ, Stewart D. The inhibitory effects of berry polyphenols on digestive enzymes. *Biofactors.* 2005;23(4):189–195.

Naemura A et al. Anti-thrombotic effect of strawberries. *Blood Coagul Fibrinolysis.* 2005 Oct;16(7):501–509.

Olsson ME, Andersson CS, Oredsson S, Berglund RH, Gustavsson KE. Antioxidant levels and inhibition of cancer cell proliferation in vitro by extracts from organically and conventionally cultivated strawberries. *J Agric Food Chem.* 2006 Feb 22;54(4): 1248–1255.

Papoutsi Z et al. Evaluation of estrogenic/anti-estrogenic activity of ellagic acid via the estrogen receptor subtypes ER alpha and ER beta. *J Agric Food Chem.* 2005;53: 7715–7720.

Rampersaud GC, Kauwell GP, Bailey LB. Folate: a key to optimizing health and reducing disease risk in the elderly. *J Am Coll Nutr.* 2003 Feb;22(1):1–8.

Skupien K, Oszmianski J, Kostrzewa-Nowak D, Tarasiuk J. In vitro antileukaemic activity of extracts from berry plant leaves against sensitive and multidrug resistant HL60 cells. *Cancer Lett.* 2006 May 18;236(2):282–291.

Spiller GA et al. Health Research Studies Center. Los Altos, CA. Unpublished, 2003 & 2005.

Stoner GD, Chen T, Kresty LA, Aziz RM, Reinemann T, Nines R. Protection against esophageal cancer in rodents with lyophilized berries: potential mechanisms. *Nutr Cancer.* 2006;54(1):33–46.

Sunflower Seeds   www.sunflowerusa.org
Allman-Farinelli MA, Gomes K, Favaloro EJ, Petocz P. A diet rich in high-oleic-acid sunflower oil favorably alters low-density lipoprotein cholesterol, triglycerides, and factor VII coagulant activity. *J Am Diet Assoc.* 2005 Jul;105(7):1071–1079.

Binkoski AE, Kris-Etherton PM, Wilson TA, Mountain ML, Nicolosi RJ. Balance of unsaturated fatty acids is important to a cholesterol-lowering diet: comparison of mid-oleic sunflower oil and olive oil on cardiovascular disease risk factors. *J Am Diet Assoc.* 2005 Jul;105(7):1080–1086.

Kapadia, GJ et al. Chemopreventive effect of resveratrol, sesamol, sesame oil and sunflower oil in the Epstein-Barr virus early antigen activation assay and the mouse skin two-stage carcinogenesis. *Pharmacol Res.* 2002 Jun;45(6): 499–505.

Sweet potatoes   www.sweetpotato.org; www.cayam.com; www.ncsweetpotato.org
Bohle K, Spiegelman D, Trichopoulou A, Katsouyanni K, Trichopoulos D. Vitamins A, C and E and the risk of breast cancer: results from a case-control study in Greece. *British Journal of Cancer.* 1999 Jan;79(1):23–27.

Cho J, Kang JS, Long PH, Jing J, Back Y, Chung KS. Antioxidant and memory enhancing effects of purple sweet potato anthocyanin and cordyceps mushroom extract. *Arch Pharm Res.* 2003 Oct;26(10):821–825.

Hagiwara A et al. Prevention by natural food anthocyanins, purple sweet potato color and red cabbage color, of 2-amino-1-methyl-6-phenylimidazo [4,5-b]pyridine (PhIP)-associated colorectal carcinogenesis in rats initiated with 1,2-dimethlyhydrazine. *J Toxicol Sci.* 2002 Feb;27(1):57–68.

Kusano S, Abe H. Antidiabetic activity of white skinned sweet potato (Ipomoea batatas L.) in obese Zucker fatty rats. *Biol Pharm Bull* 2000;23(1):23–26.

Ludvik B, Waldhausl W, Prager R, Kautzky-Willer A, Pacini G. Mode of action of ipomoea batatas (Caiapo) in type 2 diabetic patients. *Metabolism* 2003;52(7):875–880.

Pandey M, Shukla VK. Diet and gallbladder cancer: a case-control study. *Eur J Cancer Prev.* 2002 Aug;11(4):365–372.

Rabah IO, Hou DX, Komine S, Fujii M. Potential chemopreventive properties of extract from baked sweet potato (Ipomoea batatas Lam. Cv. Koganesengan.). *J Agric Food Chem.* 2004 Nov;52(23):7152–7159.

Washio M et al. Risk factors for kidney cancer in a Japanese population: findings from the JACC study. *J Epidemol.* 2005 Jun;15(2):203–211.

Tea   www.tea.co.uk; www.teausa.com

Anderson RA, Polansky MM. Tea enhances insulin activity. *J Agric Food Chem.* 2002 Nov 20;50(24):7182–7186.

Arts IC, Jacobs DR Jr, Gross M et al. Dietary catechins and cancer incidence among postmenopausal women: the Iowa Women's Health Study (United States). *Cancer Causes Control.* 2002;13(4):373–382.

Arts ICW, Hollman PCH, Feskens EJM, Bueno de Mesquita HB, Kromhout D. Catechin intake might explain the inverse relation between tea consumption and ischemic heart disease: The Zutphen Elderly Study. *Am J Clin Nutr.* 2001;74:227–232.

Cabrera C, Artacho R, Gimenez R. Beneficial effects of green tea—a review. *J Am Coll Nutr.* 2006 Apr;25(2):79–99. Review.

Conney AH, Lu Y, Lou Y-R et al. Inhibitory effect of green and black tea on tumor growth. *Proc Soc Exp Biol Med.* 1999;220:229–233.

Davies MJ, Judd JT, Baer DJ et al. Black tea consumption reduces total and LDL cholesterol in mildly hypercholesterolemic adults. *J Nutr.* 2003;133(10):3298S–3302S.

Dora I, Arab L, Martinchik A et al. Black tea consumption and risk of rectal cancer in Moscow population. *Ann Epidemiol.* 2003;13(6):405–411.

Hakim IA, Harris RB. Joint effects of citrus peel use and black tea intake on the risk of squamous cell carcinoma of the skin. *BMC Dermatol.* 2001;1:3.

Hegarty VM, May HM, Khaw K-T. Tea drinking and bone mineral density in older women. *Am J Clin Nutr* 2000;71:1003–1007.

Isemura M, Saeki K, Kimura T, et al. Tea catechins and related polyphenols as anti-cancer agents. *Biofactors.* 2000;13(1–4):81–85.

Kim W et al. Effect of green tea consumption on endothelial function and circulating endothelial progenitor cells in chronic smokers. *Circ J.* 2006 Aug;70(8):1052–1057.

Kobayashi M, Unno T, Suzuki Y, et al. Heat-epimerized tea catechins have the same cholesterol-lowering activity as green tea catechins in cholesterol-fed rats. *Biosci Biotechnol Biochem.* 2005;69(12):2455–2458.

Nagao T, Komine Y, Soga S, Meguro S, Hase T, Tanaka Y, Tokimitsu I. Ingestion of a tea rich in catechins leads to a reduction in body fat and malondialdehyde-modified LDL in men. *Am J Clin Nutr.* 2005;81:122–129.

Yang YC, Lu FH, Wu JS, et al. The protective effect of habitual tea consumption on hypertension. *Arch Intern Med.* 2004;164(14):1534–1540.

Teff   www.ethnomed.org/cultures/ethiop/teff.html

Mengesha B, Ergete W. Staple Ethiopian diet and cancer of the oesophagus. *East Afr Med J.* 2005 Jul;82(7):353–356.

Tomatoes   www.tomato.org

Basu A, Imrhan V. Tomatoes versus lycopene in oxidative stress and carcinogenesis: conclusions from clinical trials. *Eur J Clin Nutr.* 2007 Mar;61(3):295–303.

Bhuvaneswari V, Nagini S. Lycopene: a review of its potential as an anticancer agent. *Current Medicinal Chemistry—Anti-Cancer Agents.* 2005 Nov;5(6):627–635.

Das S, Otani H, Maulik N, Das DK. Lycopene, tomatoes, and coronary heart disease. *Free Radic Res.* 2005 Apr;39(4):449–455.

Dutta-Roy AK, Crosbie L, Gordon MJ. Effects of tomato extract on human platelet aggregation in vitro. *Platelets.* 2001 Jun;12(4):218–227.

Guns ES, Cowell SP. Drug insight: lycopene in the prevention and treatment of prostate cancer. *Nat Clin Pract Urol.* 2005 Jan;2(1):38–43.

Kiani F, Knutsen S, Singh P, Ursin G, Fraser G. Dietary risk factors for ovarian caner: the Adventist Health Study (United States). *Cancer Causes Control.* 2006 March;17(2): 137–146.

King JL, Lila MA, Erdman Jr, JW, Campbell JK Antiproliferation effects of tomato poly-phenols in Hepa1c1c7 and LNCaP cell lines. *J Nutr.* 2003 Nov;133(11):3858S–3859S.

La Vecchi C. Mediterranean epidemiological evidence on tomatoes and the preven-tion of digestive-tract cancers. *Proc Soc Exp Biol Med.* 1998 Jun;218(2):125–128.

Stacewicz-Sapuntzakis M, Bowen PE. Role of lycopene and tomato products in prostate health. *Biochim Biophys Acta.* 2005 May 30;1740(2):202–205.

Tomatoes, red, ripe, raw, year round average. (2005). USDA National Nutrient Database for Standard Reference. Retrieved July 20, 2006, from http://www.nal.usda .gov/fnic/foodcomp/cgi-bin/list_nut_edit.pl

Wu K, Erdman JW Jr, Schwartz SJ, Platz EA, Leitzmann M, Clinton SK, DeGroff V, Willett WC, Giovannucci E. Plasma and dietary carotenoids, and the risk of prostate cancer: a nested case-control study. *Cancer Epidemiol Biomarkers Prev.* 2004 Feb;13(2):260–269.

Turmeric http://nccqm.nih.gov/health/turmeric/

Aggarwal BB et al. Curcumin suppresses the paclitaxel-induced nuclear factor-kappaB pathway in breast cancer cells and inhibits lung metastasis of human breast cancer in nude mice. *Clin Cancer Res.* 2005 Oct 15;11(20):7490–7498.

Asai A, Miyazawa T. Dietary curcuminoids prevent high-fat diet-induced lipid accu-mulation in rat liver and epididymal adipose tissue. *J Nutr.* 2001;131:2932–2935.

Cruz-Correa M et al. Combination treatment with curcumin and quercetin of adeno-mas in familial adenomatous polyposis. *Clin Gastroenterol Hepatol.* 2006 Aug;4(8): 1035–1038.

Hong JH. The effects of curcumin on the invasiveness of prostate cancer in vitro and in vivo. *Prostate Cancer Prostatic Dis.* 2006;9(2):147–152.

Lim GP, Chu T, Yang F, Beech W, Frautschy SA, Cole GM. The curry spice curcumin reduces oxidative damage and amyloid pathology in an Alzheimer transgenic mouse. *J Neuro Sci.* 2001;21:8370–8377.

Ng TP et al. Curry consumption and cognitive function in the elderly. *Am J Epidemiol.* 2006 Nov 1;164(9):898–906.

Peschel D, Koerting R, Nass N. Curcumin induces changes in expression of genes in-volved in cholesterol homeostasis. *J Nutr Biochem.* 2007 Feb; 18(2):113–119.

Singletary K. Inhibition of 7,12-dimethylbenz[a] anthracene (DMBA)-induced mammary turmorigenisis and DMA-DNA adduct formation by curcumin. *Cancer Letters.* 1996;103:137–141.

Swiak DR et al. Curcumin-induced antiproliferative and proapoptotic effects in melanoma cells are associated with suppression of IkappaB kinase and nuclear factor kappaB activity and are independent of the B-Raf/mitogen-activated/extracellular signal-regulated protein kinase pathway and the Akt pathway. *Cancer.* 2005 Aug 15;104(4):879–890.

Villasenor IM, Simon MKB, Villanueva AMA. Comparative potencies of nutraceuticals in chemically induced skin tumor prevention. *Nutr Cancer.* 2002;44:66–70.

Wu A, Ying Z, Gomez-Pinilla F. Dietary curcumin counteracts the outcome of traumatic brain injury on oxidative stress, synaptic plasticity, and cognition. *Exp Neurol.,* 2006; 197(2): 309–317.

Walnuts   www.walnuts.org

Feldman, E.B. The scientific evidence for a beneficial health relationship between walnuts and coronary heart disease. *J Nutr.* 2002 May;132(5):1062S–1101S.

Griel AE, Kris-Etherton PM, Hilpert KF, Zhao G, West SG and Corwin RL. An increase in dietary n-3 fatty acids decreases a marker of bone resorption in humans. *Nutrition Journal.* January 2007, Volume 6, doi:10.1186/1475-2891-6-2.

Lavedrine F, Zmirou D, Ravel A, Balducci F, Alary J. Blood cholesterol and walnut consumption: a cross-sectional survey in France. *Prev Med.* 1999 Apr;28(4), 333–339.

Patel G. Essential fats in walnuts are good for the heart and diabetes. *J Am Diet Assoc.* 2005 Jul;105(7):1096–1097.

Reiter et al. Melatonin in walnuts: Influence on levels of melatonin and total antioxidant capacity of blood. *Inter J Appl Basic Nutr Sci.* 2005; 21, 920–924.

Sabate et al. Does regular walnut consumption lead to weight gain? *British Journal of Nutrition* 2005; 94, 859–846.

Zibaeenezhad MJ, Shamsnia SJ, Khorasani M. Walnut consumption in hyperlipidemic patients. *Angiology.* 2005 Sep/Oct;56(5):581–583.

Watermelon   www.watermelon.org

Ghazizadeh M, Razeghi A, Valaee N, Mirbagheri E, Tahbaz F, Motevallizadeh H, Seyedahmadian F, Mirzapour H. Watermelon juice concentrate. *Asia Pac J Clin Nutr.* 2004;13(Suppl):S162.

Jian L, Du CJ, Lee AH, Binns CW. Do dietary lycopene and other carotenoids protect against prostate cancer? *Int J Cancer.* 2005 Mar 1;113(6):1010–1014.

Lee SY, Choi KY, Kim MK, Kim KM, Lee JH, Meng KH, Lee WC. The relationship between intake of vegetables and fruits and colorectal adenoma-carcinoma sequence. *Korean J Gastroenterol.* 2005 Jan;45(1):23–33.

Wheat   www.wheatfoods.org

Adam A, Lopez HW, Tressol JC, Leuillet M, Demigne C, Remesy C. Impact of whole wheat flour and its milling fractions on the cecal fermentations and the plasma and liver lipids in rats. *J Agric Food Chem.* 2002 Oct 23;50(22):6557–6562.

Anderson JW, Gilinsky NH, Deakins DA, Smith SF, O'Neal DS, Dillon DW, Oeltgen PR. Lipid responses of hypercholesterolemic men to oat-bran and wheat bran intake. *Am J Clin Nutr.* 1991; 56:355–359.

Balint G et al. Effect of Avemar—a fermented wheat germ extract—on rheumatoid arthritis. Preliminary data. *Clin Exp Rheumatol.* 2000 May/Jun;24(3):325–328.

Carter JW, Madl R, Padula F. Wheat antioxidants suppress intestinal tumor activity in Min mice. *Nutrition Research.* 2006 Jan;26(1):33–38.

Jacobs DR, Marquart L, Slavin J, Kushi L. Whole-grain intake and cancer: An expanded review and meta-analysis. *Nutr Cancer.* 1998;130:85–96.

Jacobs DR, Pereira MA, Meyer KA, Kushi LH. Fiber from whole grains, but not refined grains, is inversely associated with all-cause mortality in older women: The Iowa women's health study. *J Am Coll Nutr.* 2000;19(3 Suppl):326S–330S.

Jenkins DJA et al. Effect of wheat bran on glycemic control and risk factors for cardiovascular disease in type 2 diabetes. *Diabetes Care.* 2002;25:1522–1528.

Jenkins DJA et al. Low glycemic response to traditionally processed wheat and rye products: bulgur and pumpernickel bread. *Am J Clin Nutr.* 1986;43:516–520.

Pereira Mark A et al. Effect of whole grains on insulin sensitivity in overweight hyperinsulinemic adults. *Nutr Cancer.* 1998;30(2):85–96.

Whey   www.wheyoflife.org; www.wheyprotein.com

Agin D, et al. Effects of whey protein and resistance exercise on body composition and muscle strength in women with HIV infection. *AIDS.* 2001 Dec 7; 15(18): 2431–2440.

Aoe S et al. A controlled trial of the effect of milk basic protein (MBP) supplementation on bone metabolism in healthy menopausal women. *Osteoporos Int.* 2005 Dec;16(12):2123–2128.

Aoe S et al. Controlled trial of the effects of milk basic protein (MBP) supplementation on bone metabolism in healthy adult women. *Biosci Biotechnol Biochem.* 2001 Apr;65(4):913–918.

Beeh M, Schlaak J, Buhl R. Oral supplementation with whey proteins increases plasma glutathione levels of HIV infected patients. *European Journal of Clinical Investigation.* 2001 Feb;31(2):171–178.

Belobrajdic D, McIntosh G, Owens J. Whey proteins protect more than red meat against azoxymethane induced ACF in Wistar rats. *Cancer Letters.* 2003;198:43–51.

Belobrajdic D, McIntosh G, Owens J. A high whey protein diet reduces body weight gain and alters insulin sensitivity relative to red meat in Wistar rats. *J Nutr.* 2004; 134:1454–1458.

Bounous G. Whey protein concentrate (WPC) and glutathione modulation in cancer treatment. *Anticancer Research.* 2000;20:4785–4792.

Bounous G et al. Immunoenhancing property of dietary whey protein in mice: role of glutathione. *Clinical Investigative Medicine.* 1989;12:154–161.

Eason R, Badger T et al. Dietary exposure to whey proteins alters rat mammary gland proliferation, apoptosis, and gene expression during post-natal development: implications for cancer protective mechanism. *J Nutr.* 2004;134(12).

Fitzgerald R et al. Hypotensive peptides from milk proteins. *J Nutr.* 2003;134:S980–S988.

Hannan M et al. Effect of dietary protein on bone loss in elderly men and women: the Framingham osteoporosis study. *Journal of Bone & Mineral Research.* 2000;15(12): 2504–2512.

Markus CR et al. The bovine protein-lactalbumin increases the plasma ratio of tryptophan to the other large neutral amino acids and in vulnerable subjects raises brain serotonin activity, reduces cortisol concentration and improves mood under stress. *American Journal of Clinical Nutrition.* 2000;71:1536–1544.

Markus CR, Olivier B, de Haan EH. Whey protein rich in alpha-lactalbumin increases the ratio of plasma tryptophan to the sum of the other large neutral amino acids and improves cognitive performance in stress-vulnerable subjects. *Am J Clin Nutr.* 2002 Jun;75(6):1051–1056.

Miller GD et al. Benefits of dairy product consumption on blood pressure in humans: a summary of the biomedical literature. *Journal of the American College of Nutrition.* 2000;19(2):147S–164S.

Wong CW et al. Effects of purified bovine whey factors on cellular immune functions in ruminants. *Veterinary Immunology and Immunopathology.* 1997;56:85–96.

Zemel MB. Mechanisms of dairy modulation of adiposity. *J Nutr.* 2003;133:252–256.

Yogurt   www.aboutyogurt.com

Bharav E, Mor F, Halpern M, Weinberger A. Lactobacillus GG bacteria ameliorate arthritis in Lewis rats. *J Nutr.* 2004 Aug;134(8):1964–1969.

Fabian E, Elmadfa I. Influence of daily consumption of probiotic and conventional yoghurt on the plasma lipid profile in young healthy women. *Annals of Nutrition & Metabolism.* 2006 Jul;50(4):387–393.

Ganji V, Kafai MR. Frequent consumption of milk, yogurt, cold breakfast cereals, peppers, and cruciferous vegetables and intakes of dietary folate and riboflavin but not vitamins B-12 and B-6 are inversely associated with serum total homocysteine concentrations in the US population. *Am J Clin Nutr.* 2004 Dec;80(6):1500–1507.

Parvez S, Malik KA, Ah Kang S, Kim HY. Probiotics and their fermented food products are beneficial for health. *J Appl Microbiol.* 2006 Jun;100(6):1171–1185.

Perdigon G, de Moreno de LeBlanc A, Vasdez J, Rachid M. Role of yoghurt in the prevention of colon cancer. *Eur J Clin Nutr.* 2002 Aug;56(Suppl 3:s65–68).

Sheu BS, Wu JJ, Lo CY et al. Impact of supplement with Lactobacillus- and Bifidobacterium-containing yogurt on triple therapy for Helicobacter pylori eradication. *Aliment Pharmacol Ther.* 2002;16(9):1669–1676.

Wang KY et al. Effects of ingesting Lactobacillus- and Bifidobacterium-containing yogurt in subjects with colonized Helicobacter pylori. *Am J Clin Nutr.* 2004 Sep;80(3): 737–741.

INDEX

335; to prevent colon cancer, 336; to prevent prostate cancer, 336; for ulcers (*H. pylori* bacteria), 335; vitamin B6 in, 335; vitamin C in, 335

ulcers (*H. pylori* bacteria): almonds for, 10; bananas for, 36; barley for, 40; broccoli for, 58; cabbage for, 64, 65; cardamom for, 68; cranberries for, 115; cumin for, 118; grapefruit for, 154; horseradish for, 173; oregano for, 220; Swiss chard for, 84; turmeric for, 335; wasabi for, 173
urinary tract infections: blueberries for, 54; cranberries for, 114; elderberries for, 131

vaccine helper: quinoa, 271
viruses: cabbage and sauerkraut for, 65; eggplant for, 124; elderberries for, 131
vision: apricots for, 22; avocado for, 32; carrots for, 75; eggs to prevent cataracts and macular degeneration, 127, 128; goji berries for, 151; kale for, 177; pistachios for, 254; romaine lettuce for, 281; spinach for, 310; Swiss chard for, 84
vitamin A: in apricots, 21, 22; in broccoli, 57; in carob, 71; in carrots, 74; in celery, 81; in cherries, 87; in chocolate, 91; in currants, 121; in elderberries, 131; in grapefruit, 154; in guava, 161; in kale, 176; in lemons, 183; in mangoes, 190; in mint, 196; in onions, 212; in papaya, 223; in passion fruit, 229; in persimmon, 246; in pumpkins, 267; in romaine lettuce, 281; in spinach, 310; in sweet potatoes, 321; in Swiss chard, 84
vitamin B1 (thiamine): in beans, 46; in celery, 81; in corn, 110; in millet, 193; in pecans, 240; in pistachios, 254
vitamin B2: in celery, 81; in eggs, 127
vitamin B3 (niacin): in carrots, 74; in millet, 193
vitamin B6: in asparagus, 28; in bananas, 36; in carrots, 74; in pineapples, 249;

in pistachios, 254; in quinoa, 270; in sweet potatoes, 321; in turmeric, 335
vitamin B12: in eggs, 127
vitamin B complex: in avocado, 32; in barley, 39; in buckwheat, 61; in carob, 71; in cherries, 87; in chocolate, 91; in currants, 121; in mushrooms, 201; in oats, 205; in peppers, 243; in quinoa, 270; in rice, brown, 277; in rye, 287; in sorghum, 300; soy for, 303; in spelt, 306; in walnuts, 339
vitamin C: in apples, 17; in apricots, 21; in artichokes, 25; in asparagus, 28; in bananas, 36; in blackberries, 50; in broccoli, 57; in cabbage, 64; in carrots, 74; in cauliflower, 77; in celery, 81; in cherries, 87; in cloves, 102; in corn, 110; in cranberries, 114; in currants, 121; in elderberries, 131; in fennel, 134; in grapefruit, 154; in grapes, 158; in guava, 161; in horseradish, 172; in kale, 176; in kiwi, 180; in lemons, 183; in mangoes, 190; in onions, 212; in oranges, 216; in papaya, 223; in parsley, 226; in passion fruit, 229; in pears, 236; in peppers, 243; in persimmon, 246; in pineapples, 249; in pomegranate, 260; in potatoes, 263–64; in raspberries, 273; in romaine lettuce, 281; in strawberries, 313; in sweet potatoes, 321; in Swiss chard, 84; in tomatoes, 331; in turmeric, 335; in wasabi, 172
vitamin D: in carob, 71; in eggs, 127; in mushrooms, 201
vitamin E: in almonds, 10; in avocado, 32; in buckwheat, 61; in hazelnuts, 164; in kiwi, 180; in oats, 205; in pecans, 240; in pistachios, 254; in rice, brown, 277; in rye, 287; in sunflower seeds, 317; in Swiss chard, 84; in walnuts, 339; in wheat, 346
vitamin K: in avocado, 32; in cloves, 102; in mangoes, 190; in plums or prunes, 257; in sauerkraut, 64; in spinach, 309; in Swiss chard, 84

ABOUT THE AUTHOR

DAVID GROTTO, RD, LDN, is a national media spokesperson for the American Dietetic Association and founder of Nutrition Housecall, LLC, a nutrition consulting firm that offers personalized at-home and group dietary services. He is a scientific advisor for *Men's Health* magazine and is the advisory chair for Produce for Kids\PBS Kids' national campaign to promote healthy eating in children. Dave lives in Chicago, Illinois, with his wife, Sharon, his daughters Chloe, Katie, and Madison, and his dogs, Gracie and Abbey.